SPORT AND EXERCISE PHYSIOLOGY TESTING GUIDELINES

Sport and Exercise Physiology Testing Guidelines is a comprehensive, practical sourcebook of principles and procedures for physiological testing in sport and exercise.

Volume I: specific guidelines for physiological testing in over 30 sports disciplines.
Volume II: guidelines for exercise testing in key clinical populations.

Each volume also represents a full reference for informed, good practice in physiological assessment, covering:

General Principles of Physiological Testing including health and safety, and blood sampling.
Methodological Issues including reliability, scaling and circadian rhythms.
General Testing Procedures for lung and respiratory muscle function, anthropometry, flexibility, pulmonary gas exchange, lactate testing, RPE, strength testing and upper-body exercise.
Special Populations including children, older people and female participants.

Written and compiled by subject specialists, this authoritative laboratory research resource is for students, academics and those providing scientific support service in sport science and the exercise and health sciences.

Edward M. Winter is Professor of the Physiology of Exercise at Sheffield Hallam University. **Andrew M. Jones** is Professor of Applied Physiology at the University of Exeter. **R.C. Richard Davison** is Principal Lecturer in Exercise Physiology at the University of Portsmouth. **Paul D. Bromley** is Principal Lecturer in Exercise Physiology at Thames Valley University and Consultant Clinical Scientist in the Department of Cardiology at Ealing Hospital, London. **Thomas H. Mercer** is Professor of Clinical Exercise Physiology and Rehabilitation, Department of Physiotherapy, School of Health Sciences, Queen Margaret University College, Edinburgh.

SPORT AND EXERCISE PHYSIOLOGY TESTING GUIDELINES

The British Association of Sport and Exercise Sciences Guide

Volume II: Exercise and Clinical Testing

Edited by Edward M. Winter,
Andrew M. Jones, R.C. Richard Davison,
Paul D. Bromley and Thomas H. Mercer

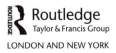
Routledge
Taylor & Francis Group

LONDON AND NEW YORK

First published 2007
by Routledge
2 Park Square, Milton Park, Abingdon, Oxon OX14 4RN

Simultaneously published in the USA and Canada
by Routledge
270 Madison Ave, New York, NY 10016

Reprinted 2007, 2008

Routledge is an imprint of the Taylor & Francis Group, an informa business

Typeset in Sabon and Futura by
Newgen Imaging Systems (P) Ltd, Chennai, India
Printed and bound in Great Britain by
TJ International Ltd, Padstow, Cornwall

British Library Cataloguing in Publication Data
A catalogue record for this book is available from the British Library

Library of Congress Cataloging in Publication Data
Sport and exercise physiology testing : guidelines : the British Association of
Sport and Exercise Sciences guide / edited by
Edward M. Winter ... [et al.]. — 1st ed.
p. cm.
Includes bibliographical references and index.
1. Physical fitness—Testing. 2. Exercise—Physiological aspects.
I. Winter, Edward M. II. British Association of Sport and Exercise Sciences.
GV436.S665 2006
613.7′1—dc22   2006011234

ISBN10: 0–415–37965–2 (hbk)
ISBN10: 0–415–37966–0 (pbk)
ISBN10: 0–203–96683–X (ebk)

ISBN13: 978–0–415–37965–6 (hbk)
ISBN13: 978–0–415–37966–3 (pbk)
ISBN13: 978–0–203–96683–9 (ebk)

CONTENTS

TABLES AND FIGURES

TABLES

FIGURES

NOTES ON CONTRIBUTORS

Greg Atkinson, Research Institute for Sport and Exercise Sciences, Liverpool John Moores University.

Anthony J. Blazevich, Centre for Sports Medicine and Human Performance, Brunel University.

Paul D. Bromley, Department of Human Sciences, Thames Valley University and Department of Cardiology, Ealing Hospital NHS Trust.

John Buckley, Centre of Exercise and Nutrition Sciences, University of Chester and The Lifestyle Exercise and Physiotherapy Centre, Shrewsbury.

Melonie Burrows, Childrens Health and Exercise Research Centre, University of Exeter.

Nigel T. Cable, Research Institute for Sport and Exercise Sciences, Liverpool John Moores University.

Dale Cannavan, Centre for Sports Medicine and Human Performance, Brunel University.

R. C. Richard Davison, Department of Sport and Exercise Science, University of Portsmouth.

Roger Eston, School of Sport and Health Sciences, University of Exeter.

Keith George, Research Institute for Sport and Exercise Sciences, Liverpool John Moores University.

David V. B. James, Faculty of Sport, Health and Social Care, University of Gloucestershire.

Graham Jarman, Faculty of Organisation and Management, Sheffield Hallam University.

Andrew M. Jones, School of Sport and Health Sciences, University of Exeter.

David A. Jones, Institute for Biophysical and Clinical Research into Human Movement, Manchester Metropolitan University and School of Sport and Exercise Sciences, University of Birmingham.

Pelagia Koufaki, Department of Metabolic and Cellular Medicine, School of Clinical Sciences, University of Liverpool.

John B. Leiper, School of Sport and Exercise Sciences, Loughborough University.

Craig A. Mahoney, School of Sport, Performing Arts and Leisure, University of Wolverhampton.

Alison McConnell, Centre for Sports Medicine and Human Performance, Brunel University.

Ron Maughan, School of Sport and Exercise Sciences, Loughborough University.

Thomas H. Mercer, School of Health Sciences, Queen Margaret University College, Edinburgh.

Alan M. Nevill, Research Institute of Healthcare Sciences, University of Wolverhampton.

Steve Olivier, School of Social and Health Sciences, University of Abertay Dundee.

Nicola Phillips, Physiotherapy Department, School of Healthcare Studies, Cardiff University.

Mike J. Price, Department of Biomolecular and Sports Science, Faculty of Health and Life Sciences, Coventry University.

Thomas Reilly, Research Institute for Sport and Exercise Sciences, Liverpool John Moores University.

Lee M. Romer, Centre for Sports Medicine and Human Performance, Brunel University.

Joan M. Round, School of Sport and Exercise Sciences, The University of Birmingham.

Leigh E. Sandals, Faculty of Sport, Health and Social Care, University of Gloucestershire.

John M. Saxton, Centre for Sport and Exercise Science, Sheffield Hallam University.

Susan M. Shirreffs, School of Sport and Exercise Sciences, Loughborough University.

Paul M. Smith, Centre for Sport and Exercise Sciences, University of Greenwich.

Neil Spurway, Centre for Exercise Science and Medicine, Institute of Biomedical and Life Sciences, University of Glasgow.

Arthur D. Stewart, School of Health Sciences, The Robert Gordon University, Aberdeen.

Gareth Stratton, REACH Group, Research Institute for Sport and Exercise Sciences, Liverpool John Moores University.

Gregory P. Whyte, Research Institute for Sport and Exercise Sciences, Liverpool John Moores University.

Craig A. Williams, Children's Health and Exercise Research Centre (CHERC), School of Sport and Health Sciences, University of Exeter.

Edward M. Winter, The Centre for Sport and Exercise Science, Sheffield Hallam University.

Dan M. Wood, Standards and quality analytical team, Department of Health.

Matthew Wyon, School of Sport Performing Arts and Leisure, University of Wolverhampton.

ACKNOWLEDGEMENTS

For the last four decades, there is one person in particular who has both guided the development of sport and exercise science in the United Kingdom and been a constant source of inspiration to its practitioners, teachers and researchers. Many of the contributors have benefited directly from his influence.

The publication of this volume has coincided with his retirement and the editors take this opportunity to extend their appreciation and thanks to Professor N.C. Craig Sharp BVMS MRCVS PhD FIBiol FBASES FafPE.

FOREWORD

It is well recognised that scientific support plays a vital part in the preparation both of elite athletes and those for whom physical activity is a goal.

As standards of performance continue their searing rate of progress while simultaneously, concerns are expressed about the activity profile of our children and adolescents, the need for evidence-based approaches to meet these challenges increases in importance. UK Sport and the British Association of Sport and Exercise Sciences have always had a close relationship and this fourth edition of Sport and Exercise Physiology Testing Guidelines provides an opportunity to underscore this relationship.

The award of the 2012 Olympic Games to London re-emphasises the link and highlights the dual aim to improve athletic performance and enhance the health of the nation. UK Sport and BASES will be working together to achieve this aim.

Sue Campbell CBE
Chair of UK Sport

FOREWORD

BASES's guidelines on the physiological assessment of all who participate in exercise and sport whether it is at the elite or recreational level of participation represents another significant contribution to the professional development of sport and exercise science in the United Kingdom.

The editorial team has brought together researchers and practitioners in the field of exercise physiology to share with us their knowledge, insight and experience. They have produced a set of guidelines that represent current knowledge and best practice in the field of physiological assessment. The guidelines will be widely regarded as the benchmark publication for all practitioners whether they work in the laboratory or in the field. Therefore, I am delighted to commend the guidelines to you because they not only serve to share more widely the available knowledge and so contribute to raising standards but also because they reassure us that the future of sport and exercise science in the United Kingdom is in safe hands.

Clyde Williams
Professor of Sports Science
Loughborough University

INTRODUCTION

Edward M. Winter, Paul D. Bromley,
R.C Richard Davison, Andrew M. Jones
and Thomas H. Mercer

It is 21 years since under the stewardship of Tudor Hale, a working group that also comprised Neil Armstrong, Adrianne Hardman, Philip Jakeman, Craig Sharp and Edward Winter produced the Position Statement on the Physiological Assessment of the Elite Competitor. This was distributed to members of the Sports Physiology Section of the then British Association of Sports Sciences (BASS).

In 1988 the document had metamorphosed into a second edition that was formally published for and on behalf of BASS by White Line Press. BASS's accreditation scheme for physiology laboratories and personnel had been established and the second edition provided a reference frame for the associated criteria. Moreover, undergraduate study of sport and exercise science had continued to gather pace and celebrated its twelfth birthday.

Nine years later in 1997, BASS had evolved into the British Association of Sport and Exercise Sciences (BASES). The addition of 'exercise' into the Association's title clearly reflected acknowledgement that there were exercise scientists whose interests were not restricted to sport. Steve Bird and Richard Davison had assumed the mantle of responsibility to revise the second edition and edited the third edition that had a simplified title: *Physiological Testing Guidelines*. These editors, together with 22 contributing authors, produced 19 chapters that were organised under 4 rubrics: General issues and procedures; Generic testing procedures; Sport-specific testing guidelines; and Specific considerations for the assessment of the young athlete.

This fourth edition shares a common feature with edition three: the nine-year gap from the previous one. These gaps should not be confused with a lack of activity by BASES members. On the contrary, sport and exercise science has undergone astonishing growth since it became degree-standard study in the United Kingdom. The fledgling discipline has developed into a major area and some 10,000 students graduate each year with a sport or exercise-related degree. More than 100 institutions of higher education offer undergraduate sport and exercise-related programmes and approximately a third of these offer masters' courses. In addition, doctoral studies feature prominently and since 1992, sport and exercise-related subjects have had their own panel in the Higher Education Funding Councils' Research Assessment Exercise.

Mirroring this growth has been the increase in vocational applications of sport and exercise science and many enjoy careers in diverse settings. These settings include sport and exercise support work with national governing bodies, professional clubs, the Home Countries' Sport Institutes, and public and private healthcare providers as well as private, governmental and voluntary organisations that are engaged in the provision of exercise for people with, or at high risk of, a myriad of diseases and disabilities. BASES' accreditation scheme for researchers and practitioners in sport and exercise science provides a gold-standard quality assurance mechanism for senior personnel while its supervised experience scheme encourages and nurtures young scientists. Currently, there are some 387 accredited scientists and 376 who are benefiting from supervised experience.

A recent development has been the use of the term physical activity rather than exercise. Physical activity is seen to be less intimidating and encompasses every-day activities like gardening, domestic tasks and walking. These are activities in which most participate at least some time during the day.

The expansion of the evidence base that underpins physiological assessments of athletes is matched by exponential growth in the fields of clinical exercise physiology and medical and health related applications of exercise assessment. Exercise testing and the interpretation of exercise test data, especially those from integrated cardiopulmonary exercise tests, has made important contributions both to research and the clinical management of patients.

In the clinical setting, exercise testing has direct relevance in several applications. It is used in the functional assessment of patients and has implications both for the diagnosis and prognosis of conditions. It helps to determine safe and effective exercise prescription and testing is also used to evaluate the effectiveness of medical, surgical or exercise interventions that are designed to be therapeutic. The use of exercise testing in patients with diseases and disabilities means that associated exercise scientists must appreciate the implications of the disorder being investigated and be able to adapt tests and procedures to take account of existing co-morbidities, for example, obesity and musculoskeletal dysfunction, that might influence performance and results.

The impetus to this fourth edition was provided by Ged Garbutt and the outcome is an ambitious attempt to address several matters in one core text. Specifically, it aims to: address both sport and exercise/physical activity applications; acknowledge psychological aspects of exercise testing; consider technical matters such as health-and-safety issues that impact on the management of laboratories and field-based work; and acknowledge the requirement to ensure that procedures abide by principles for seeking and gaining ethics approval.

The text is intended to be a reference guide for practitioners, researchers and teachers in sport and exercise science. The editorial team are well placed to appreciate the challenges that this triune presents. Moreover, the list of contributors includes many of the United Kingdom's leading sport and exercise scientists who are similarly well placed to appreciate the challenges in applying research to scientific support for sport and exercise.

REFERENCES

Bird, S. and Davison, R. (1997). *Physiological Testing Guidelines*, 3rd edn. Leeds: The British Association of Sport and Exercise Sciences.

Hale, T., Armstrong, N., Hardman, A., Jakeman, P., Sharp, C. and Winter, E. (1988). *Position Statement on the Physiological Assessment of the Elite Competitor*, 2nd edn. Leeds: White Line Press.

PART 1

GENERAL PRINCIPLES

RATIONALE

Edward M. Winter, Paul D. Bromley,
R.C. Richard Davison, Andrew M. Jones
and Thomas H. Mercer

INTRODUCTION

The physiology of exercise can be defined as the study of how the body responds and adapts to exercise and an important part of this study is the identification of physiological characteristics that explain rather than simply describe performance. This identification applies both to competitive athletes and to those whose interests are in the role of physical activity in the promotion and maintenance of health.

The continued rise in performance standards in sport underscores the need to develop knowledge and understanding of related mechanisms to optimise athletes' training. Such optimisation ensures that training maximises adaptations but not at the expense of developing unexplained underperformance syndromes – previously known as overtraining. Similarly, the frequency, intensity and duration of physical activity required to promote and sustain health is important; concerns about the possible inactivity of our children and adolescents give rise to anxiety about possible long-term problems such as diabetes and cardio-vascular disease that might ensue from hypokinesis.

It is also well recognised that exercise can be both prophylactic and therapeutic in clinical populations. Consequently, sport and exercise science graduates are increasingly in demand with such populations because of the expertise they bring to exercise testing and interpretation.

Technological advances and the development and refinement of procedures have been and continue to be a hallmark of sport and exercise science. Furthermore, there are many sports and activities to be considered along with a variety of influential factors such as the age, gender, ability and disability of participants. This presents a major challenge for physiologists: the selection and administration of tests and their subsequent interpretation is intellectually and practically exacting.

Moreover, it is now well established that effective scientific support comprises contributions from several disciplines. Consequently, researchers and practitioners have to be able to recognise the limits of their expertise and know when to seek the advice and guidance of others. Similarly, a detailed understanding of techniques and procedures to assess the validity and reproducibility of measures is an essential competency that sport and exercise scientists must possess. It is important to know the extent to which an apparent change in a measure is meaningful and does not lie within a confidence interval for error. As differences in performance can be measured in small fractions, the identification of what is meaningful can be obscured by random error.

Overarching all this is the increased support provided to athletes by most of the world's leading sporting nations. This emphasises the need for UK-based athletes to have the best possible scientific and medical support if they are to compete effectively in international competition.

WHY ASSESS?

The rationale for assessment remains as it has for some three decades: to develop knowledge and understanding of the exercise capabilities of humans. A practical outcome of this is enhanced performance and exercise tolerance of individuals who are tested.

Assessment should be preceded by a full needs analysis which in turn should be based on a triangulation of the requirements and views of the athlete, coach and scientist. Assessments should be an integral part of an athlete's training and scientific support programmes and should be conducted regularly and frequently.

Moreover, assessments should reflect the movement and other demands of the sport or activity in which the athlete or exerciser participates. Hence, the investigator should have a detailed understanding of the mechanisms of energy release that are challenged.

Specifically, reasons for undertaking physiological tests are (Bird and Davison, 1997) to:

1   Provide an initial evaluation of strengths and weakness of the participant in the context of the sport or activity in which they participate. This information can be used to inform the design and implementation of a training programme.
2   Evaluate the effectiveness of a training programme to see if performance or rehabilitation is improving and intended physiological adaptations are occurring.
3   Evaluate the health status of an athlete or exerciser. This might be part of a joint programme with clinical staff.
4   Provide an ergogenic aid. Often, in the setting of short-term goals for the improvement of fitness for example, the prospect of being tested often acts as a motivational influence.
5   Assist in selection or identify readiness to resume training or competition.

6   Develop knowledge and understanding of a sport or activity for the benefit of coaches, future athletes and scientists.
7   Answer research questions.

In the clinical domain, the utility of exercise testing has expanded from a role that simply categorised the health status of a patient or participant to one that can diagnose functional limitation, that is, whether the origin is cardiac, pulmonary or muscular. This might be in the presence of multiple pathologies where precise diagnosis requires considerable expertise.

TEST CRITERIA

It is recognised that to be effective, assessments should be specific and valid and that resulting measures should be reproducible and sensitive to changes in performance.

Specificity

Assessments should mimic the form of exercise under scrutiny. This is a key challenge for instance in multiple-sprint activities such as field-games and racquet-sports in which changes in speed and direction of movement predominate. Factors that should be considered in the design of test protocols are:

1   Muscle groups, type of activity and range of motion required.
2   Intensity and duration of activity.
3   Energy systems recruited.
4   Resistive forces encountered.

Accordingly, activity-specific ergometers should be used and these might have to be designed to satisfy local requirements. Similarly, field-based as opposed to laboratory-based procedures might provide improved characterisations of patterns of motion. It is worth noting that sacrificing specificity to reduce artefacts is a consideration that should be made test-by-test. For instance, in diagnostic testing, it might be prudent to select a mode of exercise that does not necessarily reflect daily activities. A cycle ergometer could fall into this category but its use would achieve improved signal acquisition in electrocardiographic, pulmonary and metabolic measurements.

Validity

Validity is the extent to which a test measures what it purports to measure. This applies, for instance, to the assessment of mechanisms that might explain endurance and to the appropriate use of mechanical constructs to describe in particular, the outcomes of maximal intensity, that is, all-out exercise.

Reproducibility

An important requirement for data if they are to be considered meaningful is that they must be reproducible. Enthusiastic debate continues about the metric or metrics that most appropriately assess reproducibility (Atkinson and Nevill, 1998 and elsewhere in this text). Consequently, exercise scientists need to have a keen appreciation of these metrics and their respective advantages and disadvantages. In essence, variability in measures can be attributed to technical and biological sources. The former comprise precision and accuracy of instruments coupled with the skill of the operator, hence procedures for calibration are critical. The latter comprise random and cyclic biological variation. Knowledge and understanding of the magnitude of these errors play a key role in the interpretation of measures.

As a result, an indication of error in tests is a requirement if meaningful information is to be provided. This includes comparisons of test results with norms or those of other performers.

Sensitivity

Sensitivity is the extent to which physiological measures reflect improvements in performance. Clearly, reproducibility is implicated but sensitivity is probably at the heart of the matter: it is in itself a key measure of our understanding of mechanisms and the accuracy and precision of our instruments to reflect these mechanisms.

It is highly likely that assessments of the physiological status of athletes and exercisers will continue to be an important part of scientific programmes. Similarly, it is probable that assessments will continue to undergo development and refinement as our knowledge base grows. This will increase the sensitivity with which physiological measures explains changes in performance. As a result, the rationale for assessment will strengthen so the need for knowledgeable, skilled and experienced sport and exercise scientists will increase.

REFERENCES

Atkinson, G. and Nevill, A.M. (1998). Statistical methods for assessing measurement error (reliability) in variables relevant to sports medicine. *Sports Medicine*, 26, 217–238.

Bird, S. and Davison, R. (1997). *Physiological Testing Guidelines*, 3rd edn. Leeds: The British Association of Sport and Exercise Sciences.

CHAPTER 1

HEALTH AND SAFETY

Graham Jarman

INTRODUCTION

Laboratory and field work activities present potential hazards to investigators and participants. The purpose of this chapter is to provide a guide on how to implement a risk assessment approach to health and safety management in these settings.

A DUTY OF CARE

Principal investigators and consultants need to be cognisant of their responsibility to exercise a duty of care to athletes and exercisers, participants in research studies, clients and co-workers. This duty of care is made explicit in the enabling legislation enshrined in the Health and Safety at Work Act 1974. Of particular note are the following sections of the Act:

- Section 2: General duties of employers to their employees.
- Section 3: General duties of employers and the self-employed to persons other than their employees.
- Section 7: General duties of employees at work.

The details of the 1974 Act can be found on the HealthandSafety.co.uk website. The general duties of the Act are qualified by the principle of '*so far as is reasonably practicable*', that is, steps to reduce risk need not be taken if they are technically impossible or the time, trouble and cost of measures would be grossly disproportionate to the risk (HSE, 2003). In essence, the law requires that good management and common sense are applied to identify the risks associated with an activity and that sensible measures are implemented to control those risks.

RISK ASSESSMENT

Risk assessment is the cornerstone of health and safety management practice. The Management of Health and Safety Regulations 1999 requires that risk assessments are carried out for *all* activities and that significant findings are documented. Other regulations require that specific types of assessment are made for certain work areas, for example, working with substances (COSHH), noise and manual handling. The Health and Safety Executive (HSE) publication '*A Guide to Risk Assessment Requirements*' (HSE, 1996) examines the common features of the assessments as required by the various regulations and highlights the differences between them.

Risk assessment is essentially an examination of what in the workplace could cause harm to people. It is a structured analysis of what can cause harm, an assessment of the likelihood and impact of something harmful happening and a means to identify measures that can be implemented to mitigate the occurrence of harmful incidents.

APPROACH

The HSE advocate a five-step approach to risk assessment (HSE, 1999):

- Step 1: identify the hazards;
- Step 2: decide who might be harmed and how;
- Step 3: evaluate the risk and decide whether existing precautions are adequate or more should be done;
- Step 4: record significant findings;
- Step 5: review assessment and revise if necessary.

IDENTIFYING HAZARDS

A hazard is something that has the potential to be harmful. The following is an indicative, but not exhaustive list, of typical hazards that are likely to exist in a physiology of exercise laboratory and field-based settings:

Working with equipment:

- Electrical hazard
- Entrapment hazards
- Falls or trips.

Changes in the physiological state of participants:

- Cardio-vascular complications
- Fainting

- Vomiting
- Musculo-skeletal injury.

The administration of pharmacologically active substances and nutritional supplements:

- Overdose or acute effects
- Chronic effects
- Hypersensitivity (allergic responses).

The use of hazardous materials:

- Chemicals or laboratory reagents
- Potentially infectious material (body fluids).

Modifications to the environment:

- Heat stress
- Cold stress
- Hypoxia or hyperoxia
- Other gas mixtures.

Hazard identification could be undertaken as a systematic inspection of the laboratory or could be integral to the design of an experimental protocol.

DECIDING WHO MIGHT BE HARMED

It is important to identify who might be harmed by any activity undertaken in the laboratory. As well as considering investigators, consultants and co-workers it is imperative that participants involved in investigative procedures are adequately protected from harm. When procedures involve participants from the following groups, for example, additional precautions might be needed to reduce the risk to levels that are considered to be acceptable:

- Minors
- The ageing
- Those with learning difficulties
- Those with underlying medical conditions.

Consider also members of the public or visitors to your premises if there is a chance that they could be harmed by your activities.

EVALUATING AND CONTROLLING RISKS

Risk is an appraisal of the likelihood of a hazard causing harm and the consequence of that harm if realised. This can be represented numerically by multiplying a perceived likelihood rating by a perceived consequence rating. Table 1.1 provides an example of how a simple risk rating system could operate and how this could be used as a means to prioritise actions to control and manage risks.

Managing risk is concerned with reducing likelihood and consequence associated with particular hazards to a level at which they can be tolerated. *Control measures* are actions or interventions that reduce risk to an acceptable level. In general, the following principles should be applied in the order given:

- try a less risky option, for example, substitution;
- prevent access to a hazard, for example, by guarding;
- reduce exposure, for example, by organising the work differently;

Table 1.1   An example of a 3 × 3 risk rating system

	Consequence (C)
3	Major (death or severe injury)
2	Serious (injuries requiring three days or more absence from work)
1	Slight (minor injuries requiring no or brief absence from work)
	Likelihood (L)
3	High (event is likely to occur frequently)
2	Medium (event is likely to occur occasionally)
1	Low (event is unlikely to occur)
Risk rating (C × L)	*Action and timescale*
1 (Trivial)	No action is required to deal with trivial risks
2 (Acceptable)	No further preventative action is necessary but consideration should be given to cost-effective solutions or improvements that impose minimal or no additional cost. Monitoring is required to ensure that controls are maintained
4 (Moderate)	Effort should be made to reduce the risk but the cost of prevention should be carefully measured and limited. Risk reduction measures should be implemented within three to six months depending on the number of people exposed to hazard
6 (Substantial)	Work should not be started until the risk can be reduced. Considerable resources may have to be allocated to reduce the risk. Where the risk involves work in progress, the problems should be resolved as quickly as possible
9 (Intolerable)	Work should not be started or continued until the risk level has been reduced. Whilst the control measures should be cost effective, the legal duty to reduce the risk is absolute. This means that if it is not possible to reduce the risk, even with unlimited resources, then the work must not be started or must remain prohibited

- use of personal protective equipment, for example, use of gloves in blood sampling;
- provision of welfare facilities, for example, washing facilities for removal of contamination.

The legislation requires that you must do what is reasonably practicable to make your work and workplace safe. If risks can not be reduced to an acceptable level by applying cost-effective control measures then consideration must be given to whether or not particular activities can be justified.

RECORDING OUTCOMES OF RISK ASSESSMENT

Any risk assessment that is undertaken must be *suitable and sufficient*. It is a requirement that all significant findings are recorded and there should be documentary evidence to show that:

- a proper check was made;
- consultation with those affected was undertaken if appropriate;
- all obvious hazards have been dealt with;
- precautions are reasonable and any remaining risk is low (or tolerable).

Documentation must be retained for future use and outcomes should be communicated to any individuals who could be affected by the activity. The documents should be retained as evidence that risk assessments have been undertaken, this is particularly important if any civil liability action is taken as a result of an accident. The outcomes of risk assessments can be incorporated into other laboratory documents such as manuals, codes of practice or standard operating procedures.

REVIEWING ASSESSMENTS

It is good practice to review risk assessments periodically to ensure that control measures are effective and that significant risks are being adequately managed. If there are any material changes that affect the risk assessment and control measures in operation, then a review of the assessment should be undertaken. It is important that any amended documents are version-controlled and that all individuals who are affected are informed of the revisions.

PERSONAL INJURY CLAIMS AND PROFESSIONAL INDEMNITY

Laboratory and field-based activities can never be risk free. Should an incident which causes injury or damage occur, it is important that:

- Documentary evidence can be provided to demonstrate that a duty of care has been exercised.

- That professional indemnity and public liability insurance is in place to cover any legal cost or awards of damages if, for example, a case of negligence is proven.

In the event of personal injury to a client or co-worker there is a formal process by which this is dealt. This 'Pre-action Protocol' is covered in detail on the Department for Constitutional Affairs (DCA) website; of particular interest are the lists of standard disclosure documents given in the annex.

The BASES code of conduct (BASES, 2000) states that: 'members must ensure that suitable insurance indemnity cover is in place for all areas of work that they undertake'. Care must be taken to understand the scope, limitations and exclusions associated with any insurance cover to ensure its adequacy.

OBTAINING INFORMATION AND FURTHER GUIDANCE

The earlier discussion covers the generality of risk assessment as a process. It is recommended that reference is made to the relevant approved codes of practice and related guidance leaflets that are published by the HSE. The HSE website (www.hse.gov.uk) provides a breadth of advice in the form of downloadable leaflets. Some suggested further reading on some of the specific issues and hazards encountered in the physiology of exercise laboratory are given here.

REFERENCES AND FURTHER READING

British Association of Sport and Exercise Sciences (BASES). (2000). *Code of Conduct*. http://www.bases.org.uk/newsite/pdf/Code%20of%20Conduct.pdf. Accessed 16 December 2005.

Department for Constitutional Affairs. *Pre-Action Protocol for Personal Injury Claims*. http://www.dca.gov.uk/civil/procrules_fin/contents/protocols/prot_pic.htm. Accessed 16 December 2005.

Health and Safety Executive (HSE). (1996). *A Guide to Risk Assessment Risk Assessment Requirements*. http://www.hse.gov.uk/pubns/indg218.pdf. Accessed 11 November 2005.

Health and Safety Executive (HSE). (1999). *Five Steps to Risk Assessment*. http://www.hse.gov.uk/pubns/indg163.pdf. Accessed 11 November 2005.

Health and Safety Executive (HSE). (2001). *Blood-borne Viruses in the Workplace*. http://www.hse.gov.uk/pubns/indg342.pdf. Accessed 16 December 2005.

Health and Safety Executive (HSE). (2003). *Health and Safety Regulation...A Short Guide*. http://www.hse.gov.uk/pubns/hsc13.pdf. Accessed 15 November 2005.

Health and Safety Executive (HSE). (2005). *Coshh: A Brief Guide to the Regulations*. http://www.hse.gov.uk/pubns/indg136.pdf. Accessed 16 December 2005.

Healthandsafety.co.uk. '[A guide to] The Health and Safety at Work etc Act 1974. (Elizabeth II 1974. Chapter 37)'. http://www.healthandsafety.co.uk/haswa.htm. Accessed 15 November 2005.

Medicines and Healthcare Products Regulatory Agency. (2003). *Guidance Note 8: A Guide to what is a Medicinal Product*. http://www.mhra.gov.uk/home/groups/commsic/documents/publication/con007544.pdf. Accessed 16 December 2005.

Office of Public Sector Information. *The Management of Health and Safety at Work Regulations*. http://www.opsi.gov.uk/si/si1999/19993242.htm#13. Accessed 17 November 2005.

CHAPTER 2

PSYCHOLOGICAL ISSUES IN EXERCISE TESTING

Craig A. Mahoney

INTRODUCTION

Exercise testing usually serves one of two purposes:

- health screening and diagnosis of disease;
- fitness testing for sport/exercise.

Exercise tests for the general population are normally designed to provide exercise professionals with information on disease diagnosis or prevention, rehabilitation and intensities to commence an exercise programme (de Vries and Housh, 1995). The feedback participants receive can help to establish appropriate intrinsic motivation to achieve goal outcomes. Goal determination will vary depending upon the types of test being completed, the background to the participant, the person commissioning the tests and a range of less tangible factors.

While some participants will self-refer to receive exercise testing as part of a health club membership package, an increasing number of participants do not. The latter are often asked to attend for exercise testing as part of a corporate programme offered to employees (seen by the employers as an employee benefit) though employees might not always be positive about the impact of the assessment, the imposition on their normal lives or their perceived understanding of the purpose of the tests. Many organisations now have minimum health (or fitness) standards required for continued employment; these include the ambulance service, fire service, some police forces, professional football referees and many other occupations that have a measured, objective physical component to their employment base.

For sporting populations, the ongoing assessment of fitness may be related to the process of monitoring training programmes, assessing recovery from injury or medical intervention, or be used as part of a selection process.

Undoubtedly, many athletes approach the regular (often several times per year) assessments with minimum fuss and limited concerns about their ability to perform well, and confidence in the outcomes. However, there is another group who (like employee assessment programmes) have lingering concerns about the purpose and outcomes of exercise testing. These participants often worry for some time before the tests and then present themselves in an over anxious state. This needs to be recognised, reconciled and minimised if the results of tests are to be valid and reliable for coaches, athletes and exercise professionals.

MENTAL ENERGY

Regardless of the types of physical activity in which people engage, whether it is exercise, practice for sport, sports performance or fitness testing, an individual's mental energy to concentrate attention and maintain a positive mental attitude is essential in ensuring optimum physical performances. It is very easy to waste mental energy and therefore physical energy on worry, stress, fretting over distractions and negative thoughts. This will have the combined effect of reducing enjoyment and adversely affecting results. Effective concentration will help to maintain sound technique, for example, during running on the treadmill or when performing shuttles, while enabling participants to conserve energy. Fatigue brought about by physical effort or cognitive stress will result in muscle tiredness and a downward spiral of negative thinking that will exacerbate feelings of pain, fatigue, hopelessness and defeat.

MOTIVATION

Exercise testing has a strong association with intrinsic motivation. There is anecdotal evidence to show that people who score higher than anticipated on exercise tests can become more motivated and more committed, while those who score lower than anticipated can become less motivated and less committed. This seems to be associated with Attribution Theory that attempts to explain behaviours and has been evidenced in medical settings (Rothman *et al.*, 1993).

Athletes and participants from the general population will often involve themselves in exercise testing to identify training needs, screen their health, or evaluate the effectiveness of their training plan or health programme. In the absence of improvement or at the very minimum maintenance, that is, no relapse, participants can lose momentum and the associated intrinsic motivation for training. Though testing should not be considered in isolation from other factors such as; the time of the season for an athlete or lifestyle factors for general population participants, as these additional factors can aid in ensuring training, improvement and personal commitment are all part of an holistic personal development plan for health and fitness benefits. On this basis an understanding of the performance profiling needs and personal goals of all participants should be fully understood by the exercise professional both to tailor the right testing programme and ensure that the designed training programme meets the perceived and actual needs of each participant. It is unlikely that exercise testing will in itself, result in motivation to exercise. Beginners especially, are highly susceptible to positive feedback and vulnerable to negative outcomes. New exercise participants can often display low self-efficacy and are likely to find limited motivation from the experience of exercise testing. Once they have established some skills associated with exercise, results from exercise testing may be a useful form of feedback to aid the motivation to continue.

STRESS AND ANXIETY

Just as psychological preparation for performance in sport is now a recognised part of athlete preparation, so too are psychological aspects of physiological assessment and these should be understood by the exercise professional, and arguably the participant as well. The right mental approach to exercise testing often begins when a date is established for that 'fear inducing' battery of assessments agreed between the coach(es) and the sport scientist(s), since the very thought of exercise testing can create anxiety in many. Others will see this as an opportunity to excel, show why they should be selected above others or merely gain a better understanding of their current physiological status. However, from that point forward, participants will often consciously and subconsciously worry about the types of test, the purpose of the tests, previous experience with the tests and this can result in a range of cognitive concerns, which manifest themselves as fear and trepidation.

Cognitive appraisal by participants is common in testing environments. It is not uncommon for some participants to worry considerably about being tested and the test procedures they will have to follow. Whether this is laboratory- or field-based does not seem to matter. A significant determinant of worry is the basis of the testing, for example, is it part of regular in-season assessment or does it form part of a selection process? Sometimes it can be used in association with employment criteria, for instance, to maintain minimum work standards.

SEQUENCING

The ACSM (2005) has recommended completing tests in a particular sequence, to minimise the effects of tests on one another (Heyward, 1998). The order is broadly:

- Resting blood pressure and heart rate
- Neuromuscular tension and/or stress (if included)
- Body composition
- Muscular fitness
- Cardiorespiratory endurance
- Flexibility.

This order is regardless of whether the tests are field or laboratory based. However, it is often helpful to negotiate with, and agree, particular sequencing in tests. Experience has shown that many older athletes, who have participated in fitness test batteries over many years, are often more comfortable with some tests being completed prior to others.

Some clients might be apprehensive prior to being exercise tested and will demonstrate elevated anxiety about the testing process and particular tests included in the battery. The use of the Multi Stage Fitness Test seems consistently to raise concerns in the minds of athletes prior to its completion. This usually coincides with prior experience in the test. Naive populations, such as school children or first time participants on the test, do not normally present with this anxiety. Another test frequently associated with elevated anxiety is the assessment of maximum oxygen uptake. Endurance tests often raise fear and anxiety in the minds of participants. This can be related to previous experience, but is often underpinned by an absence of training, an existing injury or a general dislike for the test or its protocols. Exercise professionals have an obligation to screen the participant fully and ensure they are in the best physical, but also mental, health to complete the testing programme. Recognition should be given, that varying the intensity of encouragement to participants will also affect results. Due to the motivational basis to the Multi Stage Fitness Test, excessive encouragement can lead to significantly improved results for some participants.

It is incumbent on test administrators to minimise the impact of anxiety in the testing process. Test anxiety can reduce the validity and reliability of test results. To ensure this is not a compounding variable in the efficacy of the test results, clients should always be put at ease upon arrival. Establishing a good rapport between the tester and participant(s) should help to achieve this. Providing a relaxed non-intimidating environment should help to foster a confident but relaxed approach to the battery of tests being used. Ensure the environment is safe, friendly, quiet, private (where appropriate) and comfortable if possible. Careful consideration of temperature and humidity should be taken in consultation with the coaching and support staff and obviously will depend on the purpose of the tests, which may form part of an acclimatisation process. Ensuring appropriate and careful calibration has been completed will also serve to reduce concerns from the group(s) being tested.

HUMAN BEHAVIOUR

How well the exercise professional understands human behaviour and personal mood variables will play an important part in the testing experience of the participant. The importance of understanding basic human behaviour cannot be overstated in an exercise test setting. The British Association of Sport and Exercise Sciences accreditation scheme, established as a gold standard in applied sport and exercise science, has recently acknowledged the need for minimum sport science knowledge from all key sciences prior to the approval of accreditation.

When testing different groups, exercise professionals will build up a strong knowledge of the individuals and the types of test most appropriate for these specialist populations. Paediatric populations are one such specialist group. Because of the dearth of knowledge that such participants might have about laboratory- or field-based testing, it is essential that those working with young people ensure a caring, compassionate and sensitive approach to their work. This is particularly relevant in understanding the goals and motivations that young people will have towards exercise testing, particularly if the procedures are invasive, intense and not fully understood by the participants (Whitehead and Corbin, 1991; Goudas *et al.*, 1994). Notwithstanding the ethical issues that will have had to be approved prior to this, young children will often need more advanced habituation to some testing procedures. If blood samples are being taken, as will often occur in paediatric studies, then demonstration might help, as might anaesthetic creams to minimise pain. The use of mouth pieces is being superseded by face masks in peak oxygen uptake testing, however if mouth pieces are to be used it will often help habituate children and minimise anxiety if they can be given a mouth piece to take home for several days prior to the test.

MODEL OF BEHAVIOUR CHANGE

When prescribing exercise programmes after laboratory- or field-based exercise testing, it is essential that exercise professionals are cognisant of adherence issues, the stages of behaviour change a participant might be demonstrating and willingness on the part of the participant. This will vary between populations. For example, professional and elite athletes would normally present themselves for testing with high intrinsic motivation to succeed and strong personal commitment to prescribed programmes if they possess confidence in the exercise professional and feel the programmes are beneficial to their personal (and usually sporting) potential. This requires the exercise professional to be able to communicate with all exercise test participants on a practical level using language, which is sincere, simple, but not degrading. Most athletes want to be confident that the exercise professional is aware of contemporary issues and training protocols, but they might not want (or need) to know the intricate detail behind the theory.

To this end, establishing clear motives for exercise testing, having an unambiguous understanding of goals that will arise from this and an awareness of the stage, in the Stages of Behaviour Change (Prochaska and DiClemente, 1986), the participant is in will be important (Figure 2.1). These are less relevant concerns when working with elite athletes, since the Governing Body, coaching staff or the athletes have probably established these themselves. However, when assessing participants from the general population who might be part of a corporate testing programme or who have simply made themselves available for testing, or who are part of a research study involving non-elite participants, these covert motives become much more relevant. The concerns arising from this include; will the participant adhere to any exercise programme arising from analysis of the test results; how will adherence

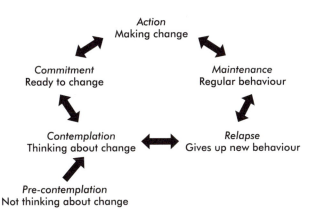

Figure 2.1   Models of the stages of behaviour

be optimised (e.g. social support, priority level, re-assessment, time allocation, SMART goals, monitoring), what factors can help them achieve their goals (or the goals of the programme funder), when re-assessment occurs will this be a positive experience for the participant?

Clearly, the whole area of exercise testing is affected by factors, which exhibit both a cognitive and a behavioural basis. To help minimise their effect on test results, exercise professionals (and participants) should have an understanding of these and be prepared to adapt testing regimens to minimise their impact wherever possible. The following is offered as guidance to participants and exercise professionals.

Guidance for participants

Prior to the day of testing, ensure good rest and sleep where possible. In the same way physical performance can be affected by under or over arousal, so too can exercise test performances. If feeling lethargic then use arousal strategies such as:

- Light exercise
- Warm up routines
- Loud music.

If participants are feeling anxious, then the following relaxation routines might help:

- Calming music
- Relaxation exercises or tape
- Imagery relaxation
- Calm movements, breathing control and tranquil thoughts
- Biofeedback (if previously developed)
- Thought awareness and positive thinking.

Guidance for exercise professionals

- Give time for habituation.
- Allow participants to take home pieces of equipment that may cause anxiety, for example, mouth pieces for VO_{2max} tests, especially children.
- Ensure all participants are supported in an equitable and consistent manner.
- Be sensitive to participant concerns related to some tests, for example, Multi Stage Fitness Test where motivation is highly significant and the test often generates considerable concerns in the minds of performers.

Exercise testing is a complex and multifaceted activity that combines the academic knowledge, practical skills, experiential awareness and personal capacity of the testing team to ensure the participant(s) have the most positive experience achievable. Where possible, exercise professionals must endeavour to ensure that all participants have a positive mental state leading up to and upon engaging in the exercise testing programme. This will increase the potential both for optimal and maximum achievable results. However, regardless of the scientific competency of the exercise physiologist undertaking the testing, sometimes no matter how effective their communication, counselling or relaxation skills, a patient with heart failure that might be progressing to end stage (i.e. death or transplant) and is being evaluated, by, for example, cardiopulmonary exercise testing, for this reason is not going to approach the test with a positive mental state. In such circumstances all we can do is manage those things that are within our control in order to minimise the potential negative experiences of testing.

REFERENCES

American College of Sports Medicine (ACSM). (2005). *ACSM's Guidelines for Exercise Testing and Prescription*, 7th edn. Philadelphia, PA: Lippincott Williams & Wilkins.

de Vries, H.A. and Housh, T.J. (1995). *Physiology of Exercise: for Physical Education, Athletics and Exercise Science*, 5th edn. Dubuque: WC Brown.

Heyward, V.H. (1998). *Advanced Fitness Assessment and Exercise Prescription*. Champaign, IL: Human Kinetics.

Goudas, M., Biddle, S. and Fox, K. (1994). Achievement goal orientations and intrinsic motivation in physical fitness testing with children. *Pediatric Exercise Science*, 6: 159–167.

Prochaska, J.O. and DiClemente, C.C. (1986). Toward a comprehensive model of change. in W.R. Miller and N. Heather (eds) *Addictive Behaviours: Processes of Change*. pp. 3–27. New York: Plenum Press.

Rothman, A., Salovey, P., Turvey, C. and Fishkin, S. (1993). Attributions of responsibility and persuasion: increasing mammography utilisation among women over 40 and with internally oriented message. *Health Psychology*, 12: 39–47.

Whitehead, J.R. and Corbin, C.B. (1991). Youth fitness testing: the effect of percentile – based evaluative feedback on intrinsic motivation. *Research Quarterly for Exercise and Sport*, 62(2): 225–231.

CHAPTER 3

BLOOD SAMPLING

Ron Maughan, Susan M. Shirreffs and
John B. Leiper

INTRODUCTION

The collection of blood samples from human subjects is required in many physiological, biochemical and nutritional investigations. The use to be made of the sample will determine the method of collection, the volume of blood required and the way in which the specimen is handled.

BLOOD SAMPLING AND HANDLING

Many different methods and sites of blood sampling can be used to collect samples for analysis, and the results obtained will be affected by the sampling site and by the procedures used in sample collection. A detailed discussion of the sampling procedures and of the consequences for measurement of various parameters is presented by Maughan *et al.* (2001).

The main sampling procedures involve collection of arterial, venous, arterialised venous or capillary blood. In most routine laboratory investigations of interest to the sports scientist, arterial blood sampling is impractical and unnecessarily invasive, and will not be considered in detail here. Where arterial blood is required, arterial puncture may be used, but in most situations, collection of arterialised venous blood as described later gives an adequate representation of arterial blood.

Venous blood

Venous blood sampling is probably the method of choice for most routine purposes: sampling from a superficial forearm or ante-cubital vein is simple, painless and relatively free from risk of complications. Sampling may be by venous puncture or by an indwelling cannula. Where repeated sampling is necessary at short time intervals, introduction of a cannula is obviously preferred to avoid repeated venous punctures. Either a plastic cannula or a butterfly-type cannula can be used. The latter has obvious limitations if introduced into an ante-cubital vein, as movement of the elbow is severely restricted. However, because it is smaller and therefore less painful for the subject, as well as being very much less expensive, it is often preferable if used in a forearm vein, provided that long-term access is not required. A 21 g cannula is adequate for most purposes, and only where large volumes of blood are required will a larger size be necessary. In most situations where vigorous movements are likely, the forearm site is preferred to the elbow. Clotting of blood in the cannula is easily avoided by flushing with sterile isotonic saline. Where intermittent sampling is performed, the cannula may be flushed with a bolus of saline to which heparin $(10–50 \text{ IU·ml}^{-1}$ of saline) is added, allowing the subject freedom to move around between samples. Alternatively where the subject is to remain static, as in a cycle or treadmill exercise test, a continuous slow infusion (about $0.3 \text{ ml·min})^{-1}$ of isotonic saline may be used, avoiding the need to add heparin. Collection of samples by venous puncture is not practical in most exercise situations, and increases the risk that samples will be affected by venous occlusion applied during puncture. If repeated venous puncture is used, care must be taken to minimise the duration of any occlusion of blood flow and to ensure that sufficient time is allowed for recovery from interruption of blood flow before samples are collected.

Flow through the superficial forearm veins is very much influenced by skin blood flow, which in turn depends on ambient temperature and the thermoregulatory strain imposed on the individual. In cold conditions, flow to the limbs and to the skin will be low, and venous blood will be highly desaturated. Where sampling occurs over time, therefore, and where the degree of arterialisation of the venous blood will influence the measures to be made, this may cause major problems. For some metabolites which are routinely measured, the difference between arterial and venous concentrations is relatively small and in many cases it may be ignored. Where a difference does occur and is of importance, the effect of a change in arterialisation of the blood at the sampling site may be critical.

Arterialised venous blood

Where arterial blood is required, there is no alternative to arterial puncture, but for most practical purposes, blood collected from a superficial vein on the dorsal surface of a heated hand is indistinguishable from arterial blood. This reflects both the very high flow rate and the opening of arterio-venous shunts in the hand. Sampling can conveniently be achieved by introduction of a butterfly cannula into a suitable vein. The hand is first heated, either by immersion up to the forearm for at least 10 min in hot (about 42°C) water (Forster *et al.*, 1972) or by insertion into a hot air box (McGuire *et al.*, 1976). If hot water immersion is used prior to exercise, arterialisation – as indicated by oxygen saturation – can be maintained for some considerable time by wearing a glove, allowing this technique to be used during exercise studies. This procedure allows large volumes of blood to be collected without problems. Capillary sampling by the fingerprick method cannot guarantee adequate volumes for many procedures.

Capillary blood

Where only small samples of blood are required, capillary blood samples can readily be obtained from a fingertip or earlobe. The use of micromethods for analysis means that the limited sample volume that can be obtained should not necessarily be a problem in metabolic studies. It is possible to make duplicate measurements of the concentrations of glucose, lactate, pyruvate, alanine, free fatty acids, glycerol, acetoacetate and 3-hydroxybutyrate as well as a number of other metabolites on a single 20 μl blood sample using routine laboratory methods (Maughan, 1982).

The sampling site should be arterialised, by immersion of the whole hand in hot (42°C) water in the case of the finger tip, and by the use of a rubefacient in the case of the earlobe. Samples can be obtained without stimulating vasodilatation, but bleeding is slower, the volumes that can be reliably collected are smaller, and the composition of the sample is more variable. It is essential that a free flowing sample is obtained. If pressure is applied, an excess of plasma over red cells will be obtained. Samples are most conveniently collected into graduated glass capillaries where only small volumes are required (typically 10–100 μl). The blood must never be expelled from these tubes by mouth, because of the obvious risks involved. Volumes greater than about 0.5 ml are difficult to obtain.

BLOOD TREATMENT AFTER COLLECTION

Analysis of most metabolites can be carried out using whole blood, plasma or serum, but the differential distribution of most metabolites and substrates between the plasma and the intracellular space may affect values. It is convenient to use whole blood for the measurement of most metabolites. Glucose, glycerol and lactate are commonly measured on either plasma or whole blood, but free fatty acid concentration should be measured using plasma or serum. The differences become significant where there is a concentration difference between the intracellular and extracellular compartments.

If plasma is to be obtained by centrifugation of the sample, a suitable anticoagulant must be added. A variety of agents can be used, depending on the measurements to be made. The potassium salt of EDTA is a convenient anticoagulant, but is clearly inappropriate when plasma potassium is to be measured. Heparin is a suitable alternative in this situation. For serum collection, blood should be added to a plain tube and left for at least 1 h before centrifugation: clotting will take place more rapidly if the sample is left in a warm place. If there is a need to stop glycolysis in serum or plasma samples (e.g. where the concentration of glucose, lactate or other glycolytic intermediates is to be measured), fluoride should be added. Where metabolites of glucose are to be measured on whole blood, the most convenient method is immediate deproteinisation of the sample to inactivate the enzymes which would otherwise alter the concentrations of substances of interest after the sample has been withdrawn.

Control of factors affecting blood and plasma volumes

Blood and plasma volumes are markedly influenced by the physical activity, hydration status and posture of the subject prior to sample collection. The sampling site and method can also affect the haemoglobin concentration, as arterial, capillary and venous samples differ in a number of respects due to fluid exchange between the vascular and extravascular spaces and to differences in the distribution of red blood cells (Harrison, 1985). The venous plasma to red cell ratio is higher than that of arterial blood, although the total body haemoglobin content is clearly not acutely affected by these factors. Haemodynamic changes caused by postural shifts will alter the fluid exchange across the capillary bed, leading to plasma volume changes that will cause changes in the circulating concentration. On going from a supine position to standing, plasma volume falls by about 10% and whole blood volume by about 5% (Harrison, 1985). This corresponds to a change in the measured haemoglobin concentration of about 7 g·l^{-1}. These changes are reversed on going from an upright to a seated or supine position. These changes make in imperative that posture is controlled in studies where haemoglobin changes are to be used as an index of changes in blood and plasma volume over the time course of an experiment. It is, however, common to see studies reported in the literature where samples were collected from subjects resting in a supine position prior to exercise in a seated (cycling or rowing) or upright (treadmill walking or running) position. The changing blood volume not only invalidates any haematological measures made in the early stages of exercise, it also confounds cardiovascular measures as the stroke volume and heart rate will also be affected by the blood volume.

SAFETY ISSUES

Whatever method is used for the collection of blood samples, the safety of the subject and of the investigator is paramount. Strict safety precautions must be followed at all times in the sampling and handling of blood. It is wise to assume that all samples are infected and to treat them accordingly. This means wearing gloves and appropriate protective clothing and following guidelines for handling of samples and disposal of waste material. Appropriate antiseptic procedures must be followed at all times, including ensuring cleanliness of the sampling environment, cleaning of the puncture site and use of clean materials to staunch bleeding after sampling. Blood sampling should be undertaken only by those with appropriate training and insurance cover, and a qualified first-aider should be available at all times. All contaminated materials must be disposed of using appropriate and clearly identified waste containers. Used needles, cannulae and lancets must be disposed off immediately in a suitable sharps bin: resheathing of used needles must never be attempted. Sharps – whether contaminated or not – must always be disposed off in an approved container and must never be mixed with other waste. Any spillage of blood must be treated immediately.

There is clearly a need for appropriate training of all laboratory personnel involved in any aspect of blood sampling and handling. Most major hospitals run courses for the training of phlebotomists, who are often individuals with no medical background. The taking of blood samples is a simple physical skill, and a medical training is not required when expert assistance is at hand. What is essential, though, is the necessary back up if something goes wrong, and a suitable training in first aid and resuscitation should be seen as a necessary part of the training for the sports scientists who collect blood samples outwith a hospital setting.

REFERENCES AND FURTHER READING

Dacie, J.V. and Lewis, S.M. (1968). *Practical Haematology*, 4th edn. London: Churchill, pp. 45–49.

Forster, H.V., Dempsey, J.A., Thomson, J., Vidruk, E. and DoPico, G.A. (1972). Estimation of arterial PO_2, PCO_2, pH and lactate from arterialized venous blood. *Journal of Applied Physiology*, 32: 134–137.

Harrison, M. (1985). Effects of thermal stress and exercise on blood volume in humans. *Physiological Review*, 65: 149–209.

Maughan, R.J. (1982). A simple rapid method for the determination of glucose, lactate, pyruvate, alanine, 3-hydroxybutyrate and acetoacetate on a single 20 µl blood sample. *Clinica Chimica Acta*, 122: 232–240.

Maughan, R.J., Leiper, J.B. and Greaves, M. (2001). Haematology. In R.G. Eston and T.P. Reilly (eds) *Kinanthropometry and Exercise Physiology Laboratory Manual*, 2nd edn. London: Spon Volume 2, pp. 99–115.

McGuire, E.A.H., Helderman, J.H., Tobin, J.D., Andres, R. and Berman, M. (1976). Effects of arterial versus venous sampling on analysis of glucose kinetics in man. *Journal of Applied Physiology*, 41: 565–573.

CHAPTER 4

ETHICS AND PHYSIOLOGICAL TESTING

Steve Olivier

WHAT IS ETHICS?

What is it to behave in an ethical manner as a researcher? The term 'ethics' suggests a set of standards by which behaviour is regulated, and these standards help us to decide what is acceptable in terms of pursuing our aims, as well as helping us to distinguish between right and wrong acts. The principal question of ethics is 'What ought I do?'

Broadly speaking, ethical actions are derived from principles and values, which are in turn derived from ethical theories. The major ethical theories are briefly introduced here for two reasons: to enable researchers to identify where principles are derived from, and to facilitate deeper thought on how potential actions may be justified.

Virtue theory focuses on being a 'good' person, and doing the right thing (e.g. being fair, honest and so on) necessarily flows from being a 'good' person. Utilitarian (consequential) theory attaches primary importance to the consequences of actions – if the 'good' consequences outweigh the 'bad' ones for all concerned by the action, then the action is right and is morally required. Lastly, Deontology holds that primacy is attached to meeting duties and obligations, that the ends do not justify the means, and that an individual's preferences, interests and rights should be respected. It is worth noting that codes of ethics are generally deontological in nature.

There are three basic principles upon which our conception of research ethics is based, namely respect for persons, beneficence (doing good) and justice. Applying these to research contexts involves consideration of autonomy (an individual's right to self-determination), obligations not to harm others (including physical, psychological or social harm), utility (producing a net balance of benefits over harm), justice (distributing benefits and harms fairly), fidelity keeping promises and contracts), privacy, and veracity (truthfulness). More specific ethical considerations would include recognition of cultural factors, preserving participant anonymity (or confidentiality, as appropriate), non-discrimination, sanctions against offenders, compliance with procedures and reports of violations (Olivier, 1995).

INFORMED CONSENT

A central feature of modern biomedical research ethics is the notion of obtaining first person, written, voluntary informed consent from research participants. Given that it is a required element of most projects, researchers need to be aware of what the concept involves.

First, 'informed' implies that potential participants (or their legal representatives) obtain sufficient information about the project. This information must be presented in such a way that it is matched to the appropriate comprehension level (see Olivier and Olivier, 2001; and Cardinal, 2000, for further details on establishing comprehension levels), enabling participants to evaluate and understand the implications of what they are about to agree to. Second, 'consent' implies free, voluntary agreement to participation, without coercion or unfair inducement.[1]

Consent can be considered to be informed when 'it is given in the full, or clear, realization of what the tests involve, including an awareness...of risk attached to what takes place' (Mahon, 1987, p. 203). Further, 'Subjects must be fully informed of the risks, procedures, and potential benefits, and that they are free to end their participation in the study with no penalty whatsoever' (Zelaznik, 1993, p. 63).

Consent is deemed ethically acceptable if the participant receives full disclosure of relevant information, if the implications are understood, if the participant voluntarily agrees to participate, if opportunities to freely ask relevant questions are present throughout the duration of the project and if the participant feels able to withdraw from the procedures at any time.

The informed consent form

The informed consent form, normally signed by the participants, should be tailored to the specific project that it relates to. The document should include the following elements:

- an explanation of the purposes of the project;
- a description of the procedures that will involve participants, including the time commitment;
- identification and description of any risks/discomforts, and potential benefits that can reasonably be foreseen, as well as any arrangements for treatment in the case of injury;
- statements regarding confidentiality, anonymity and privacy;
- identification of an appropriate individual whom the participants can approach regarding any questions about the research;

- a statement that participation is voluntary, that consent has been freely obtained and that participants may withdraw at any time without fear of sanction.

A consent form should not include language that absolves the researcher from blame, or any other waiver of legal rights releasing, or appearing to release anyone from liability (Liehmon, 1979; Veatch, 1989). The consent form should conclude with a statement that the participant has read the document and understands it, and should provide space underneath for a signature and the date. Space should also be provided for signatures of the researcher and an independent witness.

Written consent is considered to be the norm for all but the most minor of research procedures. It can serve to protect participants as well as investigators, and serves as proof that some attention has been paid to the interests of the participants. Written consent is superior to oral in that the form itself can be used as an explanatory tool and as a reference document in the communication process between researchers and participants. Also, presenting information orally as well as in written form may have the advantage of prompting participants to ask relevant questions. However, when there are doubts about the literacy level of participants, oral information should supplement proxy[2] written consent.

Witnessed consent may be particularly useful when participants are elderly or have intellectual or cultural difficulties in speech or comprehension. In these cases, an independent person, such as a nurse or a community/religious leader, should sign a document stating that the witness was present when the researcher explained the project, and that in the opinion of the witness, the participant understood the implications of the research and consented freely.

Special legal or institutional considerations may apply when the research involves, inter alia, pregnant women, foetuses, prisoners, children, wards of the state or when deception is used. Research requiring deception, or procedures carrying an unusually high risk of harm, will typically require that a researcher satisfies additional conditions.[3]

There is little unanimity concerning the practice of paying research participants, particularly when intrusive procedures are involved. Researchers should be satisfied that payment does not constitute coercion, and remuneration should not adversely affect the judgement of potential participants in respect of risk assessment. Statements on payment to participants should not deflect attention away from the other information in the informed consent form.

Obtaining informed consent at the start of a project may not be sufficient – circumstances may change and new ethical considerations might arise[4] – and researchers should be aware that consent with participants might have to be renegotiated. This might also mean that emergent issues are referred back to the original ethics committee for clearance. It is worth noting that obtaining informed consent does not ensure that a research project is ethical. The research itself must be ethical, and researchers should consider the moral issues that apply to their work.

Children as research participants[5]

When utilising children as research participants, you should consider not only their rights to choose to participate in research (and to withdraw), but also issues such as power differentials, and coercion, in the recruitment process. If you are using a gatekeeper for access (such as a coach, or teacher), that person should not recruit children on your behalf, and should not have access to any individualised data collected. Beware of obtaining proxy consent, as it is unlikely that anyone in a relatively low hierarchical position (such as pupils in a school) will refuse to participate if someone higher up (e.g. a teacher, or Head) gives permission on their behalf (Homan, 2002). You should obtain active rather than passive (assumed) consent. Passive consent involves making the assumption that non-refusal constitutes tacit agreement to participate. While this is a much easier method of recruiting, it may disregard the autonomous wishes (or voluntariness) of participants.

The Medical Research Council (2004) supports the use of children in research as long as the benefits and risks are carefully assessed. Where there is no benefit to child participants, the risk needs to be minimal (see MRC, 2004, pp. 14–15 for categories of risk). Minimal risk activities include questioning, observing and measuring children,[6] and obtaining bodily fluids without invasive intervention. This rules out more invasive procedures such as muscle biopsies.

In England and Wales, anyone who has reached the statutory age of majority (eighteen years) can consent to being a research participant in therapeutic or nontherapeutic[7] studies. For therapeutic research, the Family Reform Act 1969 provides that anyone over 16 can provide consent. Below 16, it is suggested that no one under 12 can provide individual consent (rather than assent, it should be noted), but that children over 12 can provide consent if they are deemed sufficiently mature by the researcher (Nicholson, in Jago and Bailey, 2001). For nontherapeutic work, there is no precise age below 18 at which a child acquires legal capacity, but again, for anyone over 12, an assessment of maturity must be made. The problem with this, of course, is that researchers must 'accept the possibility of prosecution if their interpretation of a child's competence to consent is deemed unacceptable' (Jago and Bailey, 2001, p. 531).

Given that most research by BASES members is nontherapeutic, what should you do? For participants under eighteen, obtain parental consent, first person consent from the participants, and proxy consent from a relevant authority figure if appropriate. If your potential participants are aged 7 to 12, obtain assent (acquiescence, or yea saying) on a simplified form, as well as parental and proxy consent as appropriate. In all cases, the language used on consent and assent forms should be tailored to the participants' comprehension levels (see Olivier and Olivier, 2001).

The ethics review process

The emphasis on research ethics in recent decades is a response to abuses perpetrated on human research participants in the past. This chapter is not the place to enumerate such details (see McNamee *et al.*, 2006), but suffice to say that the regulatory response has been to create a system of ethical review with which investigators must comply.

All funding bodies will insist, as part of the review process, that potential projects are carefully scrutinised with regard to ethical implications. Regulations in the United Kingdom are not as consistently applied as in the United States, but nevertheless, most institutions (e.g. universities, laboratories) will require formal approval of a project before data collection can proceed. Even for unfunded projects, submitting a project for ethical review has benefits for participants (protection of their rights, safety) and for researchers (evidence of compliance with proper procedures, rigour of study design). So, while some researchers view formal ethics review as a bureaucratic impediment to conducting research, it is deemed to be a valuable (if somewhat flawed) process that protects individuals and facilitates good science (Olivier, 2002).

Given that systems of ethics review vary from institution to institution and across funding bodies, it is important for the individual researcher (or team leader) to ascertain what the obligations are with regard to ethics review and compliance. Also, research managers need to be conversant with broader regulatory systems such as the Department of Health Research Governance Framework, NHS Local Research Ethics Committees and the recent introduction into UK law of the European Clinical Trials Directive (see McNamee *et al.*, 2006).

Codes of conduct and accreditation

Codes of conduct and accreditation schemes, such as those administered by BASES, are particularly useful in terms of promoting and maintaining professional competence. A code of conduct though, while promoting ethical behaviour, does not ensure it. This is because rules can conflict, because they are not exhaustive of all moral situations, because they may not take consequences of actions into account, and because they don't consider important contextual issues. Further, if rules are very specific you need an inordinate number to cover all relevant situations, and if they are general then they are likely to be of little practical use. Lastly, and perhaps most importantly, simple rule-following is mechanical, and doesn't promote moral engagement.

Researchers should adhere to the requirements of the BASES Code of Conduct, but should also carefully consider the specific ethical issues that arise from their own projects. It is incumbent on individual researchers, as human agents of moral decision-making, to personally and carefully consider ethical issues inherent in their projects, and to analyse, evaluate, synthesise and apply appropriate principles and values.

Checklist

The checklist below is designed to assist you in preparing your project for ethical review. Remember though that projects are different, and encompass a variety of ethical issues. The checklist is just a start. The challenge for all researchers is to think independently about the ethical issues presented by their work.

- Make sure that you get voluntary, written first-person informed consent. If this is deemed inappropriate, you need to justify the exception.
- Check institutional or legal guidelines about parental consent, and about obtaining a child's assent. In the case of using children as research participants, obtain the necessary parental consent, and the child's assent.
- When using vulnerable populations (e.g. the aged, wards of the state or other agencies), check that you comply with any ethical requirements specific to that group. For example, you may need witnessed consent for cognitively impaired participants.
- Satisfy yourself that participants understand the nature of the project, including any risks or potential benefits. Describing the project to them verbally will often assist in this process.
- Explain to participants that they are free to ask questions at any time, and that they can withdraw from the project whenever they want to.
- Make sure that no coercion occurs during the recruitment process. (Here you need to be clear on issues such as the researcher not being a teacher or assessor of participants' work, for example in the case of students.)
- Allow participants a 'cooling off' period to consider their participation (the time between reading the form and actually agreeing to take part).
- Assess the risk of physical, psychological or social harm to participants.
- Provide medical or other appropriate backup in the event of any potential harm in the categories mentioned earlier.
- Provide medical or other screening, as appropriate.
- Assess the risk of harm to yourself as a researcher, and any assistants (e.g. handling of body fluids, or personal safety in interview situations).
- Provide for the safe conduct of the research if anything has been identified in the preceding point (e.g. correct laboratory procedures; protection in interviews; ability to contact emergency services).
- Assess the impact of any cultural, religious, or gender issues that may pertain to your participants, and/or the dissemination of your findings.
- Provide adequate assurances regarding privacy, confidentiality, anonymity, and how you will securely store and treat your data.
- Satisfy yourself that any payments or inducements offered to participants do not adversely influence their ability to make an informed assessment of the risks and benefits of participation.
- Satisfy yourself that any funding or assistance that you receive with the research will neither result in a conflict of interest, nor compromise your academic integrity.
- If your study involves deception, state the reasons/justification, and indicate how you will debrief the participants about the deception.
- Set measures in place to provide participants with feedback/information on completion of the project.
- And of course, make sure that you have received approval to proceed from the appropriate regional, national or institutional ethics committees.

NOTES

1   I recognise that that this reduction of the concept of informed consent is simplistic, and begs the fallacy of composition (Morgan, 1974), which is the notion that one can break down complex terms into their constituents and then merely add them up as if the sum of the parts was equal to the whole. Nevertheless, it is a useful starting point for the practical application of informed consent procedures.

2   Proxy consent is consent given for an individual, by someone else, for example a parent, religious leader, etc. When seeking proxy consent, particular care should be taken to consider the issues surrounding autonomy and paternalism (see McNamee *et al.*, 2006).

3   For example, justification for deception would include that the research is important, that the results are unobtainable by other methods, that participants are not harmed, and that thorough debriefing occurs if appropriate.

4   Such as the application of new measurement procedures, for example.

5   I would like to thank Malcolm Khan, Senior Lecturer in Law at Northumbria University, for commenting on the legal accuracy of this section.

6   Such activities must be carried out in a sensitive way, with due consideration given to the child's autonomy.

7   I recognise the difficulties with this distinction in terms of describing medical research, but feel that is still useful in terms of much of the research conducted by BASES members.

REFERENCES

Cardinal, B.J. (2000). (Un)Informed consent in exercise and sport science research? A comparison of forms written for two reading levels. *Research Quarterly for Exercise and Sport*, 71(3): 295–301.

Homan, R. (2002). The principles of assumed consent: the ethics of Gatekeeping. In M. McNamee and D. Bridges (eds), *The Ethics of Educational Research*, pp. 23–40. Oxford: Blackwell.

Jago, R. and Bailey, R. (2001). Ethics and paediatric exercise science: issues and making a submission to a local ethics research committee. *Journal of Sports Sciences*, 19: 527–535.

Liehmon, W. (1979). Research involving human subjects. *The Research Quarterly*, 50(2): 157–163.

Mahon, J. (1987). Ethics and drug testing in human beings. In J.D.G. Evans (ed.), *Moral Philosophy and Contemporary Problems*. Cambridge: Press syndicate of the University of Cambridge.

Medical Research Council. (2004). *MRC Ethics Guide: Medical Research Involving Children*. http://www.mrc.ac.uk/pdf-ethics_guide_children.pdf#xml=http://www.mrc.ac.uk/scripts/texis.exe/webinator/search/xml.txt?query=children&pr=mrcall&order=r&cq=&id=422bfe0f2, accessed 7 March 2005.

McNamee, M. Olivier, S. and Wainwright, P. (2006). *Research Ethics in Exercise, Health and Sport Sciences*. Abingdon: Routledge.

Morgan, R. (1974). *Concerns and Values in Physical Education*. London: G Bell and Sons.

Nicholson, R.N. (ed.) (1986). *Medical Research with Children: Ethics, Law and Practice*. Oxford: Oxford University Press. Cited in Jago, R. and Bailey, R. (2001).

Ethics and paediatric exercise science: issues and making a submission to a local ethics research committee. *Journal of Sports Sciences*, 19: 527–535.

Olivier, S. (1995). Ethical considerations in human movement research. *Quest*, 47(2): 135–143.

Olivier, S. (2002). Ethics review of research projects involving human subjects. *Quest*, 54: 194–204.

Olivier, S. and Olivier, A. (2001). Comprehension in the informed consent process. *Sportscience*, 5(3): www.sportsci.org.

Veatch, R.M. (ed.) (1989). *Medical Ethics*. Boston, MA: Jones and Bartlett Publishers.

Zelaznik, H.N. (1993). Ethical issues in conducting and reporting research: a reaction to Kroll, Matt and Safrit. *Quest*, 45(1): 62–68.

PART 2

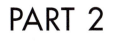

METHODOLOGICAL ISSUES

CHAPTER 5

METHOD AGREEMENT AND MEASUREMENT ERROR IN THE PHYSIOLOGY OF EXERCISE

Greg Atkinson and Alan M.Nevill

INTRODUCTION

Exercise physiologists need to make an informed choice of the most appropriate measurement tool before they start collecting data from athletes or research participants. The main criteria governing this choice are:

- the appropriate level of invasiveness and convenience of use;
- the available budget;
- the degree of test–retest measurement error;
- the degree of agreement with an alternative method, which is possibly more invasive, less convenient or more expensive.

It is important to note that the most expensive and invasive measurement tool might *not* necessarily be associated with the least test–retest measurement error. Moreover, *all* measurement methods that are employed in order to measure some aspect of human physiology have some degree of test–retest error attributable to natural biological variation. For example, use of the so-called '*gold standard*' Douglas bag method of gas analysis is still associated with substantial test–retest error due to human variability in oxygen consumption kinetics during exercise (Atkinson *et al.*, 2005a). Similarly, whilst it is conventional to compare a new automatic blood pressure monitor with sphygmomanometry, this latter method is, again, associated with substantial test–retest measurement error (Bland and Altman, 1999) that is biological in origin. This ubiquity of biological variability governs several major considerations when analysing the performance characteristics of physiological measurement tools:

- Ideally, an examination of test–retest measurement error should be inherent in any examination of the agreement between measurement tools.

Moreover, *both* measurement tools (not just the more convenient or cheaper alternative) should be appraised for test–retest measurement error. Only through such an analysis can a firm conclusion be made regarding the source of any disagreement between different methods of measurement (Bland and Altman, 2003; Atkinson *et al.*, 2005a).

- Some aspects of least-squares regression (LSR) should be used with caution to examine agreement between measurement methods relevant to exercise physiology. It is likely that both physiological measurement methods show approximately similar degrees of test–retest error due to the major component of this error being ubiquitous and biological in origin. This error, present when using either measurement method, means that an important assumption for LSR might be violated leading to biased estimates of LSR slope and intercept statistics (Ludbrook, 1997; Bland and Altman, 2003; Atkinson *et al.*, 2005a). These statistics are conventionally used to make inferences about systematic differences between methods but the slope and intercept of a LSR line is unbiased only if the 'predictor' method is associated with substantially lower levels of test–retest measurement error than the other method or is in fact a 'fixed' variable. Moreover, the prediction philosophy of regression does not sit well with the fact that most researchers desire to select, *a priori*, the best measurement tool to use throughout their investigations, rather than them aiming to predict measurements using another method as part of their study.

- Like all statistics, those used to describe error and agreement are population specific, since different populations may show different degrees of error due to biological sources. Different individuals sampled from the same population may also show different degrees of error, for example, individuals who record the highest physiological values in general might also show the greatest amount of measurement error. Therefore, whether error might differ for different individuals in the population, and whether the statistical precision of the sample error estimate is adequate, are important considerations.

There are other philosophical issues, which underpin the statistical techniques used to appraise a physiological measurement tool. Our aim is not to discuss these issues, since there are now several comprehensive reviews in which the background to the statistical analysis is explained (Atkinson and Nevill, 1998; Bland and Altman, 1999, 2003; Atkinson *et al.*, 2005a). Alternatively, we aim to summarise the most important aspects of a measurement study in the form of a checklist for exercise physiologists.

A METHOD AGREEMENT AND MEASUREMENT ERROR CHECKLIST

We present a checklist, which may be useful to exercise physiologists interested in appraising a measurement tool, either if they are performing a measurement study themselves or if they are reading a relevant paper already published in a scientific journal. By 'measurement study', we mean an investigation into either the agreement between measurement methods (a method comparison study) or test–retest measurement error (a repeatability or reliability study). We have categorised the various important points into (1) Delimitations, (2) Systematic error examination, (3) Random error examination and (4) Statistical precision.

1   Delimitations

- Ideally, the measurement study should involve at least 40 participants. If there are less than 40 participants, then scrutiny of confidence limits for the error statistics becomes even more important (see Section 4), since error estimates calculated on a small sample can be imprecise (Atkinson, 2003).

- Try to match the characteristics of the measurement study to planned uses of the measurement tool, that is, a similar population, a similar time between repeated measurements (for investigations into test–retest error), a similar exercise protocol as well as comparable resting conditions during measurements.

- Select *a priori* an amount of error that is deemed acceptable between the methods or repeated tests. This delimitation may depend on whether one wishes to use the measurement tool predominantly for research purposes (i.e. on a sample of participants) or for making measurements on individuals (e.g. for health screening purposes or for sports science support work). Atkinson and Nevill (1998) termed these considerations 'analytical goals'.

- For research purposes, the analytical goal for measurement error is best set via a statistical power calculation. One could delimit an amount of test–retest error (described by the standard deviation of the differences, for example) on the basis of an acceptable statistical power to detect a given difference between groups or treatments with a feasible sample size (Atkinson and Nevill, 2001). If a relatively large sample is feasible for future research, then a given amount of measurement error should have less impact on use of the measurement tool, and *vice versa* (Figure 5.1).

- For use of the measurement tool on individuals, one might delimit the acceptable amount of error on the basis of the 'worst scenario' individual difference, which would be allowable. This delimitation is related to the 95% limits of agreement (LOA) statistic (Bland and Altman, 1999, 2003) as well as applications of the standard error of measurement (SEM) statistic (Harvill, 1991). For example, a difference as large as 5 beat·min^{-1} between two repeated measurements of heart rate during exercise would probably still make little difference to the prescription of heart rate training 'zones' to individuals.

- The use of arbitrary 'rules of thumb' such as accepting adequate agreement between methods or tests on the basis of a correlation coefficient being above 0.9 or a coefficient of variation (CV) being below 10% is discouraged, since no relation is made between error and real uses of the measurement tool with such generalisations (Atkinson, 2003). Nevertheless, reviews (e.g. Hopkins, 2000), in

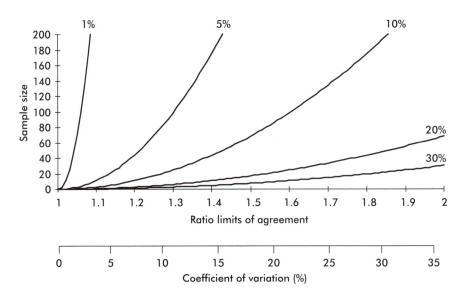

Figure 5.1 A nomogram to estimate the effects of measurement repeatability error on whether 'analytical goals' are attainable or not in exercise physiology research. Statistical power is 90%. The different lines represent different worthwhile changes of 1%, 5%, 10%, 20% and 30% due to some hypothetical intervention. The measurement error statistics, which can be utilised are the LOA and CV. For example, a physiological measurement tool, which has a repeatability CV of 5% would allow detection of a 5% change in a pre-post design experiment (using a paired *t*-test for analysis of data) and with a feasible sample size (~20 participants)

Source: Batterham, A.M. and Akthnson, G. (2005). How big does my sample need to be? A primer on the murky world of sample size estimation. *Physical Therapy in Sport* 6, 153–163.

which error statistics are cited for various measurements may be useful in establishing a 'typical' degree of acceptable error to select.[1]

2   Systematic error examination

- Compare the mean difference between methods/tests with the *a priori* defined acceptable level of agreement (see Figure 5.2 and Section 4 below on the use of confidence limits for interpretation of this mean difference).
- If systematic error is present between repeated tests using the same method (i.e. a repeatability study) and if no performance test has been administered, then be suspicious about the design of the repeatability study. Perhaps, there have been carry-over effects from previous measurements being obtained too close in time to subsequent measurements. Such a scenario could occur with measurements of intra-aural temperature, for example (Atkinson *et al.*, 2005b).
- If a performance test *is* incorporated in the protocol, then systematic differences between test and retest(s) in a repeatability study may occur due to learning effects, for example. Such information is important for advising future researchers how many familiarisation sessions might be required prior to the formal recording of physiological values.

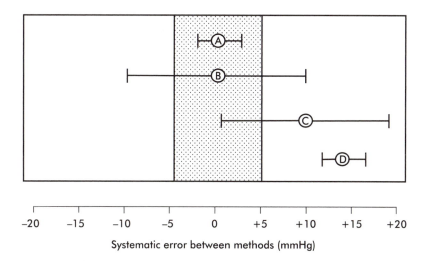

Figure 5.2 Using a confidence interval and 'region of equivalence' (shaded area) for the mean difference between methods/tests. Using the agreement between two blood pressure monitors as an example, if both of the 95% CI fall inside an *a priori* selected 'region of equivalence' of ±5 mmHg for the mean difference between methods, as is the case with point A, then we can be reasonably certain that the true systematic difference between methods is not clinically or practically important. For point D, even the lower 95% confidence limit of 10.6 mmHg for the systematic difference between methods does not lie within the designated region of equivalence, so we can be reasonably certain that the degree of systematic bias would have practical impact. The width of the CIs for points B and C suggest that the population mean bias might be practically important, but one would need more cases in the measurement study to be reasonably certain of the true magnitude, or in the case of point B, even the direction of the systematic bias for the population

- Examine whether the degree of systematic error alters over the measurement range. One can consult the Bland–Altman plot for this information (Figure 5.3). The presence of 'proportional' bias would be indicated if the points on the Bland–Altman plot show a pronounced downward or upward trend over the measurement range. If this characteristic is present, it means that the systematic difference between methods/tests differs for individuals at the low and high ends of the measurement range. Bland and Altman (1999) and Atkinson *et al.* (2005a) discuss how this proportional bias can be explored and modelled.

3   Random error examination

- Scrutinise the degree of random error between methods/tests that is present (Figure 5.3). Popular statistics used to describe random error include the SEM (Harvill, 1991), which is also known as the within-subjects standard deviation, CV, LOA and standard deviation of the differences. Each of these statistics will differ, since they are based on different underlying philosophies. For example, the LOA statistic is rooted in clinical work and can be viewed as representing the 'worst scenario' error that one might observe for an

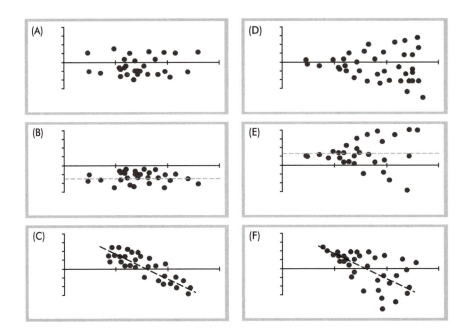

Figure 5.3 Various examples of relationships between systematic and random error and the size of the measured value as shown on a Bland-Altman plot. (A) Proportional random error. (B) systematic error present, which is uniform in nature, random errors also uniform. (C) Systematic error present, which is proportional to size of measured value, random errors uniform. (D) Proportional random error with no systematic error. (E) Uniform systematic error present with proportion random error. (F) Proportional systematic and random error

Source: Atkinson, G., Davison, R.C.R. and Nevill, A.M. (2005). Performance characteristics of gas analysis systems: what we know and what we need to know. *International Journal of Sports Medicine*, 26 (Suppl. 1): S2–S10.

individual person. The SEM statistic is popular amongst psychologists who conceptualise an average of many repeated measurements; the 'true score' for an individual (Harvill, 1991).

- Explore the relationship between random error and magnitude of measured value (Atkinson and Nevill, 1998; Bland and Altman, 1999). If the random error does increase in proportion to the size of the measured value, then a ratio statistic should be employed to describe the measurement error (e.g. CV) (Nevill and Atkinson, 1997; Bland and Altman, 1999). If the error is 'homoscedastic' (uniform over measurement range), than measurement error can be described in the particular units of measurement by calculating the LOA or SEM. Complicated relationships between magnitude of error and measured value can be analysed using non-parametric methods according to Bland and Altman (1999) or by calculating measurement error statistics for separate sub-samples within a population (Lord, 1984).

- In a repeatability study, which involves multiple retests, examine whether random error changes between separate test and retest(s). The researcher could explore whether random error reduces as more tests are administered (Nevill and Atkinson, 1998). If this is so, and in keeping with the advice above for exploration of systematic error, the researcher should communicate this learning effect on random error so that future users know exactly how many familiarisation sessions are required for total error variance to be minimised for their research.

4   Statistical precision

- Calculate the 95% confidence interval (CI) for the mean difference between methods/tests (Jones *et al.*, 1996) and compare this CI to a 'region of equivalence' for the two methods of measurement (Figure 5.2). This CI is *not* the same as the LOA statistic. Scrutiny of the lower and upper limits of this CI should not change the conclusion that has been arrived at regarding the acceptability of systematic error between methods/tests (Figure 5.2). For example, one might observe a mean difference of 10 mmHg between blood pressure measuring devices but the 95% CI might be −4 to 24 mmHg. This means that the population mean difference between methods could be as much as 4 mmHg in one direction or as much as 24 mmHg in the other direction. Only a narrower CI, mediated mostly by a greater sample size, would allow one to make a more conclusive statement regarding systematic error. Atkinson and Nevill (2001) and Atkinson *et al.* (2005a) discuss further the use of CI's and limits.

- Calculate confidence limits for the random error statistics. As above, scrutiny of the CI should not change the decision that has been made about acceptability of random error. For example, a physiological measurement method with a repeatability CV of 30% and associated CI of 25–35% indicates poor repeatability, even if the lower limit of the CI is taken into account. Bland and Altman (1999) provide details relevant to limits of agreement. Hopkins (2000) shows how to calculate confidence limits for CV and Morrow and Jackson (1993) provide details for intraclass correlation.

SUMMARY

We have presented a checklist for exercise physiologists, who are interested in examining the performance characteristics of a particular measurement tool. The most important issues to consider generally are the specific application of measurement tool (research or individual), degree of systematic and random error between methods or repeated tests, and adequate statistical precision of error estimates. All these issues cannot be encapsulated into a single statistic. Therefore, the exercise physiologist should be aware of the several statistics, which are used to measure agreement and error, especially in view of the impact error has on the validity of eventual study conclusions.

NOTE

1   One point worth noting is that several professional bodies (e.g. The British Hypertension Society) have their own evidence-based guidelines on acceptable levels of method agreement and measurement error involving the mean and standard deviation of differences statistics (O'Brien, 1998). Unfortunately, such agreed standards are rare in exercise physiology but they would be helpful.

REFERENCES

Atkinson, G. (2003). What is this thing called measurement error? In T. Reilly, M. Marfell-Jones (eds), *Kinanthropometry VIII: Proceedings of the 8th International Conference of the International Society for the Advancement of Kinanthropometry (ISAK)* pp. 3–14. London: Taylor and Francis.

Atkinson, G. and Nevill, A.M. (1998). Statistical methods in assessing measurement error (reliability) in variables relevant to sports medicine. *Sports Medicine*, 26: 217–238.

Atkinson, G. and Nevill, A.M. (2001). Selected issues in the design and analysis of sport performance research. *Journal of Sports Sciences*, 19: 811–827.

Atkinson, G., Davison, R.C.R. and Nevill, A.M. (2005a). Performance characteristics of gas analysis systems: what we know and what we need to know. *International Journal of Sports Medicine*, 26 (Suppl. 1): S2–S10.

Atkinson, G., Todd, C., Reilly, T. and Waterhouse, J.M. (2005b). Diurnal variation in cycling performance: influence of warm-up. *Journal of Sports Sciences*, 23(3): 321–329.

Bland, J.M. and Altman, D.G. (1999). Measuring agreement in method comparison studies. *Statistical Methods in Medical Research*, 8: 135–160.

Bland, J.M. and Altman, D.G. (2003). Applying the right statistics: analyses of measurement studies. *Ultrasound and Obstetrics in Gynecology*, 22: 85–93.

Harvill, L.M. (1991). An NCME instructional module on standard error of measurement. *Educational Measurement: Issues and Practice*, 10: 33–41.

Hopkins, W. (2000). Measures of reliability in sports medicine and science. *Sports Medicine*, 30: 1–15.

Jones, B. *et al.* (1996). Trials to assess equivalence: the importance of rigorous methods. *British Medical Journal*, 313: 36–39.

Lord, F.M. (1984). Standard errors of measurement at different ability levels. *Journal of Educational Measurement*, 21: 239–243.

Ludbrook, J. (1997). Comparing methods of measurement. *Clinical and Experimental Pharmacology and Physiology*, 24: 193–203.

Morrow, J.R. and Jackson, A.W. (1993). How 'significant' is your reliability? *Research Quarterly for Exercise and Sport*, 64: 352–355.

Nevill, A.M. and Atkinson, G. (1997). Assessing agreement between measurements recorded on a ratio scale in sports medicine and sports science. *British Journal of Sports Medicine*, 31: 314–318.

Nevill, A.M. and Atkinson, G. (1998). Assessing measurement agreement (repeatability) between 3 or more trials. *Journal of Sports Sciences*, 16: 29.

O'Brien, E. (1998). Automated blood pressure measurement: state of the market in 1998 and the need for an international validation protocol for blood pressure measuring devices. *Blood Pressure Monitoring*, 3: 205–211.

CHAPTER 6

SCALING: ADJUSTING PHYSIOLOGICAL AND PERFORMANCE MEASURES FOR DIFFERENCES IN BODY SIZE

Edward M. Winter

INTRODUCTION

It is well established that measures of performance and physiological characteristics are influenced by the size of the body as a whole or of its exercising segments in particular (Schmidt-Nielsen, 1984; Åstrand and Rodahl, 1986). Consequently, if the qualitative properties of tissues are to be explored meaningfully, differences in size have to be partitioned out by adjusting scores. Scaling is the technique that is used to make these adjustments and there has been a revival of interest in this area which impacts on those with interests in the physiology of exercise.

It has been suggested that in sport and exercise physiology there are four main uses of scaling techniques (Winter, 1992):

1   To compare an individual against standards for the purpose of assessment.
2   To compare groups.
3   In longitudinal studies that investigate the effects of growth or training.
4   To explore possible relationships between physiological characteristics and performance.

There is enthusiastic debate about when scaling might be appropriate and in particular, how it should be done. In heavyweight rowing for instance, in which body weight is supported, absolute measures either of performance or physiological characteristics are key and hence, do not require adjustment. Conversely, in activities such as running where body mass is unsupported and has to be carried, some form of scaling might be informative.

However, there is an intuitive attraction to adjust measures so as to develop insight into underlying mechanisms. It is at this point that serious consideration has to be given to possible methods.

RATIO STANDARDS

Traditionally, physiological characteristics such as oxygen uptake ($\dot{V}O_2$) have been scaled simply by dividing them by an anthropometric variable, for instance body mass (BM). This produces a ratio standard and the particular standard $\dot{V}O_2$/BM expressed as $ml\cdot kg^{-1}\cdot min^{-1}$ is probably the most widely used value in the physiology of exercise. However, it was suggested nearly 60 years ago by Tanner (1949) and confirmed by Packard and Boardman (1987) and Winter et al. (1991) that these standards can be misleading. Tanner (1949) stated that the ratio standard should be applied only when a 'special circumstance' has been satisfied.

For an outcome measure y and a predictor variable x, the special circumstance that allows the legitimate use of a ratio standard is given by:

$$v_x/v_y = r$$

where: v_x = coefficient of variation of x, that is $(SDx/\bar{x}) \times 100$
v_y = coefficient of variation of y, that is $(SDy/\bar{y}) \times 100$
r = Pearson's product–moment correlation coefficient.

Rarely is this special circumstance tested and arguably it is even rarer for it to be satisfied. As the disparity between each side of the equation increases, the ratio standard becomes increasingly unstable and distorts measures under consideration.

An effect of the unchallenged use of ratio standards is an apparent favourable economy in submaximal exercise in large individuals compared with those who are diminutive, whereas for maximal responses the opposite occurs. This latter observation has bedevilled researchers in the field of growth and development who see children's endurance performance capabilities increase during adolescence while simultaneously, their aerobic capabilities seemingly deteriorate.

ALLOMETRY

The preferred form of scaling is non-linear allometric modelling (Schmidt-Nielsen, 1984; Nevill et al., 1992). This modelling is based on the relationship:

$$y = ax^b$$

where: y = a performance or physiological outcome measure
x = an anthropometric predictor variable
a = the constant multiplier
b = the exponent.

The terms a and b can be identified by taking natural logarithms (ln) of both the predictor variable and outcome measure and then regressing ln y on ln x (Schmidt-Nielsen, 1984; Winter and Nevill, 2001). Groups can be compared either by analysis of covariance on the log–log regression lines or via power function ratios, that is, y/x^b. These types of ratio are created first, by raising x to the power b to create a power function and then second, by dividing y by this power function. The power function ratio presents y independent of x. As a note of caution, it should be acknowledged that this simple type of regression is not without its problems and Ricker (1973) provides a useful introduction to some of the vagaries of linear modelling.

THE SURFACE LAW

The surface area of a body is related to its volume raised to the power 0.67 and this relationship illustrates what is called the *surface law* (Schmidt-Nielsen, 1984). This means that as a body increases in mass and hence volume, there is a disproportionate reduction in the body's surface area. Conversely, as a body reduces in mass, its surface area becomes relatively greater. This is a fundamental principle which underpins for instance, the action of enzymes during digestion and partly explains differences in thermoregulation in children and adults. Heat exchange with the environment occurs at the surface of a body so thermogenesis and hence energy expenditure must occur to replace heat lost. The precise rate of thermogenesis is dependant on the temperature differences involved. For bodies that are isometric, that is, they increase proportionally, surface area increases as volume raised to the power two-thirds.

It has been suggested (Åstrand and Rodahl, 1986) and demonstrated (Nevill 1995; Welsman *et al.*, 1996; Nevill *et al.*, 2003) that maximal oxygen uptake ($\dot{V}O_{2max}$) and related measures of energy expenditure can be scaled for differences in body mass by means of the surface law; body mass can be raised to the two-thirds power and then divided into absolute values of $\dot{V}O_2$. This produces a power function which describes the aerobic capabilities of a performer with units of ml·kg$^{-0.67}$·min^{-1}. Typical values for elite athletes are presented by Nevill *et al.* (2003). They range from (mean ± SD) 192 ± 19 ml·kg$^{-0.67}$·min^{-1} for women badminton players to 310 ± 31 ml·kg$^{-0.67}$·min^{-1} for elite standard heavyweight men rowers. When their aerobic capabilities are expressed as ratio standards, the characteristics of the heavyweight men rowers appear considerably more modest yet their event demands high aerobic capability.

ELASTIC SIMILARITY

An alternative approach has been to use the power three quarters. This is based on McMahon's (1973) model of elastic similarity which acknowledges that growth in most living things is not isometric; body segments and limbs grow at different rates and hence, relative proportions change. In addition, buckling loads and other elastic properties for instance of tendons, are not accounted for in a simple surface-law approach. Moreover, in inter-species studies, animals that differ markedly in size seem to be described by a body mass exponent that approximates 0.75.

ALLOMETRIC CASCADE

However, yet another approach has recently been advanced: the allometric cascade model for metabolic rate (Darveau *et al.*, 2002). This model acknowledges two important considerations: first, the non-isometric changes in the body's segments that accompany growth and development and training induced hypertrophy; and second, the tripartite nature of $\dot{V}O_2$ and in particular, $\dot{V}O_{2max}$. The $\dot{V}O_{2max}$ is the global outcome of the rate at which the body can extract oxygen from the atmosphere via the cardiopulmonary system, transport it via the cardiovascular system and use it in skeletal muscle. The ability to release energy is as strong as the weakest part of this three-link chain.

Darveau *et al.* (2002) ascribed a weighting to each of these three facets and predicted an exponent for maximal and submaximal metabolic rate. For the former the exponent was between 0.82 and 0.92. For the latter, equivalent values were 0.76–0.79. Seemingly successful attempts have been made to validate these exponents in exercising humans (Batterham and Jackson, 2003).

RECOMMENDATIONS

In the light of these considerations and the possible confusion they create, how should the results of exercise tests be expressed? To report the results of laboratory and field-based tests which meaningfully reflect the performance and physiological status of athletes and exercisers, investigators should:

- Report absolute values of performance measures and physiological characteristics.
- Report ratio standards only when Tanner's special circumstance has been satisfied.
- For expediency, use the surface law exponent of 0.67 to scale $\dot{V}O_2$ or other related assessments of energy expenditure for differences in body mass or the size of exercising segments.
- Verify the choice of a particular exponent but acknowledge that because of sampling errors comparisons between groups might be compromised.
- For $\dot{V}O_2$ and $\dot{V}O_{2max}$ consider applying the allometric cascade model.

REFERENCES

Åstrand, P.-O. and Rodahl, K. (1986). *Textbook of Work Physiology*, 3rd edn. New York: McGraw-Hill.

Batterham, A.M. and Jackson, A.S. (2003). Validity of the allometric cascade model at submaximal and maximal metabolic rates in men. *Respiratory Physiology and Neurobiology*, 135: 103–106.

Darveau, C.-A., Suarez, R.K., Andrews, R.D. and Hochachka, P.W. (2002). Allometric cascade as a unifying principle of body mass effects on metabolism. *Nature*, 417: 166–170.

McMahon, T. (1973). Size and shape in biology. *Science*, 179: 1201–1204.

Nevill, A.M. (1995). The need to scale for differences in body size and mass: an explanation of Kleiber's 0.75 mass exponent. *Journal of Applied Physiology*, 77: 2870–2873.

Nevill, A.M., Ramsbottom, R. and Williams, C. (1992). Scaling physiological measurements for individuals of different body size. *European Journal of Applied Physiology*, 65: 110–117.

Nevill, A.M., Brown, D., Godfrey, R., Johnson, P.J., Romer, L., Stewart, A.D. and Winter, E.M. (2003). Modelling maximum oxygen uptake of elite endurance athletes. *Medicine and Science in Sports and Exercise*, 35: 488–494.

Packard, G.C. and Boardman, T.J. (1987). The misuse of ratios to scale physiological data that vary allometrically with body size. In M.E. Feder, A.F. Bennett, W.W. Burggren and R.B. Huey (eds), *New Directions in Ecological Physiology*. pp. 216–236. Cambridge: Cambridge University Press.

Ricker, W.E. (1973). Linear regressions in fishery research. *Journal of Fisheries Research Board*, Canada, 30: 409–434.

Schmidt-Nielsen, K. (1984). *Scaling: Why is Animal Size so Important?* Cambridge: Cambridge University Press.

Tanner, J.M. (1949). Fallacy of per-weight and per-surface area standards and their relation to spurious correlation. *Journal of Applied Physiology*, 2: 1–15.

Welsman, J., Armstrong, N., Nevill, A., Winter, E. and Kirby, B. (1996). Scaling peak O$_2$ for differences in body size. *Medicine and Science in Sports and Exercise*, 28: 259–265.

Winter, E.M. (1992). Scaling: partitioning out differences in size. *Pediatric Exercise Science*, 4: 296–301.

Winter, E.M. and Nevill, A.M. (2001). Scaling: adjusting for differences in body size. In: R. Eston and T. Reilly (eds), *Kinanthropometry and Exercise Physiology Laboratory Manual: Tests, Procedures and Data*, 2nd edn. *Volume 1: Anthropometry*, pp. 321–335. London: Routledge.

Winter, E.M., Brookes, F.B.C. and Hamley, E.J. (1991). Maximal exercise performance and lean leg volume in men and women. *Journal of Sports Sciences*, 9: 3–13.

CHAPTER 7

CIRCADIAN RHYTHMS

Thomas Reilly

CHRONOBIOLOGICAL BACKGROUND

Chronobiology is the science of biological rhythms. Circadian rhythms refer to cyclical fluctuations that recur regularly each solar day. The term is based on the Latin words circa (about) and dies (a day), reflecting that the endogenous rhythm (determined in constant conditions in an isolation unit) exceeds 24 h but is fine-tuned to a 24-h period by exogenous factors. These include light, temperature, habitual activity and social influences.

The circadian rhythm can be stylised by cosinor analysis. The period is predetermined as 24 h, the acrophase refers to the time when the peak occurs and the amplitude is half the distance between the highest and lowest values on the cosine curve. The trough occurs 12 h after the acrophase and after 24 h the next cycle commences. The hourly changes in core body temperature provide an example of a typical cosine function, with an acrophase around 17.50 h. Diurnal variation refers to changes within the normal daylight hours and nychthemeral conditions apply during normal habitual experiences.

The endogenous component of circadian rhythms, that is the body clock, is located in the suprachiasmatic nuclei within the hypothalamus. These nerve cells have receptors for melatonin, the hormone secreted from the pineal gland. This substance has circadian timekeeping functions due to its direct effects on the suprachiasmatic nuclei. These cells have a direct neural pathway from the retina and another input pathway through the intergeniculate leaflet. The visual receptors that enable light signals to synchronise the body clock and the environment act to assess the time of dawn and dusk according to several aspects of the quality and quantity of light.

Melatonin is secreted as darkness falls and is inhibited by light. The hormone has vasodilatory properties, causing body temperature to fall in the evening. Metabolic and other physiological functions slow down as the body prepares itself for sleep. The circadian rhythm in synthesis and release of serotonin, a substrate for melatonin and a brain neurotransmitter, is implicated in the sleep–wakefulness cycle. Whilst body temperature is regarded as a fundamental variable with which many human performance measures co-vary, the sleep–activity cycle reflects the circadian rhythm in the body's arousal system. Cells with timekeeping roles have also been located in peripheral tissues. The overall result is that the environmental light–dark cycle, the human activity–sleep cycle and the circadian system are integrated with respect to equipping the body to operate best over each day.

RHYTHMS IN PERFORMANCE

Field tests

All-out efforts such as time trials in cycling, swimming and rowing demonstrate circadian rhythms closely in phase with changes in body temperature. The evidence points to an endogenous component that combines with exogenous factors to influence the outcome (Drust *et al.*, 2005). When such tests are conducted in applied settings, time-of-day effects should be considered.

Muscle strength

The maximal capability of muscle to exert force may be measured under isometric and dynamic conditions. Traditionally isometric measures were used, the maximal voluntary contraction being recorded at a specific joint angle for purposes of replication and comparison with others. Portable dynamometers have been used for assessment of grip, back and leg strength in field conditions. Circadian rhythms have been identified for grip strength, elbow flexion, knee extension and back extension (Table 7.1). The peak time usually coincides with the acrophase in body temperature, the amplitude is 5–10% of the mean value. Observations of the quadriceps muscle after electrical stimulation suggest that peripheral more than central mechanisms are implicated in the rhythm in isometric force.

The measurement error in maximal voluntary contraction due to time of day may be corrected, provided the cosine function of the muscle group in question is known. The corrected value (MVCcorr) can be estimated by the equation:-

$$ \text{MVCcorr} = \frac{\text{MVC}t}{1 + A \times \cos^\circ(15t + 15p)} $$

where t is the time of day in decimal clock hours at which the test is performed, A is the amplitude of MVC as a per cent of the mean divided by 100, and p is the acrophase. Whilst the correction was originally designed for clinical assessments (Taylor *et al.*, 1994), the equation could be used for other strength tests that display time-of-day effects.

It is now more common to measure dynamic muscle strength in laboratory assessments rather than isometric force. Peak torque is measured under concentric and eccentric modes of muscle action and at different angular velocities using isokinetic dynamometry. Comprehensive familiarisation of subjects is required and test–retest variation may be high initially at fast angular velocities. Circadian rhythms have been reported for concentric peak torque of the knee extensors, the amplitudes and peak times being close to those reported for isometric force (see Table 7.1).

Anaerobic performance

Measures of anaerobic performance range from single, so-called explosive actions to formal measurement of maximal power output and its decline as

Table 7.1 Circadian variation in muscle strength and power from various sources. Only those publications where at least six measures have been recorded to characterise the rhythms have been cited

Muscle performance	Peak time (decimal clock hours)	Amplitude (% mean value)	Reference
Isometric strength			
Grip strength			
Left	18.00	6.4	Atkinson *et al.*, 1993
Left	17.80	6.5	Atkinson *et al.*, 1994
Right	17.90	4.7	Atkinson *et al.*, 1994
Leg strength	18.20	9.0	Coldwells *et al.*, 1994
	18.25	7.6	Atkinson *et al.*, 1994
(90° extension)	17.80	7.1	Taylor *et al.*, 1994
Back strength	16.88	10.6	Coldwells *et al.*, 1994
	18.30	6.9	Atkinson *et al.*, 1994
Dynamic strength			
(Concentric mode)			
Knee extensors			
1.05 rad·s^{-1}	15.47	3.7	Bambaeichi *et al.*, 2004
1.05 rad·s^{-1}	18.64	6.2	Atkinson *et al.*, 1995
1.57 rad·s^{-1}	18.00	4.6	Atkinson and Reilly, 1996
3.14 rad·s^{-1}	17.86	8.2	Atkinson *et al.*, 1995
Knee flexors			
3.14 rad·s^{-1}	19.76	7.2	Atkinson *et al.*, 1995
Anaerobic power			
Broad jump	17.75	3.4	Reilly and Down, 1986
Stair run	17.26	2.1	Reilly and Down, 1992
Flight time	20.30	2.4	Atkinson *et al.*, 1994

exercise is sustained. The Wingate test entails exercise on a cycle ergometer for 30 s, allowing peak anaerobic power, anaerobic capacity and a 'fatigue index' to be recorded. Peak power and mean power over the 30 s have been reported to be 8% higher in the evening (15.00 and 21.00 h) compared with night-time (03.00 h) (Hill and Smith, 1991). A higher circadian amplitude in peak and mean power output was found when the test was adapted for use on a swim bench (Reilly and Marshall, 1991). The large amplitude was attributed to the complex simulated swimming action compared to the grosser movement engaged in arm cranking. These rhythms are evident after prior activity so a systematic warm-up does not eliminate the circadian effect on anaerobic performance.

Power production can also be monitored in a stair-run and in jump tests (Atkinson and Reilly, 1996). The circadian rhythm in the standard stair-run test peaked at 17.26 h, the amplitude being 2.1% of the 24-h mean (see Table 7.1). Similar findings apply to standing broad jump (amplitude 3.4%) and flight time in a vertical jump (2.4%). Bernard et al. (1998) showed that flight time and jump power ($W \cdot kg^{-1}$) were greater in the afternoon and evening (14.00 and 18.00 h) than in the morning (09.00 h), the difference between means amounting to 7.0% and 2.6%, respectively. Such variations can have pronounced effects on global performance in training or competition, highlighting the need to reduce measurement error to a minimum when anaerobic performance is assessed.

PHYSIOLOGICAL RESPONSES

Rest

Circadian rhythms are evident in a range of endocrine, respiratory, digestive and renal functions. There is close correspondence between the circadian rhythm in core temperature and that in oxygen consumption ($\dot{V}O_2$) and minute ventilation ($\dot{V}E$), the change in temperature accounting for 37% and 24% of the variation in these metabolic measures, respectively (Reilly and Brooks, 1982). The amplitude of the rhythm in $\dot{V}E$ is greater than that of $\dot{V}O_2$; over and above the reduced requirement for oxygen at night-time, bronchoconstriction decreases the flow of air through the respiratory passages. Resting values are recorded over 10 min in order to reduce measurement error and, if a pre-exercise resting value is needed, it is acceptable to have the subject on the ergometer to be used, for example sitting motionless and comfortable on a cycle or rowing ergometer.

Heart rate at rest tends to be recorded in assessments of athletes, notably in endurance specialists whose training regimens lead to low resting values. The rhythm in heart rate tends to occur earlier in the afternoon than does that of $\dot{V}O_2$ or $\dot{V}CO_2$, this phase lead being attributed in part to changes in catecholamines whose peaks occur around 13.00 h. Adrenaline and noradrenaline have been linked with diurnal variations in alertness rather than enslaved to the rhythm in body temperature, although some dependence is likely (see Reilly *et al.*, 1997).

Submaximal exercise

In the main, the circadian rhythms evident at rest persist during light and moderate exercise. The rhythm in $\dot{V}O_2$ parallels that in $\dot{V}CO_2$, indicating stability in the respiratory exchange ratio. A standard light snack is recommended, at least 3 h prior to testing, to avoid circadian influences in substrate utilisation. It seems also that the energy cost of locomotion and the net mechanical efficiency are constant with time of day. When running economy is employed, the resting $\dot{V}O_2$ value should be subtracted, otherwise 'economy' would appear to be improved at night-time.

The rhythms in $\dot{V}O_2$ and $\dot{V}CO_2$ tend to fade as exercise is intensified. In contrast the rhythm in $\dot{V}E$ is accentuated and is reflected in a circadian rhythm in the ventilation equivalent of oxygen (Reilly and Brooks, 1990). The rhythm in $\dot{V}E$ may partly explain the mild dyspnoea sometimes associated with exercising in the early morning and the elevated perceived exertion noted at this time. The rhythm in heart rate persists for both arm and leg exercise, but decreases as exercise approaches maximal effort. Psychophysical methods also display circadian rhythmicity, expressed in the self-chosen work-rate. This value determines the pace individuals set for sustaining continuous exercise.

The 'anaerobic threshold' is used as a submaximal index of aerobic capacity. Forsyth and Reilly (2004) used the Dmax method to indicate 'lactate threshold' in rowers and reported a circadian rhythm for $\dot{V}O_2$ and heart rate at the threshold; the higher values for both variables were in phase with the rectal temperature data. When lactate threshold is used as a marker of performance change, tests should be conducted at the same time of day to eliminate circadian influences.

Maximal responses

The amplitude of the resting rhythm in $\dot{V}O_2$ would represent <0.3% of the $\dot{V}O_{2max}$ in a typical endurance athlete; a variation of this magnitude at maximal exercise is hard to detect. When subjects exercise to voluntary exhaustion, the highest $\dot{V}O_2$ value is referred to as peak rather than maximal if standard physiological criteria are not fulfilled. Arm exercise does not generally yield a plateau in $\dot{V}O_2$ before subjects desist in an incremental test to voluntary exhaustion, so a circadian rhythm reflects the influence of the total work done rather than innate physiological capacity. When subjects failing to demonstrate a plateau in $\dot{V}O_2$ during leg exercise to exhaustion in an incremental test were recalled for repeat testing, $\dot{V}O_{2max}$ was found to be stable (Reilly and Brooks, 1990).

The rhythm in submaximal heart rate is evident at exhaustion, albeit reduced in amplitude. The lowered values at night-time may be attributed to a decreased sympathetic drive. The variation is insufficient to affect cardiac output which, like $\dot{V}O_{2max}$, is a stable function. Whilst field performance tests display circadian variation, the effect cannot be explained by fluctuations in the transport or delivery of oxygen to the active muscles.

OVERVIEW

The evidence that circadian rhythms influence many physical fitness and performance measures is comprehensive. Therefore, serial tests on an individual athlete should be conducted at the same time of day for results to be compared.

The influence of individual differences on human circadian rhythms seems to be small. Lifestyle factors, such as morning or evening types, have no major effects on rhythm characteristics, nor has personality type. The phasing of the rhythm is relatively advanced with ageing, shifting towards a more morning-type profile. Fitness does not affect the acrophase of circadian rhythms but may increase their amplitude by means of a lowered trough. The rhythm is influenced by menstrual cycle phase, the decreased amplitude in muscle performance during the luteal compared to the follicular phase being linked to fluctuations in reproductive steroid hormones (Bambaeichi *et al.*, 2004).

Sports scientists must consider the time of day when planning and conducting fitness tests. This recommendation applies to both laboratory and field measures. Such care should be part of an overall preparation for administering test protocols that commence with familiarising the individual with the test procedures. Reduction in measurement error is paramount if changes between tests are to be identified and interpreted properly. This attention to detail is an essential part of quality control.

REFERENCES

Atkinson, G. and Reilly, T. (1996). Circadian variation in sports performance. *Sports Medicine*, 21: 292–312.

Atkinson, G., Coldwells, A. and Reilly, T. (1993). A comparison of circadian rhythms in work performance between physically active and inactive subjects. *Ergonomics*, 36: 273–281.

Atkinson, G., Coldwells, A., Reilly, T. and Waterhouse, J. (1994). An age-comparison of circadian rhythms in physical performance measures. In S. Harris, H. Suominen, P. Era and W.S. Harris (eds), *Towards Healthy Aging: International Perspectives Part 1. Physical and Biomedical Aspects Volume 3, Physical Activity, Aging and Sports*, pp. 205–216, Albany, NY: Center for Study of Aging.

Atkinson, G., Greeves, J., Reilly, T. and Cable, N.T. (1995). Day-to-day and circadian variability of leg strength measured with the LIDO isokinetic dynamometer. *Journal of Sports Sciences*, 13: 18–19.

Bambaeichi, E., Reilly, T., Cable, N.T. and Giacomoni, M. (2004). The isolated and combined effects of menstrual phase and time-of-day on muscle strength of eumenorrheic women. *Chronobiology International*, 21: 645–660.

Bernard, T., Giacomoni, M., Gavarry, O., Seymat, M. and Falgairette, G. (1998). Time-of-day effects in maximal anaerobic leg exercise. *European Journal of Applied Physiology*, 77: 133–138.

Coldwells, A., Atkinson, G. and Reilly, T. (1994). Sources of variation in back and leg dynamometry. *Ergonomics*, 37: 79–86.

Drust, B., Waterhouse, J., Atkinson, G., Edwards, B. and Reilly, T. (2005). Circadian rhythms in sports performance: an update. *Chronobiology International*, 22: 21–44.

Forsyth, J.J. and Reilly, T. (2004). Circadian rhythms in blood lactate concentration during incremental ergometer rowing. *European Journal of Applied Physiology*, 92: 69–74.

Hill, D.W. and Smith, J.C. (1991). Circadian rhythms in anaerobic power and capacity. *Canadian Journal of Sports Science*, 16: 30–32.

Reilly, T. and Brooks, G.A. (1982). Investigation of circadian rhythms in metabolic responses to exercise. *Ergonomics*, 25: 1093–1107.

Reilly, T. and Brooks, G.A. (1990). Selective persistence of circadian rhythms in physiological responses to exercise. *Chronobiology International*, 7: 59–67.

Reilly, T. and Down, A. (1986). Circadian variation in the standing broad jump. *Perceptual and Motor Skills*, 62: 830.

Reilly, T. and Down, A. (1992). Investigation of circadian rhythms in anaerobic power and capacity of the legs. *Journal of Sports Medicine and Physical Fitness*, 32: 342–347.

Reilly, T. and Marshall, S. (1991). Circadian rhythms in power output on a swim bench. *Journal of Swimming Research*, 7: 11–13.

Reilly, T., Atkinson, G. and Waterhouse, J. (1997). *Biological Rhythms and Exercise.* Oxford: Oxford University Press.

Taylor, D., Gibson, H., Edwards, R.H.T. and Reilly, T. (1994). Correction of isometric strength tests for time of day. *European Journal of Experimental Musculoskeletal Research*, 3: 25–27.

PART 3

GENERAL PROCEDURES

CHAPTER 8

LUNG AND RESPIRATORY MUSCLE FUNCTION

Alison McConnell

INTRODUCTION

The following section will describe briefly the structure and function of the healthy respiratory system, as well as considering why the assessment of lung and respiratory muscle function is relevant to sport and exercise science. The final section will describe the equipment and procedures for undertaking basic lung function and respiratory muscle assessments.

PHYSIOLOGY OF BREATHING

A detailed description of the physiology of the respiratory system is beyond the scope of this section, and the reader is referred to West (1999) for this information. However, in order to place the assessment of the respiratory system into context, it is necessary to provide a very brief overview of the act of breathing.

The principal function of the respiratory system is the exchange of the respiratory gases, oxygen and carbon dioxide. The movement of air into and out of the lungs is brought about by the contraction of skeletal muscles, which are activated by both automatic and conscious control mechanisms. The structure of the lungs provides for a huge interface between air and capillary blood; it has been estimated that the combined alveolar surface area of both adult lungs is equivalent to that of half a tennis court. Each alveolus is surrounded by a dense network of capillaries. The large surface area of the gas/blood interface, combined with the high affinity of haemoglobin for oxygen, and the sigmoid shape of its dissociation curve, ensure the complete equilibration of the respiratory gases across the respiratory membrane. Accordingly, arterial oxygen saturation remains around 97%, even during heavy exercise (see later for exceptions), and oxygen transport in healthy human beings at sea level is not generally considered to be limited by the diffusing capacity of their lungs.

The precise mechanisms that control the level of breathing (minute ventilation, $\dot{V}_E$) in response to changing metabolic demand remain relatively poorly understood. However, it is known that the control is more closely linked to carbon dioxide production than to oxygen uptake (Wasserman et al., 1978). As well as ensuring the maintenance of oxygen delivery during exercise, the respiratory system plays a crucial role in acid–base homeostasis. Stimulation of the carotid chemoreceptors by hydrogen ions drives up $\dot{V}_E$, and facilitates the removal of carbon dioxide (in excess of metabolic demand), which increases pH (Wasserman et al., 1975). The ventilatory compensation for a metabolic acidosis ensures that exercise can be sustained above the lactate threshold for much longer than would otherwise be the case.

WHY ASSESS LUNG AND RESPIRATORY MUSCLE FUNCTION?

Minute ventilation displays a more than 10-fold increase between rest and peak exercise, with typical resting values of 8–10 $l \cdot min^{-1}$ and values approaching 150–200 $l \cdot min^{-1}$ during maximal exercise. The highest values for $\dot{V}_E$ are recorded in athletes such as rowers, where it is not uncommon for $\dot{V}_E$ to reach 250 $l \cdot min^{-1}$ at peak exercise in elite, open-class oarsmen.

The relevance of lung function to elite endurance performance remains a topic of debate, since it is well known that there is no ventilatory (diffusion) limitation to performance in healthy human beings at sea level. The exceptions to this received wisdom are elite endurance trained individuals; 40–50% of this group show arterial oxygen desaturation at peak exercise, which is indicative of a diffusion limitation to oxygen transport (Powers et al., 1993). However, the aetiology is multifactoral, and the phenomenon is not explained totally by mechanical constraints upon breathing.

Notwithstanding these observations of diffusion limitation in endurance athletes, the apparent excess capacity of the ventilatory system has led to the assumption that there is no ventilatory limitation to exercise performance. However, it is a common observation that endurance athletes tend to have large lung volumes, even when body size is taken into account. Other evidence from untrained individuals also points to a relationship between lung function and maximal oxygen uptake that cannot be explained by body size (Nevill and Holder, 1999). The reasons for these observations are currently unknown.

Other evidence also points to a potential ventilatory limitation to exercise performance. Breathing is brought about by the action of muscles, which can demand as much as 16% of oxygen uptake during maximal exercise (Harms, 2000). The inspiratory muscles (which undertake the majority of the mechanical work of breathing) have been shown in numerous studies to exhibit fatigue after both short, high intensity bouts of exercise (Johnson et al., 1993; Babcock et al., 1996; McConnell et al., 1997; Volianitis et al., 2001a; Romer et al., 2002a, 2004; Lomax and McConnell, 2003), and prolonged moderate intensity exercise such as marathon running (Loke *et al.*, 1982; Hill *et al.*, 1991). This is suggestive of a system that is working at the limits of its capacity. The fact that pre-fatigue of the respiratory muscles impairs performance (Mador and Acevedo, 1991), and that specific inspiratory muscle training improves performance (Volianitis *et al.*, 2001a; Romer *et al.*, 2002a,b) adds further weight to the argument that the ventilatory system exerts a limitation to exercise performance.

Whilst it is debatable whether superior lung function is associated with superior endurance performance, it is well recognised that impaired lung function has a detrimental influence upon exercise performance (Aliverti and Macklem, 2001). Although impairment of lung function may not necessarily result in a compromise to gas exchange, studies on people with lung disease demonstrate that the breathlessness associated with lung function impairment becomes an exercise-limiting factor (Hamilton *et al.*, 1996). Similarly, high levels of respiratory muscle work and inspiratory muscle fatigue have been implicated in impairment of exercise performance due to blood flow 'stealing' by the respiratory muscles (Harms, 2000).

Accordingly, the routine assessment of lung function and respiratory muscle function in athletes is worthwhile, and essential in any athlete who reports inappropriate levels of breathlessness during training or competition. The source of inappropriate breathlessness is most likely to be exercise-induced asthma. Data from the GB team that competed in the Athens Olympics indicated that 21% of the squad had exercise-induced asthma that qualified for treatment under International Olympic Committee criteria (Dickinson *et al.*, 2005 (in press). Prevalence rates were highest in the sports of swimming and cycling (over 40%). The prevalence rate in Team GB as a whole was more than twice that in the UK general population (8%).

ROUTINE ASSESSMENT AND INTERPRETATION OF LUNG FUNCTION

The guidance below is based upon a variety of sources, but principally the recommendations of the American Thoracic Society (American Thoracic Society, 1995) and European Respiratory Society (Quanjer *et al.*, 1993), as well as extensive practical experience.

A 'classic', global test of breathing capacity is the maximum voluntary ventilation (MVV) test. The capacity to move air in and out of the lungs is influenced by the participants' physical size, age, gender and race. All other things being equal (e.g. age, gender, etc.), the outcome of an MVV test is also influenced by the condition of the respiratory muscles (weakness and susceptibility to fatigue), narrowing of the airways (e.g. asthma), loss of lung elastic recoil (e.g. emphysema), as well as the distensability of the lungs and thoracic cage (e.g. scoliosis). The MVV is therefore a somewhat 'blunt instrument' that should lead on to more specific tests in the presence of a relatively poor performance.

The MVV requires the participant to breathe in and out as hard as possible for a predetermined time, usually 15 s (MVV_{15}). The test is most easily performed using an electronic spirometer that measures flow rate directly, and most proprietary spirometry systems have a function that permits MVV testing. It is important that the equipment has a low resistance to airflow, as a back pressure will impair the validity of the measurements. The test can also be performed for longer durations (e.g. 4 min, discussed later), but then requires supplemental carbon dioxide to prevent severe hypocapnia. The participant requires strong encouragement throughout the test, which shows a task learning effect. During serial assessments of MVV_{15} (repeated to obtain a reliable value (two values should be within 10% or 20 $l \cdot min^{-1}$)), at least 3 min should be allowed between tests. Because the manoeuvre results is some hypocapnia it is also helpful to instruct the participant to hold their breath at the end of the test in order to allow normocapnia to be restored more rapidly.

The 4-min MVV ($MVV_{4\,min}$, also known as the maximum sustained ventilation) gives an index of the fatigue resistance of the respiratory muscles, since the progressive decline in flow rate is due to muscle fatigue. There is also a task learning effect in the assessment of $MVV_{4\,min}$, which should not be repeated for at least an hour; visual feedback of a target $\dot{V}_E$ is also helpful. Most healthy untrained people can sustain 60–70% of their MVV_{15} for 4 min, and trained individuals over 80% (Anholm et al., 1989), that is, $MVV_{4\,min}$ is 60–80% of MVV_{15}. At peak exercise, healthy people achieve a $\dot{V}_E$ of 70–80% of their MVV_{15} (Hesser et al., 1981); thus, $MVV_{4\,min}$ and peak exercise $\dot{V}_E$ are broadly equivalent.

STATIC LUNG FUNCTION

After the MVV, the most basic assessment of lung function involves the measurement of lung volumes (static lung volumes), which are measured in litres and expressed under BTPS conditions. Figure 8.1 illustrates the static lung volumes, definitions of which are provided below:

- *Total lung capacity (TLC).* The volume of air in the lungs at full inspiration. This cannot be measured without access to specialised equipment.
- *Vital capacity (VC).* The maximum volume that can be exhaled/inhaled between the lungs being completely inflated and the end of a full expiration. VC can be measured during either a 'forced' (with maximal effort; FVC) or relaxed manoeuvre (VC). The relaxed manoeuvre is more appropriate for patients with lung disease whose airways tend to collapse during a forced manoeuvre.
- *Residual volume (RV).* The volume of air remaining in the lungs at the end of a full expiration. This cannot be measured without access to specialised equipment.
- *Functional residual capacity (FRC).* The volume of air remaining in the lungs after a resting tidal breath. This changes during exercise, when it becomes known as end expiratory lung volume (EELV).
- *Expiratory and inspiratory reserve volumes (ERV/IRV).* The volumes available between the beginning or end of tidal breath and TLC and RV, respectively.

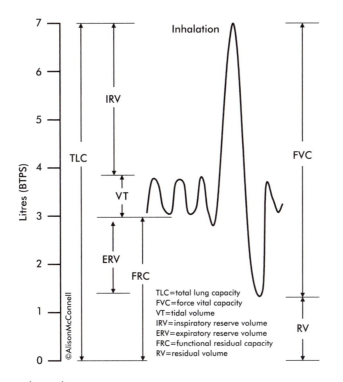

Figure 8.1   Static lung volumes

Lung function is influenced by a number of physiological and demographic factors, as well as by the presence of disease. For example, there is a strong influence of body size, gender and age, as well as ethnicity. For this reason, there are population-specific prediction equations that assist in the interpretation of measured values (see Lung Function Reference Values in the Reference section). Generally, lung volumes are greater in larger individuals, are lower in women, and decrease with age. A component of the effect of gender appears to be independent of the effect of body size (Becklake, 1986).

A description of the breathing manoeuvres required to assess lung volumes is given in the next section.

DYNAMIC LUNG FUNCTION

The condition of the airways (as distinct from the measurement of lung volumes) can be assessed using a technique known as spirometry (dynamic lung function). Obstructive lung diseases such as asthma are diagnosed by measuring the rate of expiratory airflow during forced expiratory manoeuvres. By plotting either volume against time (Figure 8.2 (A) or flow against volume (by integration of the flow signal) (Figure 8.2 (B)), a 'spirogram' is constructed. Figure 8.2 (A) and (B) illustrate each of these approaches and identifies a number of parameters that provide information about airway function (see legend for details). The most commonly used index of airway calibre is the forced expiratory volume in 1 s (FEV_1), which can be assessed using either a bellows (also known as wedge) spirometer, or using electronic spirometry. Electronic spirometers allow the construction of so-called flow volume loops (Figure 8.2 (B)).

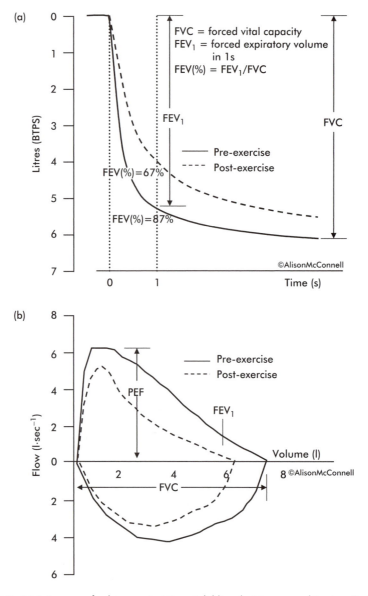

Figure 8.2 (a) Spirogram of volume against time. Solid line depicts a normal tracing. Dashed line depicts the response of an individual with EIA after an exercise challenge (bronchoconstriction). Note the decline in the ratio of FEV_1 to FVC in the presence of bronchoconstriction. (b) Spirogram of volume against flow. Line coding as above

A method that many asthma patients use to self-monitor their airway function is peak expiratory flow (PEF) measurement. Whilst this is easily assessed, using very inexpensive equipment (e.g. Mini Wright Peak Flow Meter), it is highly effort dependent and its reliability is poor. Accordingly, PEF is satisfactory for patient self-monitoring, but not for diagnostic testing (Quanjer *et al.*, 1997).

Because FEV_1 is influenced by vital capacity, it is expressed as a fraction of vital capacity (FEV%). In the presence of normal airways, FEV% should exceed 80% for individuals under 30 years, and 75% up to late middle age.

Conducting a dynamic lung function test

The description here is for conducting a forced flow volume loop, but the basic principles are the same for static lung volume assessment and FEV_1 measured using a bellows spirometer.

1   Ensure that your equipment is calibrated and working properly (e.g. check for leaks in hoses).
2   Ensure that all equipment that will come in contact with the participant (e.g. mouthpiece), or that he/she will inhale through (tubing), is sterile, and/or protected by a disposable viral filter.
3   Complete any necessary consent documentation.
4   Measure the particpant's stature.
5   Explain to the participant exactly what you wish them to do before starting the test.
6   Measurements can be made seated or standing, but ensure that no clothing restricts the thorax, and that the neck is slightly extended.
7   For a manouvre, explain that the manoeuvre must be performed 'forcefully'. Then fit the nose clip, instruct the participant to go onto the mouthpiece, and to inhale 'until [your] lungs are as full as they can possibly be'.
8   When it is clear that they have achieved this (don't hesitate at this point), instruct them to 'blow out as hard and fast as [you] can...keep going, out, out, squeeze out'. Encourage them to keep going until they cannot squeeze any more air from their lungs. During this latter phase, encourage them to keep breathing 'out, out, squeeze out'.
9   As soon as it is clear that their lungs are empty instruct them to 'breathe in as fast as [you] can...big deep breath, keep going'. You can describe this manoeuvre as being like a huge gasp. If you are measuring FEV_1 using a bellows spirometer, there is no requirement to undertake the inspiratory part of the manoeuvre (stop at the end of 8).
10 Take the mouthpiece out of the participant's mouth (having a piece of tissue ready for saliva). Leave the nose clip in place and allow around 15–30 s rest before repeating the procedure.
11 If there were deficiencies in the quality of the manoeuvre, for example, he/she didn't exhale fully, explain what went wrong and what can be done to improve things on the next attempt.

12   Once you have three measurements of FVC and FEV_1 that were technically satisfactory and are within 5% (or 100 ml) of each other you can stop (it may take as many as eight attempts to achieve this).

13   Remove the mouthpiece (having a piece of tissue ready for saliva) and nose clip.

14   Report the largest of the three technically satisfactory measurements (best of three).

15   If eight manoeuvres are performed without achieving the 5% criterion, then record the highest value measured.

Common faults

- Incomplete inspiration or expiration;
- initiation of the manoeuvre before the participant is attached to the mouthpiece;
- leakage of air around the lip/mouthpiece interface;
- coughing.

Most modern electronic spirometers will store the data within a built-in database, and will also calculate 'percent predicted values' by referencing the participant's measured values to appropriate prediction equations (see Lung Function Reference Values).

It is relatively rare to encounter an otherwise healthy physically active person who has clear evidence of abnormal lung function in a rested state. However, it is possible to have normal lung function in a rested state, and to have an airway responsiveness to exercise, or exercise-induced asthma (EIA). People with EIA generally complain of breathlessness following exercise, or during repeated bouts of exercise that are interspersed with rest. If EIA is suspected, then lung function should be assessed post-exercise, preferably after an activity that typically provokes symptoms. Measurement should be repeated 3, 5, 10, 15, 20 and 30 min after exercise has ceased (this is to take account of the individual variation in the time of the nadir of the response). A fall in FEV_1 of >10% is indicative of EIA. Specialist EIA testing facilities are available at the Olympic Medical Institute and some English Institute of Sport Centres. If lung function assessment identifies an individual with apparently abnormal lung function, they should be referred to their GP with a copy of their test results for confirmation and treatment, as appropriate.

One might imagine that it is very rare to identify an athlete with EIA, who was unaware that they had the condition. However, routine EIA screening of Team GB prior to the Athens Olympics identified seven athletes with no previous diagnosis of EIA (Dickinson *et al.*, 2005 (in press)). This represented ~10% of the symptomatic athletes who were referred for testing, and 2.6% of the entire squad. Measurement of lung function is therefore recommended as a routine part of athlete profiling (Dickinson *et al.*, 2005 (in press)).

ASSESSMENT AND INTERPRETATION OF RESPIRATORY MUSCLE FUNCTION

Unlike lung function, which can be predicted with reasonable accuracy on the basis of stature, gender and age, respiratory muscle function shows much less predictability. This makes interpretation of one-off measurements largely meaningless, unless there is gross weakness. However, the observation that some forms of exercise are associated with inspiratory muscle fatigue (IMF), and that specific inspiratory muscle training (IMT) abolishes IMF and improves performance, has led to an interest in this method of assessment. The role of the expiratory muscles in exercise limitation currently remains unknown.

Thus, assessment of respiratory muscle function is recommended for diagnosis of exercise induced IMF, as well as for monitoring the influence of IMT. In 2002, the American Thoracic Society and European Respiratory Society published an extensive set of guidelines for respiratory muscle assessment (ATS/ERS, 2002). Readers wishing to know more about respiratory muscle assessment in general are referred to this source. Below is a practical guide to assessing just one aspect of muscle function, namely, respiratory muscle strength.

For obvious reasons, it is not possible to obtain a direct measurement of respiratory muscle force output. Accordingly, surrogate measurements are used to provide an index of global respiratory muscle strength. The maximal respiratory pressures measured at the mouth provide simple indices that are very reliable when performed by competent 'technicians' (Romer and McConnell, 2004). Respiratory pressures are measured against an occluded airway (incorporating a 1 mm diameter leak to maintain an open glottis) at prescribed lung volumes (discussed later). The equipment required is portable and hand-held (mouth pressure meter).

Because maximum respiratory pressures are indices of maximal strength, they are highly effort-dependent and require well-motivated participants. Efforts must be sustained for at least 1.5 s in order that an average pressure over 1 s can be calculated (by the measuring instrument). This averaging enhances the reliability of the measurement. The measurements must also be made at predetermined lung volumes. This is because of the length–tension relationship of the respiratory muscles. Maximal inspiratory pressure (MIP) is measured at residual volume and maximal expiratory pressure (MEP) at total lung capacity.

Care must also be taken to ensure that any task learning and other effects are expressed fully before recording measured values. It has been shown that there is a considerable effect of repeated measurement upon MIP, even in experienced participants. This effect is large enough to mask changes in MIP due to the effects of inspiratory muscle fatigue. After 18 repeated trials, MIP was 11.4% higher than the best of the first three measurements made (Volianitis et al., 2001b). However, this learning effect can be overcome to a large extent by a bout of sub-maximal inspiratory loading prior to the assessment of MIP (two sets of 30 breaths against an inspiratory threshold load equivalent to

40% of the best MIP measured during the first three efforts). Following this prior loading, the difference between the best of the first three efforts and the 18th measurement was only 3%. Thus, the time taken to obtain reliable measurements of MIP can be curtailed considerably by implementing a bout of prior loading.

For reasons given earlier, it is difficult to offer typical values for MIP and MEP, and the reader is cautioned against using reference values within the literature, because their predictive power and functional relevance is questionable. Notwithstanding this, it is possible to offer some 'ball park' estimates of values that should be expected in healthy young people; males range MIP = 110–140 cmH$_2$O; females range MIP = 90–120 cmH$_2$O. Values for MEP are typically 30% higher than MIP.

After strenuous exercise, MIP can fall by between 10% and 30%. (McConnell et al., 1997; Volianitis et al., 2001a; Romer et al., 2002a; Lomax and McConnell, 2003), depending upon the intensity of exercise and its modality (swimming appears to be a very potent stimulus to IMF, see Lomax and McConnell, 2003). Following a 4–6 week programme of inspiratory muscle training (IMT), improvements in MIP in the order of 25–35% could be observed (Volianitis et al., 2001a; Romer et al., 2002a,b).

Conducting a MIP and MEP test

"Contraindications – MIP and MEP efforts produce large changes in thoracic, upper airway, middle ear and sinus pressures. This is contraindicated in people with a history of spontaneous pneumothorax, recent trauma to the rib cage, a recently perforated eardrum (or other middle ear pathology), or acute sinusitis (until the condition has resolved). Urinary incontinence is also a contraindication for MEP, but not MIP testing."

1 Ensure that your equipment is calibrated and working properly.
2 Ensure that all equipment that will come in contact with the participant (e.g. mouthpiece), or that he/she will inhale through, is sterile, and/or protected by a disposable viral filter.
3 Complete any necessary consent documentation.
4 Explain to the participant exactly what you wish them to do before starting the test. During the measurement of MIP and MEP the participant will be unable to generate any airflow against the mouth pressure meter, which contains only a small (1 mm) leak; they must be prepared for this.
5 Measurements can be made seated or standing, but ensure that no clothing restricts the thorax, and that a nose-clip is in place.
6 Because of the length–tension relationship of the respiratory muscles, inspiratory pressures (MIP) are measured at residual volume and expiratory pressures (MEP) at total lung capacity.
7 Ideally, MIP measurements should be preceded by a bout of prior loading to reduce the effect of repeated measurement (discussed earlier, and Volianitis et al., 2001b). If suitable equipment is not available for this procedure, up to 18 repeated trials may be necessary to establish reliable data (Volianitis et al., 2001b). However, a pragmatic compromise between rigour and time constraints is to record up to 10 efforts.

8   For MIP assessment, ensure that the participant 'squeezes out slowly' to residual volume.

9   Then instruct them to 'breathe in hard...pull, pull, pull' holding the effort for at least 2 s, and no more than 3 s, and maintaining encouragement throughout. Then instruct the participant to 'relax and come off the mouthpiece' (having a piece of tissue ready for saliva).

10   Take the meter from the participant and record the measured value.

11   Leave the nose-clip in place and allow at least 30 s rest before repeating.

12   If there were deficiencies in the quality of the manoeuvre, for example, he/she did not sustain the effort for long enough, explain what went wrong and what can be done to improve things on the next attempt.

13   For MEP assessment, ensure that the participant breathes in fully to total lung capacity.

14   Then instruct them to 'breathe out hard...push, push, push' holding the effort for no more than 3 s (then as in 9 earlier). During the expiratory effort there is a tendency for air to leak around the lips/mouthpiece. Leaks can be prevented if the participant pinches their lips in place around the mouthpiece by encircling them with the thumb and forefinger.

15   Serial measurements of MIP or MEP should not differ by more than 10%, or 10 cmH$_2$O (which ever is the smallest), and should be repeated until three measurements meet the criterion. At least five measurements should be made.

16   Report the largest of the three technically satisfactory measurements (best of three).

17   If 10 manoeuvres are performed without achieving the 10% criterion, then record the highest value measured.

Common faults

- Incomplete inspiration or expiration
- Not maintaining the effort for long enough.

ACKNOWLEDGEMENT

I am grateful to Dr Lee Romer for his advice during the preparation of this manuscript. I also declare a beneficial interest in the POWERbreathe® inspiratory muscle trainer (royalty share of licence income).

REFERENCES

Aliverti, A. and Macklem, P.T. (2001). How and why exercise is impaired in COPD. *Respiration*, 68(3): 229–239.

American Thoracic Society. (1995). ATS statement – standardization of spirometry. 1994 update. *American Review of Respiratory Disease*, 152(5): 1107–1136.

American Thoracic Society/European Respiratory Society. (2002). ATS/ERS Statement on respiratory muscle testing. *American Journal of Respiratory and Critical Care Medicine*, 166(4): 518–624.

Anholm, J.D., Stray-Gundersen, J., Ramanathan, M. and Johnson, R.L. Jr (1989). Sustained maximal ventilation after endurance exercise in athletes. *Journal of Applied Physiology*, 67(5): 1759–1763.

Babcock M.A., Pegelow D.F., Johnson B.D., Dempsey J.A. (1996). Aerobic fitness effects on exercise-induced low-frequency diaphragm fatigue. *Journal of Applied Physiology,* 81(5): 2156–2164.

Becklake, M.R. (1986). Concepts of normality applied to the measurement of lung function. *American Journal of Medicine*, 80: 1158–1164.

Casaburi, R., Whipp, B.J., Wasserman, K. and Stremel, R.W. (1978). Ventilatory control characteristics of the exercise hyperpnea as discerned from dynamic forcing techniques. *Chest*, 73 (Suppl. 2): 280–283.

Dickinson, J.W., Whyte, G.P., McConnell, A.K. and Harries, M.G. (2005). The impact of changes in the IOC-MC asthma criteria: a British perspective. *Thorax* 60(8): 629–632.

Hamilton, A.L., Killian, K.J., Summers, E. and Jones, N.L. (1996). Symptom intensity and subjective limitation to exercise in patients with cardiorespiratory disorders. *Chest*, 110(5): 1255–1263.

Harms, C.A. (2000). Effect of skeletal muscle demand on cardiovascular function. *Medicine and Science in Sports and Exercise*, 32(1): 94–99.

Hesser, C.M., Linnarsson, D. and Fagraeus, L. (1981). Pulmonary mechanisms and work of breathing at maximal ventilation and raised air pressure. *Journal of Applied Physiology*, 50(4): 747–753.

Hill, N.S., Jacoby, C. and Farber, H.W. (1991). Effect of an endurance triathlon on pulmonary function. *Medicine and Science in Sports and Exercise*, 23(11): 1260–1264.

Johnson, B.D., Babcock, M.A., Suman, O.E. and Dempsey, J.A. (1993). Exercise-induced diaphragmatic fatigue in healthy humans. *Journal of Physiology*, 460: 385–405.

Loke, J., Mahler, D.A. and Virgulto, J.A. (1982). Respiratory muscle fatigue after marathon running. *Journal of Applied Physiology*, 52(4): 821–824.

Lomax, M.E. and McConnell, A.K. (2003). Inspiratory muscle fatigue in swimmers after a single 200 m swim. *Journal of Sports Science*, 21(8): 659–664.

McConnell, A.K., Caine, M.P. and Sharpe, G.R. (1997). Inspiratory muscle fatigue following running to volitional fatigue: the influence of baseline strength. *International Journal of Sports Medicine*, 18(3): 169–173.

Mador, M.J. and Acevedo, F.A. (1991). Effect of respiratory muscle fatigue on subsequent exercise performance. *Journal of Applied Physiology*, 70(5): 2059–2065.

Nevill, A.M. and Holder, R.L. (1999). Identifying population differences in lung function: results from the Allied Dunbar national fitness survey. *Annals of Human Biology*, 26(3): 267–285.

Powers, S.K., Martin, D. and Dodd, S. (1993). Exercise-induced hypoxaemia in elite endurance athletes. Incidence, causes and impact on VO_{2max}. *Sports Medicine*, 16(1): 14–22.

Quanjer, P.H., Tammeling, G.J., Cotes, J.E., Pedersen, O.F., Peslin, R. and Yernault, J.C. (1993). Lung volume and forced ventilatory flows. Report Working Party Standardization of lung function tests; Official Statement European Respiratory Society. *European Respiratory Journal*, 6 (Suppl. 16): 5–40.

Quanjer, P.H., Lebowitz, M.D., Gregg, I., Miller, M.R. and Pedersen, O.F. (1997). Peak expiratory flow: conclusions and recommendations of a Working Party of the European Respiratory Society. *European Respiratory Journal* (Suppl. 24): 2S–8S.

Romer, L.M. and McConnell, A.K. (2004). Inter-test reliability for non-invasive measures of respiratory muscle function in healthy humans. *European Journal of Applied Physiology*, 91(2–3): 167–176.

Romer, L.M., McConnell, A.K. and Jones, D.A. (2000a) Inspiratory muscle fatigue in trained cyclists: effects of inspiratory muscle training. *Medicine and Science in Sports and Exercise*, 34(5): 785–792.

Romer, L.M., McConnell, A.K. and Jones, D.A. (2002b). Effects of inspiratory muscle training upon recovery time during high intensity, repetitive sprint activity. *International Journal of Sports Medicine*, 23(5): 353–360.

Romer, L.M., Bridge, M.W., McConnell, A.K. and Jones, D.A. (2004). Influence of environmental temperature on exercise-induced inspiratory muscle fatigue. *European Journal of Applied Physiology*, 91(5–6): 656–663.

Volianitis, S., McConnell, A.K., Koutedakis, Y., McNaughton, L., Backx, K. and Jones, D.A. (2001a). Inspiratory muscle training improves rowing performance. *Medicine Science Sports Exercise*, 33(5): 803–809.

Volianitis, S., McConnell, A.K. and Jones, D.A. (2001b). Assessment of maximum inspiratory pressure. Prior submaximal respiratory muscle activity ('warm-up') enhances maximum inspiratory activity and attenuates the learning effect of repeated measurement. *Respiration*, 68(1): 22–27.

Wasserman, K. (1978). Breathing during exercise. *New England Journal of Medicine*, 298(14): 780–785.

Wasserman, K., Whipp, B.J., Koyal, S.N. and Cleary, M.G. (1975). Effect of carotid body resection on ventilatory and acid-base control during exercise. *Journal of Applied Physiology*, 39(3): 354–358.

West, J.B. (1999). Respiratory Physiology, 6th edn. London: Lippincott, Williams & Wilkins.

LUNG FUNCTION REFERENCE VALUES

Adults

Crapo, R.O., Morris, A.H. and Gardner, R.M. (1981). Reference spirometric values using techniques and equipment that meet ATS recommendations. *American Review of Respiratory Disease*, 123: 659–664.

Knudson, R.J., Lebowitz, M.D., Holberg, C.J. and Burrows, B. (1983). Changes in the normal maximal expiratory flow-volume curve with growth and aging. *American Review of Respiratory Disease*, 127: 725–734.

Quanjer, P.H., Tammeling, G.J., Cotes, J.E., Pedersen, O.F., Peslin, R. and Yernault, J.C. (1993). Lung volume and forced ventilatory flows. Report Working Party Standardization of lung function tests; Official Statement European Respiratory Society. *European Respiratory Journal*, 6 (Suppl. 16): 5–40.

Children/adolescents

Quanjer, P.H., Borsboom, G.J.J.M., Brunekreef, B., Zach, M., Forche, G., Cotes, J.E., Sanchis, J. and Paoletti, P. (1995). Spirometric reference values for white European children and adolescents: Polgar revisited. *Pediatric Pulmonology*, 19: 135–142.

Wang, X., Dockery, D.W., Wypij, D., Fay, M.E. and Ferris, B.G. (1993). Pulmonary function between 6 and 18 years of age. *Pediatric Pulmonology*, 15: 75–88.

CHAPTER 9

SURFACE ANTHROPOMETRY

Arthur D. Stewart and Roger Eston

INTRODUCTION

Anthropometry is defined as 'measurement of the human body'. Surface anthropometry may therefore be defined as the science of acquiring and utilising surface dimensional measurements which describe the human phenotype. Measurements of mass, stature, skeletal breadths, segment lengths, girths and skinfolds are used, either as raw data or derived ratios or predicted values to describe human size, proportions, shape, composition and symmetry. Historically, anthropometry draws from diverse disciplines including anatomy, physiology, nutrition and medicine, and the multiplicity of methodologies which prevail have caused some confusion for the exercise scientist in practice today.

Previous attempts to standardise surface anthropometric measures did not achieve widespread recognition (Lohman *et al.*, 1988; Reilly *et al.*, 1996). Nevertheless, the recommendation by Reilly *et al.* (1996) to ensure inclusion of the thigh measurement with the four commonly used upper body skinfolds (biceps, triceps, subscapular and iliac crest) (Durnin and Womersley, 1974) to provide a more valid estimate of body fat has recently been confirmed in healthy young men and women (Eston *et al.*, 2005). The publication of 'Anthropometrica' (Norton and Olds, 1996) was a significant advance in the anthropometric sciences, particularly for the application of surface anthropometry techniques. This text has formed the basis of the content of the accreditation courses approved by the International Society for the Advancement of Kinanthropometry (ISAK). The general procedures and location of the various sites are also described and illustrated by Hawes and Martin (Hawes and Martin, 2001), however the current definitive guide for all anthropometric procedures is ISAK's standards manual (ISAK, 2001) (revised 2006). The purpose of this chapter is to summarise key principles and methods for measuring the most commonly used skinfolds and girths.

MEASUREMENT PRE-REQUISITES

For all measurements, subjects require appropriate information in advance, and informed written consent should be obtained. Anthropometry requires a spacious (minimum 3 m × 3 m) well-illuminated area, affording privacy. Subjects should present for measurement in suitable apparel, recovered from previous exercise, fully hydrated and voided. Clothing should conform to the natural contours of the skin and allow easy access for landmarking and measurement. For males, running shorts or swimwear is ideal, and for females, either a two-piece swimming costume, or running shorts and a sports top which exposes the shoulders and abdominal area, are suitable. (One-piece swimwear, rowing suits or leotards are *not* suitable.) Some subjects may prefer a loose fitting shirt which can be lifted to access measurement sites. All measurements (except hip girth, which is measured over close fitting clothing for reasons of modesty) are performed on clean, dry unbroken skin. Cultural differences may preclude the acquisition of some or all measurements in some subjects. Measurement of females or children by male anthropometrists requires particular sensitivity and the individual's entitlement to a chaperone. It is always advisable to have another adult (preferably female) present in such circumstances.

RECOMMENDED EQUIPMENT

Stadiometer – (e.g. Holtain, Crosswell, Crymych, UK) mounted on wall or stand with sliding headboard and accurate to 0.1 cm.

Weighing scales – calibrated and graduated to 100 g suggested range to be up to 150 kg (e.g. SECA, Birmingham, UK).

Skinfold calipers – Harpenden (British Indicators, c/o Assist Creative Resources, Wrexham, UK) calibrated to 10 g·mm^{-2}, scale to 80 mm in new models, 40 mm in old ones, which can be read to 0.1 mm by interpolation. Holtain (Crosswell, Crymych, UK) calipers are of similar quality and can be used with equal precision.

Anthropometric tape – Metal, with a stub extending several centimetres beyond the zero line. The Rosscraft anthropometric tape (Rosscraft Innovations Inc, Vancouver, Canada) is a modified version of the Lufkin W606PM (Cooper Industries, USA). Both can be read to 0.1 cm, and are recommended.

Segmometer – A flexible metal tape with rigid sliding branches for identifying lengths and landmark locations (Rosscraft Innovations Inc, Vancouver, Canada) read to 0.1 cm.

Anthropometric box – These are not commercially available, but should be made from plywood or a strong fibre-board equivalent capable of supporting an individual who may weigh 150 kg. The box should be 30 cm × 40 cm × 50 cm, to facilitate ease of measuring subjects of differing size.

PROCEDURES

Stature is measured to 0.1 cm without footwear and with the head in the Frankfort plane (orbitale and tragion are horizontally aligned). The heels are together and touching the scale of the stadiometer. The subject inspires for measurement, and the recorder brings down the headboard to compress the hair.

Body mass is measured to 0.1 kg. The subject wears exercise apparel or light clothing but no footwear. If nude mass is required, clothing could be weighed separately.

Landmarking. Skeletal Landmarks (bony locations defining measurement sites) are located via palpation of overlying soft tissue. Because some measurements vary considerably over a short distance, landmarking the correct site is essential for reproducible measurements. Landmarks should be located generally and then released. They should then be re-located specifically before marking, as the skin can move several centimetres in relation to underlying bone. Skinfold locations are marked with a cross, with two lines intersecting at right angles. A longer line should represent the orientation of the skinfold, and the shorter line should define the finger and thumb placement. Bony edges are commonly marked with a short (0.5 cm) line, while points (e.g. the inferior tip of the scapula) are marked with a dot, from which linear measurements are made.

Protocol. Measurements should be made on the *right* side of the body. Left-handed subjects may have greater muscle mass on the left limb, in which case girths on both sides can be recorded. Subjects are encouraged to relax their muscles before measurement to reduce discomfort and improve reproducibility. Measurements should be made in series – moving from one site to the next until the entire protocol is complete.

Skinfolds. Ensure the skin is dry and unbroken, and the landmark is clearly visible. The anthropometrist's left hand approaches the subject's skin surface at 90°. The skinfold is raised at the marked site, with the shorter line visible at the edge of the anthropometrist's forefinger and thumb. The fold is grasped firmly in the required orientation, following natural cleavage lines of the skin and raised far enough (but no further) so the fold has parallel sides. Palpation helps avoid incorporating underlying muscle into the grasp. The near edge of the caliper blades are applied to the raised fold 1 cm away from the thumb and forefinger, at a depth of mid-fingernail (see Figure 9.1).

The calipers are held at 90° to the skinfold, the spring pressure is released and the measurement value recorded 2 s afterwards. In the case of large skinfolds, the needle is likely to be moving at this time, but the value is recorded nonetheless. The calipers are removed before the skinfold is released.

Skinfold locations are illustrated in Figure 9.2. and described in Table 9.1.

Girths. A cross-handed technique is used with the stub held in the left hand, and the case in the right hand. Approaching from the side of the subject, the stub is passed around the body segment, grasped by the right hand, and then passed back to the left hand which pulls it to the appropriate tension. The middle fingers of both hands can then be used for 'pinning' the tape, and moving it a short distance up or down and maintaining its orientation 90° to the long

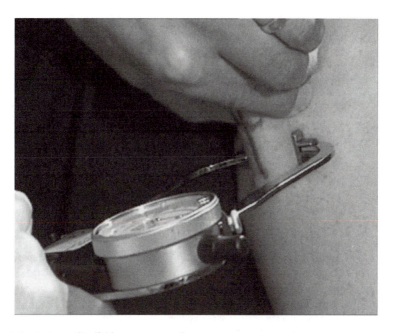

Figure 9.1   A triceps skindfold measurement illustrating appropriate technique

axis of the segment. There should be no visible indentation of the skin at the measurement. In the case of maximal measurements it is necessary to measure lesser measurements superior and inferior to the final measurement site. If the skin surface is concave, the tape spans the concavity in a straight line. For torso sites, measurements should be made at the end of a normal expiration (Table 9.2).

MEASUREMENT PROFORMA

The *mean* of duplicate or the *median* of triplicate measures (when the first two measures differ by more than 5% for skinfolds and 1% for other measures) is recommended. In some situations only a single set of measures is possible, and the error of the measurer needs to be quantified as this governs the meaning and implication of the data (Pederson and Gore, 1996). This should be in the form of *Technical Error of Measurement (TEM)*, and expressed as a percentage of the measurement value.

$$\text{TEM} = [\Sigma(x_2 - x_1)^2] \cdot 2n^{-1}$$

$$\% \, \text{TEM} = 100 \cdot \text{TEM} \cdot m^{-1}$$

where x_1 and x_2 are replicate pairs of measures, n is the number of pairs and m is the mean value for that measure across the sample.

Table 9.1   Skinfold measurements

Skinfold	*Location and landmarking*	*Orientation*	*Body position for measurement*
Triceps[a]	Mid-point of a straight line between the acromiale and the radiale on the posterior aspect of the arm	Vertical	Standing Shoulder slightly externally rotated
Subscapular	2 cm lateral and 2 cm inferior to the inferior angle of the scapula	Oblique – ~45° dipping laterally	Standing
Biceps[a]	Mid-point level of a straight line between the acromiale and the radiale on the Anterior aspect of the arm	Vertical	Standing Shoulder slightly externally rotated
Iliac crest	Immediately superior to the crest of the ilium, on the ilio-axilla line	Near horizontal	Standing Right arm placed across torso
Supraspinale	The intersection of a horizontal line drawn from the crest of the ilium, with a line joining the anterior superior iliac spine and the anterior axillary fold	Oblique	Standing
Abdominal	5 cm lateral of the midpoint of the umbilicus	Vertical	Standing
Thigh[a]	Mid-point of the perpendicular distance between the inguinal crease at the mid-line of the thigh and the mid-point of the posterior border of the patella when seated with the knee flexed to 90°	Longitudinal	Sitting with leg extended and foot supported, the subject extends the knee and clasps hands under hamstrings and lifts gently for measurement
Medial calf	The most medial aspect of the calf, at the level of maximum girth, with subject standing and weight evenly distributed	Vertical	Standing, foot on box, with knee at 90°

Note

a These sites ideally require a wide-spreading caliper or segmometer to locate, because curvature of the skin surface affects site location if a tape is used

Error magnitude varies with the recorder, the measurement type and site. For serial measurements, a statistical basis for detecting real change should be included. Because the TEM equates to the standard error of a single measurement, then overlapping standard errors indicate no significant change in serial measures – either at the 68% (for 1SE) or 95% (for 2SE) level. Clearly, experienced anthropometrists with low TEMs are several times more likely to detect real change than others.

The conversion of raw data into indices may be justified in terms of fat patterning (Stewart, 2003b; Eston *et al.*, 2005) (skinfold ratios) corrected girths (Martin *et al.*, 1990), proportions (the ratio of segment lengths or

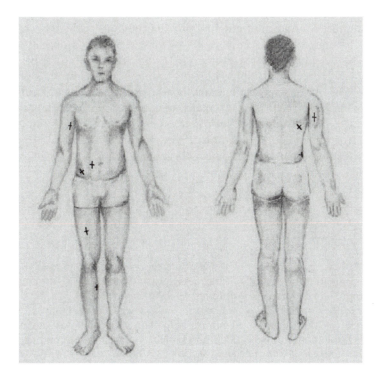

Figure 9.2 Skinfold locations
Source: M. Svensen

Table 9.2 Girth measurements

Girth	Location	Body position	Notes
Chest	At level of mid-sternum	Arms abducted slightly	Measure at the end of a normal expiration
Waist	Narrowest circumference between thorax and pelvis	Arms folded	Mid-point between iliac crest and 10th rib, if no obvious narrowing
Hip	At the level of maximum posterior protuberance of buttocks	Relaxed, feet together	Measure from the side, over clothing
Upper arm	Mid acromiale-radiale	Arm abducted slightly, elbow extended	
Forearm	Maximum	Shoulder slightly flexed, elbow extended	
Mid-thigh	Mid trochanterion – tibiale laterale level	Weight equally distributed	
Calf	Maximum	Weight equally distributed	

anthropometric somatotype (Heath and Carter, 1967). Corrected girths involve subtracting the skinfold multiplied by pi from the limb girth, and are a useful surrogate for muscularity. Predicting tissue masses of fat (Sinning *et al.*, 1985; Stewart, 2003c) or muscle (Martin *et al.*, 1990; Stewart, 2003a) has obvious appeal but is problematic. Numerous methodological assumptions govern the conversion of linear surface measurements into tissue mass, and sample-specificity restricts the utility of many equations. If used, they should be accompanied by the standard error of the estimate or confidence limits, as well as total error of prediction equations (Stewart and Hannan, 2000), although the use of raw anthropometric data is becoming more accepted and is to be encouraged.

REFERENCES

Durnin, J.V.G.A. and Womersley, J. (1974). Body fat assessment from total body density and its estimation from skinfold thickness: measurements on 481 men and women aged from 16 to 72 years. *British Journal of Nutrition*, 32: 77–97.

Eston, R.G., Rowlands, A.V., Charlesworth, S., Davies, A. and Hoppitt, T. (2005). Prediction of DXA-determined whole body fat from skinfolds: importance of including skinfolds from the thigh and calf in young, healthy men and women. *European Journal of Clinical Nutrition*, 59: 695–702.

Hawes, M. and Martin, A. (2001). Human body composition. In Eston, R.G. and Reilly, T. (eds), *Kinanthropometry and Exercise Physiology Laboratory Manual: Tests, Procedures and Data. Volume 1: Anthropometry*. Routledge, London, pp. 7–46.

Heath, B.H. and Carter, J.E.L. (1967). A modified somatotype method. *American Journal of Physical Anthropology*, 27: 57–74.

International Society for the Advancement of Kinanthropometry. (2001). International standards for anthropometric assessment. North West University (Potchefstroom Campus), Potchefstroom 2520, South Africa: ISAK (revised 2006).

Lohman, T.G., Roche, A.F. and Martorell, R. (eds) (1988). *Anthropometric Standardization Reference Manual*. Champaign, IL. Human Kinetics.

Martin, A.D., Spenst, L.F., Drinkwater, D.T. and Clarys, J.P. (1990). Anthropometric estimation of muscle mass in men. *Medicine and Science in Sports and Exercise*, 22: 729–733.

Norton, K. and Olds, T. (eds) (1996). *Anthropometrica*. Sydney: University of New South Wales Press, pp. 77–96.

Pederson, D. and Gore, C. (1996). Anthropometry measurement error. In K. Norton and T. Olds (eds), *Anthropometrica*. Sydney: University of New South Wales Press, pp. 77–96.

Reilly, T., Maughan, R.J. and Hardy, L. (1996). Body fat consensus statement of the steering groups of the British Olympic Association. *Sports Exercise and Injury*, 2: 46–49.

Sinning, W.E., Dolny, D.G., Little, K.D., Cunningham, L.N., Racaniello, A., Siconolfi, S.F. and Sholes, J.L. (1985). Validity of 'generalised' equations for body composition analysis in male athletes. *Medicine and Science in Sports and Exercise*, 17: 124–130.

Stewart, A.D. (2003a). Fat patterning – indicators and implications. *Nutrition*, 19: 568–569.

Stewart, A.D. (2003b). Anthropometric fat patterning in male and female subjects. In T. Reilly and M. Marfell-Jones (eds), *Kinanthropometry VIII*. London, Routledge, pp. 195–202.

Stewart, A.D. (2003c). Mass fractionation in male and female athletes. In T. Reilly and M. Marfell-Jones (eds), *Kinanthropometry VIII*. London, Routledge, pp. 203–210.

Stewart, A.D. and Hannan, W.J. (2000). Body composition prediction in male athletes using dual X-ray absorptiometry as the reference method. *Journal of Sports Sciences*, 18: 263–274.

CHAPTER 10

MEASURING FLEXIBILITY

Nicola Phillips

Flexibility has been defined as 'the intrinsic property of body tissues, which determines the range of motion achievable without injury at a joint or group of joints' (Holt *et al.*, 1996, p. 172). However the term flexibility has historically involved some confusion or contention. Inconsistencies in terminology used by varying disciplines has been a major factor, where the term often means different things to different disciplines. For example, Kisner (2002) defined flexibility as the ability of a muscle to relax and yield to stretch. This definition emphasises the contractile component of soft tissue structures around a joint rather than the movement available at a specific joint or joints.

Before considering appropriate measures of flexibility it is therefore important to clarify what is meant by flexibility, which type of flexibility you want to measure and whether a test is appropriate for that measure. Accuracy and reliability of testing has been discussed in general in previous chapters but the type of flexibility being measured will have a major impact on the validity of any specific test. When measuring flexibility, it should not be thought of as a whole body component but as a joint or body segment specific issue. Flexibility will often be joint-specific in different sports and measurement should therefore reflect those variations.

STATIC AND DYNAMIC TESTS

Static flexibility is a measure of range of movement, usually passive, around one or more joints in a body segment. Static flexibility is thought to be primarily limited by an individual's ability to tolerate stretch and could therefore be affected by factors such as varying tolerance of discomfort or state of relaxation. Physiotherapists and other health professionals might also assess limits of motion through 'end-feel' of the movement (Norkin and White, 1995), which is a subjective measure of resistance to the limits of movement. Although a fairly sensitive measure when performed by an experienced individual, the subjective nature with limited scope to attribute a figure to the outcome poses definite limitations to this technique.

Dynamic flexibility is considered by some disciplines as the range of motion usually achieved through active movement involving muscle contraction. Following this definition, test movements would be made specific to functional movements required in various sporting activities (MacDougall *et al.*, 1991). The measures would thus be the same as for passive stretching but would follow a different strategy for achieving the range of movement. However other disciplines would regard dynamic flexibility as something entirely different. Gleim and McHugh (1997) discuss dynamic flexibility in terms of measuring increasing stiffness in a muscle as range is increased and it is put on a stretch, either actively or passively. It has been argued that this is the more objective way of measuring flexibility. In view of the lack of consensus in current literature regarding dynamic flexibility, this chapter will be restricted to measuring range of movement to that reflecting passive flexibility.

EQUIPMENT

There is a wide variety of measuring tools available and some will be more applicable in certain sports than others. They also vary in complexity of use and cost. The simplest and cheapest would probably be the standard tape measure, whereas the more costly would be use of a digital camera and appropriate software for angular measurement. Goniometers or digital inclinometers are also used to measure joint angles. The procedures described in the regional sections of this chapter could be used interchangeably with most of the equipment listed. However, it is important to decide on a specific piece of equipment for each test and to use it consistently for flexibility measures to be meaningful.

PROCEDURES

The following procedures are essential for flexibility measurement as each of the conditions below has been shown to affect flexibility.

- The environment should be standardised, especially regarding temperature and whether measurements are made inside or outside.
- Any warm up should also be standardised as this could have major effects on muscle extensibility.
- Starting positions should be recorded carefully to allow repetition on subsequent occasions for meaningful comparison.
- Instructions should also be standardised, particularly if there is a likelihood of different testers taking measurements over a training/competitive season.

- The actual protocol should be the same each time, including the number of attempts as there is likely to be a learning as well as a warm up effect with many of the tests. It would be usual to decide on a mean or the best of three attempts.
- An appropriate battery of tests should be selected for an individual sport as different sports will have very different flexibility requirements and will be joint or region specific.

SPECIFIC MEASURES

The following sections describe commonly used tests of flexibility. Some tests measure single joint movement, whereas others measure multi-joint segments. It is by no means a comprehensive list but provides a sufficient battery of tests to be able to assess most frequently measured segments. There are also numerous variations of the tests described which have been modified for sport specificity. It is beyond the scope of this chapter to discuss the myriad adaptations, therefore the tests described will provide a standard starting point from which to develop a sports-specific testing protocol as appropriate.

UPPER LIMB

Shoulder flexion

- The subject lies supine with knees bent and back flattened (Figure 10.1).
- The arm is raised above head with elbow straight.
- The angle between the humerus and trunk is then measured using a goniometer, inclinometer or motion analysis software package.

Tip – make sure that the lumbar spine does not come away from the support surface giving an appearance of additional shoulder range of movement.
   Some sports, for example, gymnastics, swimming, racket or throwing activities involve greater range of movement than this test allows. An alternative test could be used for these sports:

- The subject lies prone with chin or forehead resting on support surface and arms stretched above head.
- The arm is lifted from the support surface.
- The distance of the arm from the support surface can then be measured using a tape measure.

Tip – ensure that the head remains in contact with the support surface to standardise range of movement measured.

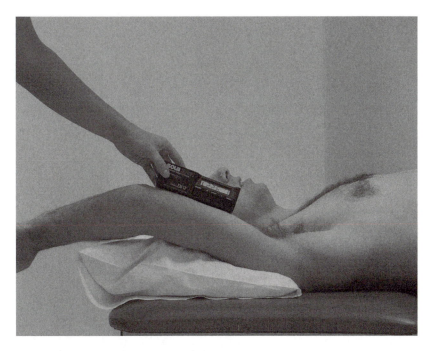

Figure 10.1   Measuring shoulder flexion in supine

Reach behind back – combined rotation, adduction and extension

Part 1

- The subject stands with arms by their side (Figure 10.2).
- The subject is instructed to raise one arm behind their head and reach down their spine as far as possible.
- The distance of the middle finger from the 7th Cervical vertebra is measured with a tape measure.
- The distance can then be compared to the contralateral side.

Part 2

- The subject stands with arms by their side.
- The subject is instructed to take their arm behind their back and reach up as far as possible.
- The distance of the middle finger from the 7th Cervical vertebra is measured with a tape measure.

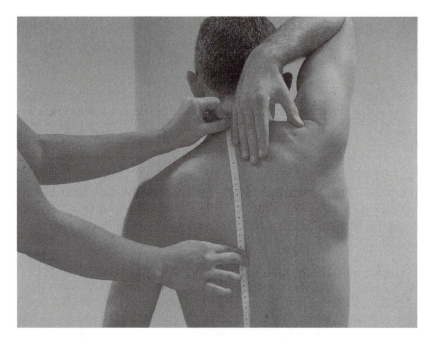

Figure 10.2   Measuring combined elevation and external rotation (back scratch)

Shoulder rotation

Although the reach tests incorporate rotation, isolated internal or external rotation are important measures in some sports. For instance, Tyler *et al.* (1999) reported a significant relationship between shoulder internal rotation and posterior shoulder tightness in baseball pitchers. The following tests are options for more specific measures.

Internal rotation

- The subject lies supine with knees bent and back flattened and with shoulder to be tested held at 90° abduction and elbow in 90° flexion (Figure 10.3).
- The tester fixes the scapula by placing the hand over the acromion.
- The subject can be asked to actively internally rotate or moved into the range passively, depending on the testing protocol chosen. (The choice of procedure should be recorded to ensure accurate repetition on subsequent testing.)
- The angle of rotation of the forearm can be measured with a goniometer, inclinometer or motion analysis software.

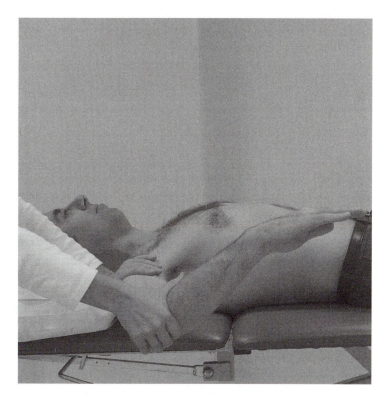

Figure 10.3 Measuring shoulder internal rotation at 90° abduction in supine

External rotation

- The subject lies supine with knees bent and back flattened and with shoulder to be tested held at 90° abduction and elbow in 90° flexion.
- The tester fixes the scapula by placing the hand over the acromion.
- The subject can be asked to actively internally rotate or moved into the range passively, depending on the testing protocol chosen. (The choice of procedure should be recorded to ensure accurate repetition on subsequent testing.)
- The angle of rotation of the forearm can be measured with a goniometer, inclinometer or motion analysis software.

Tip – make sure the trunk or the scapula does not lift from the support surface and that elbow flexion/extension remains constant to avoid giving an appearance of additional shoulder range of movement.

It should be noted that less range of movement would be expected when the scapula is fixed as described earlier than when the subject is asked to freely move into internal or external rotation. The technique described earlier is designed to control accessory scapulothoracic motion and is therefore thought to be more representative of glenohumeral movement (Awan *et al.*, 2002). However, there is a learning element for the measurer in this test, which could affect standardisation on subsequent testing.

LOWER LIMB

Straight leg raise

The straight leg raise is a commonly used test, although there are varied reports about its validity for hamstring flexibility measurement because of the influence of concurrent sciatic nerve stretch during the test. Varied recommendations have been made by previous authors as to whether the contralateral leg should remain straight or flexed during the test (Gajdosik, 1991; Kendall *et al.*, 1997). The test described here uses a straight leg but providing testing remains consistent, either could be used.

- The subject lies supine, arms at side and legs straight (Figure 10.4).
- The tester lifts the leg to be measured, keeping the knee straight.
- Maximum movement is measured as an angle between the leg and the support surface using a goniometer, inclinometer or motion analysis software.

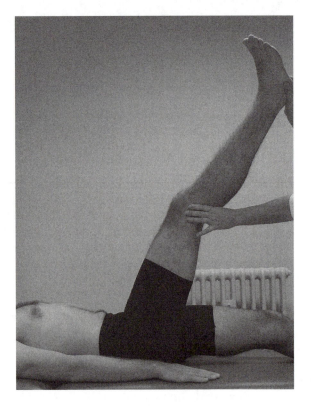

Figure 10.4 Measuring hamstring flexibility using the straight leg raise

Active knee extension test/passive knee extension test

This test is considered to be more specific to hamstrings as opposed to the straight leg raise where neural structures are often a limiting factor (Sullivan *et al.*, 1992; de Weijer *et al.*, 2003). The active knee extension (AKE) was proposed by Gajdosk and Lusin (1983) as a modification of the straight leg raise but there has been some argument about its inter- tester reliability (Worrell *et al.*, 1991). Consequently the test has since been modified to a passive version and both intra-and inter-tester reliability has been reported elsewhere (Gajdosik *et al.*, 1993).

- The subject to be tested lies supine with to be tested held at 90° hip flexion and 90° knee flexion. The contralateral leg is straight.
- AKE – the subject actively extends the knee whilst maintaining the hip at 90° or
- Passive knee extension (PKE) – the subject's knee is passively extended whilst maintaining the hip at 90°.
- Range of movement is measured by the angle of knee flexion using goniometer, inclinometer or motion analysis software.

Hip abduction – adductors/groin

- The subject lies supine with legs straight.
- The tester fixes the opposite hip over the pelvis.
- The subject then slides their leg out to the side as far as possible whilst keeping their toes pointed upwards.
- The angle of abduction can then be measured from the midline using a goniometer, inclinometer or motion analysis software.

Tip: Rotation of the pelvis or the hip can alter the range of movement significantly and therefore need to be standardised between tests.

Hip adduction – tensor fascia latae and iliotibial band

The iliotibial band is a structure that can become shortened in a variety of sports involving running. Adduction of the hip is therefore a useful movement to assess the length of tensor fascia latae and the iliotibial band.

- The subject lies on their side with the leg to be tested uppermost and with their back close to the edge of the testing surface.
- The upper leg is dropped off the edge of the surface, behind the body.
- The angle of drop can be measured using a goniometer, inclinometer or motion analysis software.

Tip: Anything less than 10° of movement is generally regarded as abnormal (Kendall *et al.*, 1997).

Thomas test

The Thomas test is a specific test for hip flexor flexibility as described by Kendall *et al.* (1997). It can be modified through altering knee flexion to include or exclude rectus femoris as a component in the range. Maintaining a straight knee excludes rectus femoris. Adding knee flexion in the test position will assess the length of rectus femoris following assessment of the hip flexors.

- The subject leans back against the edge of a treatment couch or table.
- The non-test thigh is held firmly as closely to the chest as possible.
- The subject lowers into a supine position on the treatment couch or table, whilst maintaining the hip position of the non-test leg.
- The angle of the test thigh to the floor can be measured using a goniometer, inclinometer or motion analysis software (Figure 10.5).
- Rectus femoris range can then be measured by passively flexing the knee.
- The knee angle can then be measured using a goniometer, inclinometer or motion analysis software.

Note that the Thomas test is a sensitive test but requires an appropriate testing surface that is not always possible when testing in the field. The following test also assesses hip flexor movement.

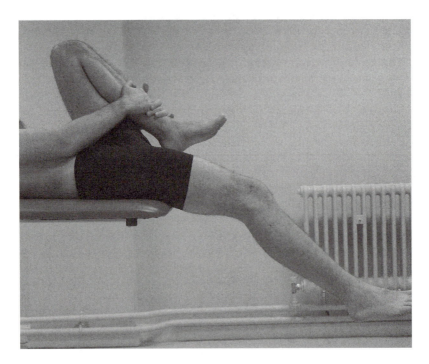

Figure 10.5   Measuring hip flexor length using the Thomas test

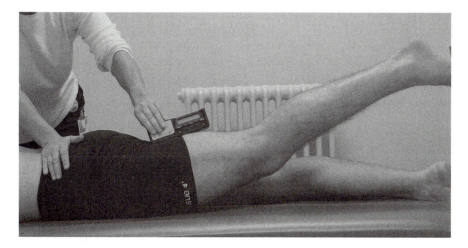

Figure 10.6 Measuring hip flexor length in prone lying

Prone hip extension

- The subject lies prone on the test surface.
- The test leg is lifted whilst keeping the knee in extension.
- The angle of the leg to the test surface can then be measured using a goniometer, inclinometer or motion analysis software (Figure 10.6).
- Adding knee flexion to this movement will introduce rectus femoris as an additional component in the test.

Tip: Ensure that the pelvis is kept in contact with the test surface to prevent the subject from rotating the trunk in order to compensate for any lack of movement. Typical range of movement would be 10°.

Hip rotation

Isolated hip rotation is a useful measure for some sports, particularly when links have been made with limited hip movement through the kinetic chain to upper limb injuries, particularly in sports involving throwing (Kibler, 1995, Kraemer, *et al.*, 1995). The following test is useful for isolating hip movement easily but a limitation is that it will be most transferable to sporting activities that happen in some flexion, which is not the case for throwing activities. However, limitations of hip rotation in a throwing position are often still highlighted by testing in this position but adaptation of the test to be performed in supine might need to be considered for some screening situations.

Internal rotation

- The subject lies supine with the test hip and knee at 90° and the foot relaxed.
- The hip is moved into internal rotation (foot away from midline of body).
- The angle of rotation can be measured using a goniometer, inclinometer or motion analysis software.

External rotation

- The subject lies supine with the test hip and knee at 90° and the foot relaxed.
- The hip is moved into external rotation (foot towards midline of body).
- The angle of rotation can be measured using a goniometer, inclinometer or motion analysis software.

Knee extension

Although knee flexion is frequently measured as an outcome measure following injury and also during function to assess efficacy in activities such as landing, it is not usually regarded as a measure of flexibility and knee measurement has therefore been restricted to extension for these purposes.

Knee extension, or more importantly hyperextension, is a commonly used measure of general flexibility in athletes.

- The subject lies supine with knees straight.
- Extension, or hyperextension is then performed passively or actively, depending on the required protocol.
- The angle is then measured from the tibia to the horizontal using a goniometer, inclinometer or motion analysis software.

Tip: This test can also be performed in standing but care should be taken to standardise hip and ankle positions, which can confound the readings.

Ankle dorsiflexion

The ankle joint has two major plantar flexors, gastrocnemius and soleus. The former is a two joint muscle, extending over the knee, whilst the latter is a single joint muscle originating from the tibia. It is therefore important that both the following dorsiflexion tests are completed to ensure assessment of the flexibility of both muscles.

Ankle dorsiflexion with straight knee – gastrocnemius bias

- The subject is in stride standing and leans forward onto arms (Figure 10.7).

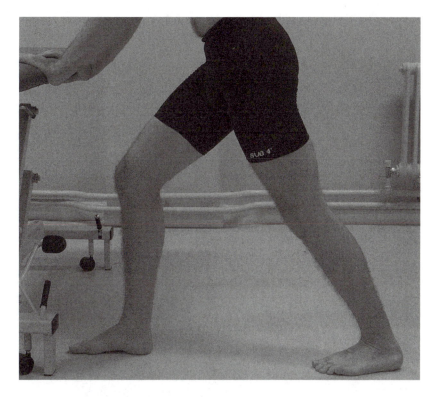

Figure 10.7 Measuring gastrocnemius length in stride standing

- The pelvis is kept in posterior tilt, the hip and knee in extension.
- The rear foot is taken as far back as possible whilst still keeping the heel on the floor.
- The angle of the lower leg to the foot is then measured from the horizontal or the dorsum of the foot, using a goniometer, inclinometer or motion analysis software.

Ankle dorsiflexion with bent knee – soleus bias

- The subject is in stride standing and leans forward onto arms (Figure 10.8).
- The pelvis is kept in posterior tilt, the hip in extension.
- The rear foot is taken as far back as possible whilst still keeping the heel on the floor additional dorsiflexion can then be achieved through knee flexion.
- The angle of the lower leg to the foot is then measured from the horizontal or the dorsum of the foot, using a goniometer, inclinometer or motion analysis software.

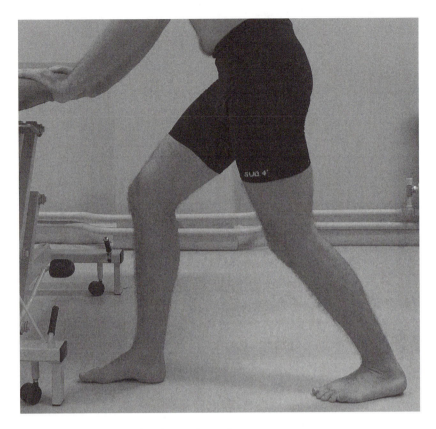

Figure 10.8   Measuring soleus length in stride standing

Ankle dorsiflexion with bent knee – soleus bias – alternative method

- The subject is in stride standing and leans forward onto arms.
- The test leg is placed up against a wall.
- The foot is then placed as far from the wall as possible whilst still being able to maintain the knee in contact with the wall and the heel on the floor.
- The maximal distance where this position can be achieved is then recorded with a tape measure.

Ankle plantar flexion

- The subject lies supine with knees straight. A rolled towel may need to be put under the calf or the feet placed over the edge of a bed to allow heel movement.
- The toes are pointed down, either actively or passively depending on the chosen protocol.

- The angle of the dorsum of the foot to plantigrade (90° to the tibia) using a goniometer, inclinometer or motion analysis software.

TRUNK

Sit and reach

The sit and reach test has traditionally been used as a field test for hamstring flexibility as it requires minimal equipment. However, it is significantly limited by lumbar spine and scapulothoracic flexibility and has therefore been placed in the trunk section. It has been established that anthropometric differences have a significant effect on sit and reach scores (Shephard *et al.*, 1990) making the test inappropriate for comparing between individuals, although it might still be useful for intra-subject comparison.

- The subject is positioned in long sitting, with knees straight and feet placed up against the sit and reach box (Figure 10.9).
- The arms are stretched out, elbows extended, palms down onto the top surface of the box.
- The bar on the sit and reach scale is pushed forward as far as possible by leaning the trunk, whilst maintaining the straight leg position. The movement should be a slow steady stretch with no bouncing permitted.
- The end position is held for 3 s and the scale recorded in centimetres from the sit and reach box.

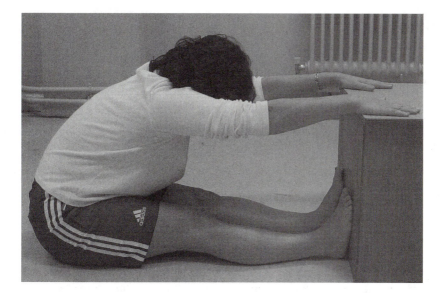

Figure 10.9   Measuring hamstring flexibility using the sit and reach test

Lumbar spine flexion

Lumbar spine flexion in standing is another test frequently used as a measure of general flexibility. There are a variety of tests used but two are described later.

Hands to floor

- The subject starts in a standing position, knees straight, arms by their side.
- The subject leans forward, letting arms drop towards the floor with fingers extended.
- The distance between floor and finger tips is measured with a tape measure.

Tip: In sports requiring higher degrees of flexibility, this test can be performed on a box and the distance from the base of support down to the fingertips below can be measured with a tape measure.

The earlier test is easily conducted but only provides a very gross measure of trunk flexibility as it is impossible to tell whether range has been achieved through lumbar spine of hamstring flexibility, much like the sit and reach test.

The following test provides a more specific measure of lumbar spine flexion (Modified Schrobers).

- The subject starts in a standing position, knees straight, arms by their side.
- The base of a tape measure is held over the 1st sacral vertebra and extended to the 1st lumbar vertebra and the length recorded.
- The subject leans forward, letting arms drop towards the floor.
- The increase in length between the two points described earlier is used as the measure of lumbar spine movement.

Tip: Surfacing marking the skin over the above points will help accuracy. Note that this test requires an element of palpation skill in highlighting fixed anatomical points for measurement.

Lumbar spine extension

This movement is even more difficult to standardise and is likely to need to be adapted for sports that require a very high degree of lumbar extension, such as gymnastics. The following test is more appropriate for general use.

- The subject starts in a standing position, knees straight, arms by their side.
- The subject is instructed to slide their hands down the back of their legs whilst arching backwards.
- The distance from fingertips to the floor can be measured with a tape measure.

Tip: Side flexion of the lumbar spine is less frequently measured in general screening as opposed to situations of injury. It can be measured in a similar way by asking the subject to slide one hand down the side of the same leg and measuring from the floor as above.

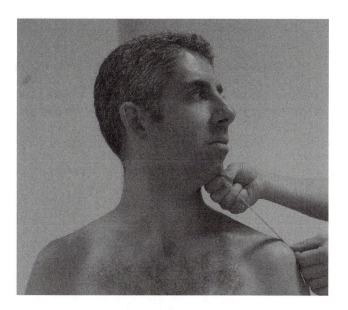

Figure 10.10 Measuring cervical spine rotation in sitting

Cervical spine flexion

- The subject starts in upright sitting with shoulders back.
- The subject drops their head forward and looks down.
- The distance between the chin and the sternal notch can be measured with a tape measure.

Tip: Extension can be measured in a similar way by recording the increase in distance from chin to sternal notch or alternatively the distance between occiput and 7th cervical spine (Figure 10.10).

Cervical spine rotation

Rotation is more likely to be useful as a routine cervical spine movement measure than flexion and extension, particularly in sports such as swimming.

- The subject starts in upright sitting with shoulders back.
- The subject then turns their head to look over one shoulder.
- The distance from the chin to acromion can be measured with a tape measure.

ACKNOWLEDGEMENTS

Thanks to Matthew Townsend and Michelle Evans for their assistance in producing the figures.

REFERENCES

Awan, R., Smith J. and Boon, A.J. (2002). Measuring shoulder internal rotation range of motion: a comparison of 3 techniques. *Archives of Physical Medicine and Rehabilitation*, 83(9): 1229–1234.

de Weijer, V.C., Gorniak, G.C. and Shamus, E. (2003). The effect of static stretch and warm-up exercise on hamstring length over the course of 24 hours. *Journal of Orthopedics and Sports Physical Therapists*, 33(12): 727–733.

Gajdosik, R.L. (1991). Passive compliance and length of clinically short hamstring muscles of healthy men. *Clinical Biomechanics*, 6: 239–244.

Gajdosik, R. Lusin (1983). G. Hamstring muscle tightness. Reliability of an active-knee-extension test. *Physical Therapy*, 7: 1085–1090.

Gajdosik, R.L., Rieck, M.A., Sullivan, D.K. and Wightman, S.E. (1993). Comparison of four clinical tests for assessing hamstring muscle length. *Journal of Orthopedics and Sports Physical Therapists*, 18: 614–618.

Gleim, G.W. and McHugh, M.P. (1997). Flexibility and its effects on sports injury and performance. *Sports Medicine*, 24(5): 289–299.

Holt, J., Holt, L.E. and Pelham, T.W. (1996). Flexibility redefined. In T. Bauer (ed.), *Biomechanics in Sports XIII*, pp. 170–174. Thunder Bay, Ontario: Lakehead University.

Kendall, F.P., McCreary, E.K. and Provance, P.G. (1997). Muscle testing and function, 5th edn. London: Lipincott, William and Wilkins.

Kibler, W.B. (1995). Biomechanical analysis of the shoulder during tennis activities. *Clinical Sports Medicine*, 14(1): 1–8.

Kisner, C. and Colby, L.A. (2002). Therapeutic exercise: Foundation and techniques, 4th edn. F.A. Davis Company.

Kraemer, W.J., Triplett, N.T. and Fry, A.C. (1995). An in depth sports medicine profile of women collegiate tennis players. *Journal of Sports Rehabilitation*, 4: 79–88.

MacDougall, J.D., Wenger, H.A. and Green, H.J. (eds) (1991). Physiological testing of the high-performance athlete, 2nd edn. IL: Human Kinetics Books.

Magnusson, S.P., Simonsen, E.B., Aagaard, P., Buesen, J., Johannson, F. and Kjaer, M. (1997). Determinants of musculoskeletal flexibility: viscoelastic properties, cross-sectional area, EMG and stretch tolerance. *Scandinavian Journal of Medicine, Science and Sports*, 7: 195–202.

Magnusson, S.P., Simonsen, E.B., Aagaard, P., Sorensen, H. and Kajer, M. (1996). A mechanism for altered flexibility in human skeletal muscle. *Journal of Physiology*, 487: 291–298.

Norkin, C.C. and White, D.J. (1995). Measurement of joint motion: a guide to goniometry, 2nd edn. Philadelphia, PA: F.A. Davis.

Shephard, R.J., Berridge, M. and Montelpare, W. (1990). On the generality of the 'sit and reach' test: an analysis of flexibility data for an aging population. *Research Quarterly for Exercise and Sport*, 61(4): 326–330.

Sullivan, M.K., Dejulia, J.J., and Worrell, T.W. (1992). Effect of pelvic position and stretching on hamstring muscle flexibility. *Medicine and Science in Sports and Exercise*, 24(12): 1383–1389.

Tyler, T.F., Roy, T., Nicholas, S.J. and Gleim, G.W. (1999). Reliability and validity of a new method of measuring posterior shoulder tightness. *Journal of Orthopedics and Sports Physical Therapy*, 29(5): 262–269.

Worrell, T.W., Perrin, D.H., Gansneder, B.M. and Gieck, J.H. (1991). Comparison of isokinetic strength and flexibility measures between hamstring injured and non-injured athletes. *Journal of Orthopedics and Sports Physical Therapy*, 13: 118–125.

CHAPTER 11

PULMONARY GAS EXCHANGE

David V.B. James, Leigh E. Sandals,
Dan M. Wood and Andrew M. Jones

INTRODUCTION

Pulmonary gas exchange (PGE) variables include oxygen uptake ($\dot{V}O_2$) and carbon dioxide output ($\dot{V}CO_2$). However, variables representing ventilation, for example expired minute ventilation ($\dot{V}_E$), and derived variables, for example respiratory exchange ratio, will also be considered in this chapter. Gas exchange variables are routinely measured at rest or during exercise to determine the following:

- resting metabolic rate
- work efficiency or economy
- maximal oxygen uptake
- gas exchange thresholds
- gas exchange kinetics.

Such information is routinely used in an exercise context to:

- determine performance potential
- recommend exercise training intensities
- examine the effect of exercise training
- establish causes for exercise intolerance.

With the increased availability of semi-automated PGE measurement systems, and software to determine PGE parameters, it may be tempting to avoid asking too many questions about the quality of the data. However, in this measurement area the quality of the data should always be questioned, not least because measurement errors may be compounded through necessary calculations. This has been nicely summed up previously by Haldane (1912, preface) who in his paper stated that, 'the descriptions are given in considerable detail, as attention to small matters of detail is often of much importance'.

Despite the proliferation of semi-automated on-line measurement systems, the traditional 'off-line' Douglas bag based approach is still recognised by many as the 'gold standard' in the measurement of PGE. An advantage of the Douglas bag method derives from the transparency of the steps in determining PGE variables, so this approach is very useful when attempting to systematically identify potential sources of error. Once such errors have been quantified and minimised, other measurement systems may be compared to the gold standard (for further discussion see Lamarra and Whipp, 1995).

In the first part of this chapter we consider key potential measurement errors when using the Douglas bag technique in normal ambient conditions (i.e. 20.9% O_2), and approaches to quantify and minimise the systematic errors (accuracy) and random errors (precision). The range of applications of the Douglas bag technique will be considered, raising the question about suitable approaches when PGE is changing rapidly. With the increased availability of rapidly responding gas analysers and flow measurement, breath-by-breath determination of PGE is possible. We have chosen not to consider on-line systems involving mixing chambers due to their decreasing popularity, and numerous, often problematic, assumptions (Atkinson *et al.*, 2005). Throughout the chapter we suggest an approach that is uncompromising, and might be considered best practice.

The basic calculation of $\dot{V}O_2$ is:

$$\dot{V}O_2 = \dot{V}_I \times F_IO_2 - \dot{V}_E \times F_EO_2$$

where $\dot{V}_I$ and $\dot{V}_E$ are the rate at which air is inspired and expired respectively, and F_IO_2 and F_EO_2 are the fractions of oxygen in the inspired and expired air, respectively.

The basic calculation of $\dot{V}CO_2$ is:

$$\dot{V}CO_2 = \dot{V}_E \times F_ECO_2 - \dot{V}_I \times F_ICO_2$$

where F_ECO_2 and F_ICO_2 are the fractions of carbon dioxide in the expired and inspired air, respectively. However, due to the small quantity of CO_2 in the inspired gas under normal atmospheric conditions, without introducing any meaningful systematic error, the equation may be rewritten as:

$$\dot{V}CO_2 = \dot{V}_E \times F_ECO_2$$

The volume of a gas varies depending on its temperature (Charles' Law), pressure (Boyle's Law) and content of water vapour. Further calculations to standardise $\dot{V}_I$ and $\dot{V}_E$ are therefore necessary in order that comparisons can be made between data collected in different circumstances. For example, expirate collected in a Douglas bag, which is then allowed to cool to room temperature, is in the form Ambient Temperature and Pressure Saturated (ATPS). Further calculations may be used to convert this volume of expirate into Body Temperature and Pressure Saturated (BTPS) or Standard Temperature and Pressure Dry (STPD) forms.

Through the following section, where relevant, procedures to minimise potential sources of measurement error are presented for each term in the earlier calculations. In addition, the resulting precision (95% confidence limits) of the measurement, and the impact on the precision of $\dot{V}O_2$ itself, is presented. To determine the influence of measurement precision on $\dot{V}O_2$ precision, certain assumptions were necessary. Assumptions include a 45 s collection of expirate during *heavy* intensity exercise, where the following values are used in the calculation: $F_EO_2 = 0.165$; $F_ECO_2 = 0.041$; $\dot{V}_E$ (BTPS) $= 80.0 \; l \cdot min^{-1}$; $\dot{V}O_2 = 3.616 \; l \cdot min^{-1}$; $\dot{V}CO_2 = 3.226 \; l \cdot min^{-1}$.

Commonly, neither off-line (Douglas bag) nor commercially available on-line PGE systems directly measure $\dot{V}_I$. Instead, $\dot{V}_I$ is determined using a nitrogen correction factor that 'converts' $\dot{V}_E$ into $\dot{V}_I$. The assumption on which this correction factor is based is that nitrogen (N_2) is metabolically inert, such that the volume of N_2 expired and the volume of N_2 inspired is equal. This can be represented by the following equation:

$$\dot{V}_I \times F_IN_2 = \dot{V}_E \times F_EN_2$$

where F_IN_2 and F_EN_2 are the fractions of N_2 in inspired and expired air, respectively.

This equation can then be rearranged to calculate $\dot{V}_I$ from $\dot{V}_E$. Although neither F_IN_2 nor F_EN_2 are typically measured when the Douglas bag method is used, it is assumed that inspired air is composed only of O_2, CO_2 and N_2, so with values for O_2 and CO_2, N_2 may be determined:

$$F_IN_2 = 1 - F_IO_2 - F_ICO_2$$

This assumption is valid because the trace gases (i.e. argon, neon, helium, etc.) that comprise ~0.93% of inspired air are metabolically inert and can, therefore, be combined with N_2. Errors may be made if it is assumed that inspired gas fractions are equivalent to outside gas fractions when working in a laboratory, even when the laboratory is well ventilated. Sandals (2003) found the mean (95% confidence limits) for F_IO_2 and F_ICO_2 in a well-ventilated laboratory (with one exercising subject and two experimenters) to be 0.20915 (± 0.00035) and 0.0007 (± 0.0003), respectively over 38 tests. For heavy intensity exercise, the difference between actual inspired and assumed inspired (i.e. outside) gas fractions translates into a systematic error of 0.18% and 0.99% for $\dot{V}O_2$ and $\dot{V}CO_2$, respectively. The only way to correct for such systematic errors is to determine average inspired gas fractions over a series of exercise tests in the normal laboratory conditions. The precision of the $\dot{V}O_2$ and $\dot{V}CO_2$ determination is $\pm 0.88\%$ and $\pm 0.74\%$, respectively. The only way to improve precision further is to determine inspired gas fractions during *each* exercise test.

If it is assumed that expired air is composed only of O_2, CO_2 and N_2, an expression for F_EN_2 that involves F_EO_2 and F_ECO_2, both of which are typically measured, can be used:

$$F_EN_2 = 1 - F_EO_2 - F_ECO_2$$

On-line systems, based on mass spectrometers for determination of gas fractions, directly measure all inspired (F_IN_2, F_IO_2, F_ICO_2) and expired (F_EN_2, F_EO_2, F_ECO_2) gas fractions, thereby reducing the number of necessary assumptions for these systems. It is of relevance to both on-line and Douglas bag methods that although the assumption that N_2 is inert has been challenged in the past (Dudka *et al.*, 1971; Cissik *et al.*, 1972), the assumption is generally considered appropriate, particularly during exercise when minute ventilation is elevated (Wilmore and Costill, 1973).

DOUGLAS BAG METHOD

The discrete nature, and often prolonged duration, of expired gas collections into a Douglas bag suggests that this technique is most suited to determining steady state gas exchange. The technique may also appropriately be employed when PGE variables are changing systematically in a predictable way, for example, during exercise with a progressively increasing work rate (or speed).

The required duration for each discrete collection of expired gas into a Douglas bag should be determined by how quickly the bag becomes filled, which in turn depends on the minute ventilation. It is this requirement that determines sampling frequency, and therefore limits the utility of this technique in examining PGE kinetics. The need to 'fill' the bag is partly related to the need to average over a number of breaths, so it is important to only include a *whole* number of breaths in each collection of expirate. However, the need to adequately fill the bag is also related to minimising several potential sources or error. An obvious source of error is inaccurate timing. One approach to ensure accurate timing is the addition of timer switches to the Douglas bag valves. Before considering the other sources of error, it is perhaps worth pointing out that any leak in the collection apparatus will induce an error, and that it is therefore important to check for leaks in the Douglas bag itself, the two-way valve, the connecting tubing and the three-way breathing valve.

The accuracy and precision of the determined volume of expired gas (expirate) may be affected by the volume measuring device, the determination of ambient pressure, the determination of gas temperature and the volume of any sample removed for determination of gas fractions. Volume is often determined by evacuating collected expirate through a dry gas meter in off-line systems, although traditionally various spirometers have been used. Calibration of the dry gas meter ensures accurate gas volume determination, and calibration is normally undertaken by exposing the dry gas meter to a range of known volumes. To ensure a valid calibration approach, these known volumes should be delivered to the dry gas meter in exactly the same way that expirate would normally be delivered (for further information, see Hart and Withers, 1996). In this regard, a syringe is normally used to pass known volumes of gas into a Douglas bag through the normal collection assembly. The known gas volumes are then passed through the dry gas meter with the help of a vacuum pump. The flow rate of the vacuum pump must be set to that used when evacuating expirate to ensure a valid calibration. A regression equation is then produced to correct the volume meter reading to the actual volume. Sandals (2003) has determined the precision of such a calibration approach to be ±0.057 l. When this level of precision is considered for $\dot{V}O_2$ determination, a value for $\dot{V}O_2$ precision of $\pm0.86\%$ is calculated.

Ambient pressure is normally determined with a mercury barometer via a Vernier scale. Barometers should be regularly checked for their accuracy. This is possible by applying the following equation (WMO, 1996):

$$P_{B_{LAB}} = P_{B_{SL}}/(H/29.27T_{LAB})$$

where $P_{B_{SL}}$ is the barometric pressure (P_B) at sea-level, $P_{B_{LAB}}$ is the P_B for the laboratory (and both pressures are in hPa where 1 mm Hg = 1.33 hPa), H is the laboratory elevation in metres (from ordinance survey map), and T_{LAB} is the laboratory temperature in Kelvin.

A good quality barometer will normally have a resolution of 0.05 mmHg, and it can be assumed that measurement can be accurately made to within ±0.2 mmHg. When this level of precision is considered for $\dot{V}O_2$ determination, a value for $\dot{V}O_2$ precision of $\pm0.03\%$ is calculated (Sandals, 2003).

Expired gas temperature is normally determined at the inlet port of the dry gas meter with the use of a thermistor probe. Commonly available probes have a resolution of 0.1°C, and are normally factory calibrated with maximum accuracy in the region of ±0.2°C. Errors in the measurement of expired gas temperature may have a cumulative effect on $\dot{V}_E$ translation from ATPS to STPD (and therefore $\dot{V}O_2$ determination) via both the determination of gas temperature itself, and the use of gas temperature in the determination of the partial pressure of water vapour in the gas (P_{H_2O}). Taking a maximum possible error of ±0.2°C in the determination of gas temperature, this translates into a precision of $\pm0.07\%$ in the conversion of $\dot{V}_E$ from ATPS to STPD. This is further compounded by a ±0.2 mmHg error in P_{H_2O} determination, resulting in an accumulated precision of $\pm0.1\%$ in the conversion of $\dot{V}_E$ from ATPS to STPD and hence $\dot{V}O_2$ determination (Sandals, 2003).

The sample volume removed for determination of gas fractions should be accurately determined. This is normally done by removing gas from the Douglas bag at a known flow rate. The accuracy of the flow rate may be checked by filling a bag with a known gas volume, and timing the emptying of the bag. Sandals (2003) has noted significant discrepancies in the actual flow rate and that at which flow controllers are set. Once flow rate is known, the precision of determination of sample volume has been shown to be ±0.007 l·min^{-1}. When this level of precision is considered for $\dot{V}O_2$ determination, a value for $\dot{V}O_2$ precision of $\pm0.11\%$ is calculated (Sandals, 2003).

Having considered factors that might influence the accuracy and precision of the determined volume of expirate, factors that influence the accuracy and precision of the gas fractions are now considered. Due to the influence of gas fraction determination on $\dot{V}O_2$ and $\dot{V}CO_2$, the importance of accurate and precise determination of expired fractions of oxygen (F_EO_2) and carbon dioxide (F_ECO_2) cannot be overemphasised. Table 11.1, produced by Sandals (2003), demonstrates just how influential errors in F_EO_2 and F_ECO_2 can be in the determination of $\dot{V}O_2$ and $\dot{V}CO_2$. For example, in the heavy exercise intensity

Table 11.1 Effect of a 1% increase in F_EO_2 and F_ECO_2 on the error incurred in the calculation of $\dot{V}O_2$ and $\dot{V}CO_2$ at three levels of exercise intensity

Exercise intensity	1% increase in F_EO_2		1% increase in F_ECO_2	
	% error in $\dot{V}O_2$	% error in $\dot{V}CO_2$	% error in $\dot{V}O_2$	% error in $\dot{V}CO_2$
Moderate	−3.07	0.00	−0.21	+1.01
Heavy	−4.61	0.00	−0.24	+1.01
Severe	−7.94	0.00	−0.30	+1.01

domain, a 1% overestimation for F_EO_2 converts to a 4.61% underestimation of $\dot{V}O_2$. This is because the F_EO_2 variable is used twice in the calculation of $\dot{V}O_2$ and the error incurred at the first stage of the calculation is in the same direction as that which is introduced at the second stage. In the calculation of $\dot{V}CO_2$ no variable is used twice so this amplification effect does not occur. However, since similar factors will influence the determination of $\dot{V}O_2$ and $\dot{V}CO_2$, errors in both calculations should be minimised.

A potential source of error that is often ignored is the contamination of expirate with any residual gas in the bag after evacuation. Whilst vacuum pumps are commonly employed to thoroughly evacuate Douglas bags, residual gas remains mainly in the non-compressible part of the bag (the neck) between the bag and the two-way valve. Minimising the volume of the 'neck' of the bag is an important part of minimising this potential error. However, it is also possible to quantify the volume of the 'neck' of the bags, and correct for the contamination effect of residual gas (Prieur *et al.*, 1998). A correction may be performed by knowing the volume and the concentration of the gas contained in the 'neck' of the bag following evacuation. Flushing the bags with room air of known concentration prior to evacuation allows for such a correction. If this procedure is followed, one may have increased confidence in measurement of the oxygen fraction (F_EO_2), and carbon dioxide fraction (F_ECO_2) in the expirate. Sandals (2003) has calculated that with such a correction the precision is ±0.031 l for the residual volume, which translates to ±0.05% for $\dot{V}O_2$ determination.

When using partial pressure analysers, water vapour partial pressure presents a gas fraction diluting effect, which may lead to a further source of error (Beaver, 1973; Norton and Wilmore, 1975). The water vapour is evident (as water droplets) as the expirate cools to room temperature in the bag. Partial pressure analysers are commonly used in off-line PGE systems, whereas on-line systems are increasingly incorporating mass spectrometry to determine gas fractions. Mass spectrometers are not influenced by water vapour partial pressure. When using partial pressure gas analysers, water vapour should be dealt with consistently when calibrating the analysers (when using dry bottled gases and moist air) and when analysing the expirate (when using saturated air). A possible approach is to first saturate all gas presented to the analysers using Nafian tubing (e.g. MH Series Humidier; Perma Pure Inc, New Jersey, USA) immersed in water, and then cool and dry the gas using a condenser (e.g. Buhler PKE3; Paterson Instruments, Leighton Buzzard, UK) to a consistent saturated water vapour pressure (e.g. 6.47 mmHg at 5.0°C; see Draper *et al.*, 2003). When adopting this approach, the calibration of the analysers and the resulting accuracy of the expired gas fraction measurement are improved.

A two-point calibration (zero and span) is commonly used for the O_2 and the CO_2 analyser. In each case, adjusting the zero setting is equivalent to altering the intercept of a linear function relating the analyser reading to the output from the sample cell, while adjusting the span is equivalent to altering the slope of this relationship. For both analysers, the zero setting is adjusted to ensure that the reading on the analyser is zero when gas from a cylinder of N_2 is passed through the analyser (the zero gas). For the O_2 analyser the span setting is adjusted to ensure that the reading on the analyser is 0.2095 when outside air is passed through the analyser. For the CO_2 analyser the span setting is adjusted to ensure that the reading on the analyser is the same as the gas fraction of a gravimetrically prepared cylinder (normally 0.0400 CO_2). Precise measurements of the atmospheric O_2 fraction since 1915 have been in the range of 0.20945–0.20952 (Machta and Hughes, 1970) and recent data suggest that a realistic current value for the CO_2 fraction would be ~0.00036 (Keeling *et al.*, 1995). It is not clear why the 0.2093 and 0.0003 values for F_IO_2 and F_ICO_2, respectively, have been so widely adopted in the physiological literature. However, it is plausible that they arose from Haldane's investigations of mine air at the start of the twentieth century and have been assumed to be constant over time (Haldane, 1912). The data from the meteorological literature show that the O_2 fraction in fresh outside (atmospheric) air is relatively constant, varying by ~0.00002 over a year (Keeling and Shertz, 1992). The precision of the gravimetrically prepared gas mixtures is reported to be within ±0.0001 of the actual nominal gas fraction (BOC Gases, New Jersey, USA). Taking the worst-case scenario, a precision of ±0.0001 for the measured expired gas fractions, translates into a precision of ±0.34% for $\dot{V}O_2$.

Table 11.2 presents an overview showing that after careful consideration of potential sources of error, and taking action to minimise each potential error, the degree of precision may be quantified. Sandals (2003) has calculated that when each source of uncertainty is combined in the calculation of $\dot{V}O_2$, an overall value for precision may be derived. Whilst we have presented precision for each potential source of error based on certain assumptions (e.g. heavy intensity exercise and 45 s collection of expirate), Sandals (2003)

Table 11.2 Effect of measurement precision on the determined $\dot{V}O_2$ for heavy intensity exercise with 45 s expirate collections

Measurement	Precision in $\dot{V}O_2$ (%)
Volume (with dry gas meter)	0.86
Ambient pressure (with barometer)	0.03
Expired gas temperature (with thermistor probe)	0.10
Sample volume (with flow controller)	0.11
Residual volume	0.05
Expired gas fractions (gas analysers)	0.34

Table 11.3 Total precision in the calculation of $\dot{V}O_2$ and $\dot{V}CO_2$ at three levels of exercise intensity and for four collection periods

Exercise intensity	Total % precision in $\dot{V}O_2$				Total % precision in $\dot{V}CO_2$			
	Collection period (s)				Collection period (s)			
	15	30	45	60	15	30	45	60
Moderate	6.0	3.3	2.4	2.0	6.2	3.5	2.6	2.1
Heavy	3.2	1.8	1.4	1.1	3.4	1.9	1.4	1.2
Severe	1.9	1.2	0.9	0.8	1.8	1.1	0.8	0.7

has determined overall precision for a range of assumptions (see Table 11.3). For the assumptions made earlier in this chapter, the overall precision of $\dot{V}O_2$ determination is calculated to be 1.4%. Of particular note is the finding that the degree of precision is increased as exercise intensity increases (for a given collection period) or the expirate collection duration increases (for a given exercise intensity).

BREATH-BY-BREATH METHOD

Although the Douglas bag method is still regarded by many as the 'gold standard' in the measurement of PGE, the requirement for collection of expired air over relatively lengthy periods (typically 30–60 s) essentially limits its use to steady-state exercise conditions. However, a great deal of important information concerning the integrated pulmonary–cardiovascular–muscle metabolic response to exercise can be gleaned under non-steady-state conditions. For example, the breath-by-breath measurement of PGE during ramp incremental exercise tests in which the external work rate is increased rapidly until the participant reaches exhaustion (typically in 10–12 min) permits not only the determination of the peak $\dot{V}O_2$, but also estimates of 'delta efficiency' (from the slope of the relationship between $\dot{V}O_2$ and work rate) and the lactate threshold (from the associated non-linear responses of $\dot{V}CO_2$ and $\dot{V}_E$) (Whipp *et al.*, 1981). These and other derived PGE variables are useful not only in the evaluation of exercise capacity in athletes and healthy volunteers but also in defining the physiological limitations to exercise performance in disease (Wasserman *et al.*, 1999). Furthermore, the breath-by-breath measurement of PGE in the abrupt transition from rest (or, more often, very light exercise) to a higher constant work rate can provide important information on the dynamic adjustment of oxidative metabolism following a 'step' increase in metabolic demand. The rate at which $\dot{V}O_2$ rises (i.e. the $\dot{V}O_2$ kinetics) during such exercise is another parameter of aerobic fitness, which is relevant both in health and disease and which can also be used to differentiate central versus peripheral limitations to exercise performance (Jones and Poole, 2005).

The principles of measuring PGE continuously (i.e. breath-by-breath) are essentially the same as those outlined earlier except that both flow and the concentration of the expirate are sampled continuously and the necessary calculations are performed 'on-line' by a microcomputer. Typically, commercial metabolic carts integrate a measurement of flow (by directing the expirate through a turbine or ultrasonic flowmeter) with a measurement of the gas concentration profiles (by directing samples of the expirate at the mouth into the gas analysers). One important consideration here is the accurate time-alignment of the gas concentration with the flow signals: the determination of the gas concentration will be delayed relative to that of flow owing to the transit time for the gas sampled at the mouth to arrive at the gas analysers and the subsequent response dynamics of those analysers. This delay is typically measured during the semi-automated calibration procedures of most commercially available systems and 'corrected' during subsequent exercise testing so that the concentration and flow signals measured at the mouth are appropriately aligned. However, greater care must be taken if exercise testing is to be conducted under conditions of hypoxia or hyperoxia because changes in gas viscosity will alter the transit time of the gas from the sample probe to the analysers.

The validity of PGE measurements with metabolic carts is ideally checked by simultaneous measurement of PGE using the Douglas bag technique (assuming that error in the latter is both known and minimised; see earlier). Ideally, PGE should be measured with both systems in the 'steady-state' over a wide range of exercise intensities (from rest to maximum) in a variety of subjects. A difference of less than approximately 5% in measurements of PGE and $\dot{V}_E$ is generally considered acceptable in such comparisons (Lamarra and Whipp, 1995). The accuracy of PGE and $\dot{V}_E$ measurement in the non-steady-state can be ascertained in a similar fashion by comparing the average values obtained by the two systems over the first 2 or 3 min following a step change in work rate. It is recommended that these checks be carried out at least every few weeks.

Despite careful attention to calibration and system maintenance, breath-by-breath PGE measurements are inherently 'noisy'; that is, there is considerable breath-to-breath variability in measures of PGE even in the steady-state. One solution to this is to average the PGE values over 10-s or 15-s periods, and this approach is very effective during incremental exercise tests and in situations where only steady-state PGE values are of interest. During exercise transients, however, such an approach is likely to obscure important events such as the Phase I–Phase II transition. Therefore, in the study of PGE kinetics, it is customary to reduce breath-to-breath noise by converting breath-by-breath values into second-by-second values and then averaging together an appropriate number of like-transitions. Just how many such transitions are required to sufficiently reduce breath-to-breath noise and increase confidence in the parameters derived from subsequent curve-fitting procedures depends on the extent of the noise (this can vary substantially from subject to subject), the amplitude of the PGE response above baseline (which will depend upon the imposed work rate and therefore, to some extent, the fitness of the subject), and the desired confidence level (Lamarra et al., 1987; Lamarra, 1990).

A portion of the breath-to-breath variability in PGE can be attributed to changes in the lung gas stores so that PGE measured at the mouth will not necessarily represent alveolar gas exchange for any given breath. This will be especially true during the first few seconds of a transition from a lower to a higher metabolic rate. Several algorithms have been developed to enable 'correction' of PGE measurements made at the mouth for changes in lung gas stores (Aunchincloss et al., 1966; Wessel et al., 1979; Beaver et al., 1981). Cautero et al. (2003) have recently suggested that the methods of Gronlund (1984), in which the respiratory cycle is defined as the time elapsing between two equal O_2 fractions in two subsequent breaths, are more appropriate for the determination of 'true' alveolar gas exchange. However, as recently summarised by Whipp et al. (2005), this approach presents as many problems as it solves.

CONCLUSIONS

The measurement and interpretation of the PGE response to exercise is an essential component of the physiological evaluation of subjects across the entire spectrum of fitness and physical activity (from elite athletes to patients with a variety of disease states). Determination of one or more of the parameters of aerobic fitness ($\dot{V}O_2$ peak, work efficiency, lactate/gas exchange threshold and gas exchange kinetics) is likely to be of value in work with sportspeople, except for those who participate exclusively in very short-duration (<60 s) sprint or power events. The same aerobic fitness parameters will determine tolerance to the activities of daily living in elderly and patient populations. However, the measurement of PGE is fraught with the potential for serious error, irrespective of whether 'off-line' or 'on-line' systems are used, and this can lead to flawed, and potentially dangerous, data interpretation. It is important, therefore, that investigators work diligently first to identify, and then to minimise, the errors associated with their measurement systems. PGE data can only be interpreted appropriately in the light of the known error margins.

REFERENCES

Atkinson, G., Davison, R.C.R. and Nevill, A.M. (2005). Performance characteristics of gas analysis systems: what we know and what we need to know. *International Journal of Sports Medicine*, 26 (suppl. 1): S2–S10.

Auchincloss, J.H., Gilbert, R. and Baule, G.H. (1966). Effect of ventilation on oxygen transfer during exercise. *Journal of Applied Physiology*, 21: 810.

Beaver, W.L. (1973). Water vapour corrections in oxygen consumption calculations. *Journal of Applied Physiology*, 35: 928–931.

Beaver, W.L., Lamarra, N. and Wasserman, K. (1981). Breath-by-breath measurement of true alveolar gas exchange. *Journal of Applied Physiology*, 51: 1662–1675.

Cautero, M., di Prampero, P.E. and Capelli, C. (2003). New acquisitions in the assessment of breath-by-breath alveolar gas transfer in humans. *European Journal of Applied Physiology*, 90: 231–241.

Cissik, J.H., Johnson, R.E. and Rokosch, D.K. (1972). Production of gaseous nitrogen in human steady-state conditions. *Journal of Applied Physiology*, 32: 155–159.

Draper, S., Wood, D.M. and Fallowfield, J.L. (2003). The $\dot{V}O_2$ response to exhaustive square wave exercise: influence of exercise intensity and the mode. *European Journal of Applied Physiology*, 90: 92–99.

Dudka, L.T., Inglis, H.J., Johnson, R.E., Pechinski, J.M. and Plowman, S. (1971). Inequality of inspired and expired gaseous nitrogen in man. *Nature*, 232: 265–268.

Gronlund, J. (1984). A new method for breath-to-breath determination of oxygen flux across the alveolar membrane. *European Journal of Applied Physiology and Occupational Physiology*, 52: 167–172.

Haldane, J.S. (1912). *Methods of Air Analysis*. London, Griffin and Co.

Hart, J.D. and Withers, R.T. (1996). The calibration of gas volume measuring devices at continuous and pulsatile flows. *Australian Journal of Science and Medicine in Sport*, 28: 61–65.

Jones, A.M. and Poole, D.C. (eds). (2005). Oxygen Uptake Kinetics in Sport, Exercise and Medicine, London and New York: Routledge.

Keeling, C.D., Whorf, T.P., Wahlen, M. and van der Plicht, J. (1995). Interannual extremes in the rate of rise of atmospheric carbon dioxide since 1980. *Nature*, 375: 666–670.

Keeling, R.F. and Shertz, S.R. (1992). Seasonal and interannual variations in atmospheric oxygen and implications for the global carbon cycle. *Nature*, 358: 723–727.

Lamarra, N. (1990). Variables, constants and parameters: clarifying the system structure, *Medicine and Science in Sports and Exercise*, 22: 88–95.

Lamarra, N. and Whipp, B.J. (1995). Measurement of pulmonary gas exchange, in P.J. Maud, and C. Foster (eds). *The Physiological Assessment of Human Fitness*, Champaign, IL: Human Kinetics, pp. 19–35.

Lamarra, N., Whipp, B.J., Ward, S.A. and Wasserman, K. (1987). Effect of interbreath fluctuations on characterizing exercise gas exchange kinetics. *Journal of Applied Physiology*, 62: 2003–2012.

Machta, L. and Hughes, E. (1970). Atmospheric oxygen in 1967 and 1970. *Science*, 168: 1582–1584.

Norton, A.C. and Wilmore, J.H. (1975). Effects of water vapour on respiratory gas measurements and calculations. *The NSCPT Analyser*, 9: 6–9.

Prieur, F., Busso, T., Castells, J., Bonnefoy, R., Bennoit, H., Geyssant, A. and Denis, C. (1998). Validity of oxygen uptake measurements during exercise under moderate hyperoxia. *Medicine and Science in Sports and Exercise*, 30: 958–962.

Sandals, L.E. (2003). Oxygen uptake during middle-distance running. Unpublished PhD thesis, University of Gloucestershire.

Wasserman, K., Hansen, J.E., Sue, D.Y., Casaburi, R. and Whipp, B.J. (1999). *Principles of Exercise Testing and Interpretation. Maryland*, 3rd edn. USA: Lippincott, Williams and Wilkins.

Wessel, H.U., Stout, R.L., Bastanier, C.K. and Paul, M.H. (1979). Breath-by-breath variation of FRC: effect on VO$_2$ and VCO$_2$ measured at the mouth. *Journal of Applied Physiology*, 46: 1122–1126.

Whipp, B.J., Davis, J.A., Torres, F. and Wasserman, K. (1981). A test to determine parameters of aerobic function during exercise. *Journal of Applied Physiology*, 50: 217–221.

Whipp, B.J., Ward, S.A. and Rossiter, H.B. (2005). Pulmonary O$_2$ uptake during exercise: conflating muscular and cardiovascular responses. *Medicine and Science in Sports and Exercise*, 37: 1574–1585.

Wilmore, J.H. and Costill, D.L. (1973). Adequacy of the Haldane transformation in the computation of exercise $\dot{V}O_2$ in man. *Journal of Applied Physiology*, 35: 85–89.

WMO: World Meteorological Organisation. (1996). Guide to meteorological instruments and methods of observation. *WMO Publication*, 8: 1–21.

CHAPTER 12

LACTATE TESTING

Neil Spurway and Andrew M. Jones

THEORETICAL BACKGROUND

Lactate production by muscle during sub-maximal exercise was traditionally ascribed to a shortfall in oxygen supply, forcing vigorously active muscles to resort in part to anaerobic metabolism for their ATP requirements. However, work in the past 15–20 years (review: Spurway, 1992) has shown that fully aerobic muscle produces lactate when operating above ~50% maximal work rates. Connett *et al.* (1990) propose that this lactate production may be explained by three steps:

1   NADH builds up in mitochondria to drive their electron transport chains faster;
2   in turn, this build-up is reflected in the cytoplasmic NADH pool;
3   elevated cytoplasmic NADH increases the rate of reduction of pyruvate to lactate.

Other suggestions about the mechanism have been made, particularly in terms of changes in the activity of pyruvate dehydrogenase. On all accounts, however, the muscle's ATP production remains essentially the result of *aerobic* glycolysis, so the old concept of a major resort to anaerobic metabolism must be dropped. Even on a conservative view, therefore, the lactate production must be considered to represent an upper bound estimate of the total anaerobic activity, and it is almost certainly a very considerable over-estimate.

Nevertheless, increases in muscle oxidative capacity as a result of training diminish the need for NADH build-up to drive electron transport, and so result in reduced lactate production at any given work rate (Holloszy and Coyle, 1984; Jones and Carter, 2000). Thus in qualitative terms, *though not in quantitative ones*, the consequence for muscle lactate production on the new account remains much as the traditional concept would have predicted.

During exercise there is not a one-to-one relationship between lactate in muscle and lactate in blood, but lactate concentration ([lactate]) in the blood does give an indirect yet reproducible indication of the aerobic capacity of the working muscles. Lactate accumulation curves can therefore be used to assess changes in aerobic fitness and (by empirical rule of thumb) as guides to training intensity. The tests have obvious relevance for endurance athletes, but are also appropriate on the same sort of rule-of-thumb basis for players of multiple sprint games, who need to remove lactate quickly during recovery periods and even during support running.

GENERAL NOTES ON LACTATE METHODOLOGY

When assessing any individual there is a need for careful standardisation of repeat tests (exercise protocol and procedures for lactate sampling and assay). Capillary sampling from fingertips is generally utilised for safety and ease, but earlobe sampling is preferred by some laboratories, and is especially useful where the hands are in use, as on rowing, canoeing, skiing or arm crank ergometers. However, it should be noted that differences in blood [lactate] do occur according to the form of blood used (venous vs. arterial vs. capillary), the site of sampling and the post-sampling treatment and assay method. Likewise, there are substantial differences between plasma, whole blood and lysed blood. The most crucial practical implication of these differences is that any longitudinal study of a single athlete must adopt rigorously identical procedures for every sample. Other implications are in extrapolating any laboratory results to the field where different methods may be used, in the interpolation of performance at various blood lactate reference values, and in making comparisons between data from different laboratories and different individuals. In any case, calibration of lactate analysers and checking with standards of known concentration are essential and, when reporting results, details of the methodology used must be included.

TERMINOLOGY

Blood lactate concentrations are typically found to be significantly higher than resting values at work rates of 55–70% VO_{2max}. At higher work rates than these, blood concentrations are greater still. The work rate above which the blood [lactate] consistently exceeds the resting or baseline value (~ 1 mmol$\cdot$l^{-1}) has been given various names, including *Lactate Threshold* and *Anaerobic Threshold*. The latter term embodies an implicit assumption, namely the historical view that blood lactate accumulation reflected lactate production by the muscles resorting to anaerobic metabolism in conditions of hypoxia. As it is now recognised that fully aerobic muscles can produce lactate (see *Theoretical background*), the term Anaerobic Threshold is misleading. By contrast, the designation Lactate Threshold (LT) embodies no such assumptions, and simply represents what is observed; its use is therefore recommended. A blood [lactate] of 2 mmol·l^{-1} is accepted in some laboratories as a rough guide to the location of LT, but direct identification of the first 'break-point' on a blood lactate accumulation curve is greatly preferable (Figure 12.1).

A further frequently encountered term is *Onset of Blood Lactate Accumulation (OBLA)*. Though sometimes confused with LT, OBLA was initially approximated by the substantially higher reference value, 4 mmol·l^{-1}, and so was clearly not intended to represent the same functional intensity. Leading laboratories now note that, when blood [lactate] measured at the end of a 3–4 min exercise period is somewhere in the vicinity of 4 mmol·l^{-1}, it will not stay steady at that level but will *rise continually over time thereafter*. Thus it might reach 6 mmol·l^{-1} after 30 min *at the same work rate*. By contrast, a value of 2.5 mmol·l^{-1} at 4 min will typically fall to 2 or 1.5 mmol·l^{-1} if the same work rate is maintained for 30 min. 'OBLA' is thus intended to represent the minimum work rate at which a rise, rather than a fall, occurs over this kind of timescale. It will be evident that exactly defining this in practice is not easy.

The dynamics of blood lactate accumulation during constant-work-rate exercise are perhaps better embodied in the *Maximal Lactate Steady State (MLSS)* concept. The MLSS may be determined from 4 to 5 exercise bouts, each of up to 30 min duration and performed on separate days, with blood [lactate] determined at rest and after every subsequent 5 min of exercise (Figure 12.2). MLSS is defined as the highest work rate (or speed of running, etc.) at which blood [lactate] is elevated above baseline but is stable over time; in theoretical terms, therefore, it can be regarded as being infinitesimally lower than OBLA. In practice the MLSS is considered to have been exceeded when the increase in blood [lactate] between 10 and 30 min of exercise is greater than 1.0 mmol·l^{-1}. The assessment of MLSS is both time- and labour-intensive and, while remaining the 'gold standard', the MLSS is rarely directly measured but is often

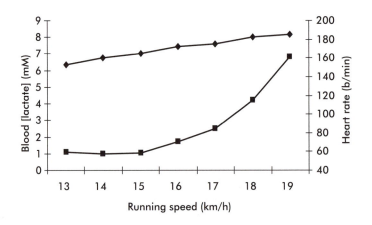

Figure 12.1 Typical blood lactate (closed squares) and heart rate (closed diamonds) responses to a multi-stage incremental treadmill test in an endurance athlete. In this example, the LT occurs at 15 km·h^{-1} while the LTP occurs at 17 km·h^{-1}

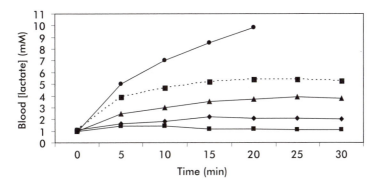

Figure 12.2 Determination of the running speed at the MLSS in an endurance athlete (the same as in Figure 12.1). This athlete completed five treadmill runs of up to 30 min duration at different running speeds (14, 15, 16, 17 and 18 km·h^{-1}) on different days. At 14 and 15 km·h^{-1}, blood [lactate] did not increase appreciably above that measured at rest; at 16 and 17 km·h^{-1}, blood [lactate] reached a delayed but elevated steady-state; and at 18 km·h^{-1}, blood [lactate] did not attain a steady state but increased inexorably until the athlete became exhausted. The running speed at the MLSS is therefore 17 km·h^{-1}

estimated using a variety of more practicable methods (Jones and Doust, 2001). Recent studies indicate that the work rate or speed at the *Lactate Turnpoint* (LTP), a second 'sudden and sustained' increase in blood [lactate] during incremental exercise (Figure 12.1), provides a good approximation of the work rate or speed at the MLSS (Smith and Jones, 2001; Pringle and Jones, 2002). Note, however, that the blood [lactate] measured at the LTP (~3 mmol·l^{-1}) will typically under-estimate the blood [lactate] at the MLSS (~4–6 mmol·l^{-1}).

A new term *Lactate Minimum Running Speed* (and hence by extrapolation to other sports, *Lactate Minimum Work Rate*), was introduced by Tegtbur *et al.* (1993). Though originally presented in a manner strongly suggestive of MLSS, the lactate minimum work rate has since been found to depend critically upon the test protocol and, as defined by certain interpretations of the original procedure, to relate more closely to LT than to MLSS. Since no approach to consensus has yet been reached, procedural details are not presented here.

DETERMINATION OF LT, LTP AND BLOOD LACTATE REFERENCE VALUES

The general procedures for an incremental protocol permitting the assessment of LT, LTP and various blood lactate reference values are described later. The reasons for selecting this protocol are three-fold: first, only 5–8 blood samples are usually required; second, it takes a minimum amount of time; and, finally, each exercise stage is sufficiently long for measurements of 'steady-state' oxygen uptake (VO$_2$) and heart rate (HR) to be made, so that exercise economy can be evaluated and training can be prescribed. This also enables the LT (for example) to be described as a metabolic rate (i.e. units of VO$_2$), which is technically correct. However, in situations where the relationship between blood [lactate] and work rate or exercise speed are not relevant, such as in patient populations, the LT can be conveniently determined (or estimated using non-invasive gas exchange procedures) to a close approximation with fast, non-steady-state, incremental protocols (Wasserman *et al.*, 1994). One other advantage to the protocol described later is that, if the test is continued to exhaustion, the measured peak VO_2 provides a close approximation of the VO_2 max (to within ~5%).

Protocol

The individual should report to the laboratory rested (i.e. having performed no strenuous exercise in the preceding 24–48 h), euhydrated and at least 3 h following the consumption of a light carbohydrate-based meal. No warm-up other than stretching is needed, as the initial exercise intensity should require no more than about 40% VO_{2max}. However, some individuals will prefer to complete 5–10 min of light exercise in preparation for the test, and this is strongly recommended for people with limited experience on the test ergometer. In this period, the test procedures along with safety considerations can be emphasised.

The protocol consists of exercising on an ergometer (treadmill, cycle, rowing, etc.), with the intensity (work rate, running speed, etc.) being increased every 4 min until the individual approaches or attains volitional exhaustion. Individual investigators may have a personal preference for the use of continuous or discontinuous protocols, although short breaks in exercise to facilitate 'clean' blood sampling do not seem to have a major influence on the derived blood lactate accumulation curve (Gullstrand *et al.*, 1994). [Lactate] is measured in blood samples obtained at the end of each 4-min stage for the subsequent determination of the work rate or exercise speed equivalent to LT, LTP and appropriate blood lactate reference concentrations (e.g. 2, 3, 4 mmol·l^{-1}). For children between 11 and 15 years and for well-trained athletes in whom a steady-state is reached more rapidly, exercise stages of 3-min duration are recommended. It is important that the exercise intensity selected for the first exercise stage is sufficiently low that it does not cause blood [lactate] to be appreciably elevated above the resting value; one should therefore 'err on the side of caution' in selecting this first intensity. The increment in exercise intensity between stages should be selected to allow the completion of a minimum of 5 and a maximum of 9 stages, with the number of stages being determined largely by the precision required in the determination of LT, LTP and the fixed blood lactate reference values. For example, in treadmill tests the increment will typically lie between 0.5 and 1.5 km·h^{-1} and in cycle or rowing ergometer tests the increment will typically lie between 20 and 50 W.

Expired air may be analysed continuously using an on-line system, or collected in Douglas bags between minutes 3–4, 7–8, 11–12, etc. for normal healthy adults, and between minutes 2–3, 5–6, 8–9 and 11–12 for children and trained athletes. The HR should be recorded during the final minute of each stage.

Blood sampling

Samples of capillary blood are obtained at rest – more than 2 h after previous exercise – and immediately after each 4-min stage; that is to say, after the cardio-respiratory measurements, but before the exercise intensity is increased. Blood sampling procedures should adhere to the appropriate health and safety guidelines (see Chapter 3).

Treatment of the blood lactate data

A graph of exercise intensity against blood [lactate] should be constructed. From this, the LT and LTP can be determined and/or the exercise intensities equivalent to appropriate blood lactate reference values can be interpolated. Plotting the HR response to the incremental test on a second y-axis enables the HR at the various 'thresholds' to be easily determined (Figure 12.1) and possibly used in the prescription of appropriate training intensities. Finally, it can also be useful to plot blood [lactate] against the relative exercise intensity (as $\%VO_{2max}$).

Reliability and sensitivity

Test-retest comparisons of ± 0.2 mmol·l^{-1} (i.e. error of $< \pm 10\%$) are generally considered to be acceptable in the assessment of blood [lactate] at a specific absolute work rate or exercise speed. The various lactate 'thresholds' are known to be very sensitive to improvements in aerobic capacity resulting, in particular, from endurance exercise training. A 'rightward shift' in the blood lactate curve when plotted against exercise intensity (along with a corresponding rightward shift in the HR response to exercise) is the expected outcome when an individual is re-tested following the commencement or continuation of an endurance training programme. In well-trained athletes, changes in the sub-maximal blood [lactate] profile can occur in the absence of any change in VO_{2max}. However, it is important to remember that the absolute blood [lactate] is also sensitive to factors such as muscle glycogen depletion and various dietary interventions, so that care should be taken to ensure that tests are carried out under standardised conditions (both laboratory- and individual-specific).

A NOTE ON THE ASSESSMENT OF BLOOD [LACTATE] FOLLOWING MAXIMAL-INTENSITY EXERCISE

Although this chapter has focused on the use of blood [lactate] measurement in the assessment of sub-maximal exercise performance, it should be noted that such measurements can also be valuable in other contexts. For example, the

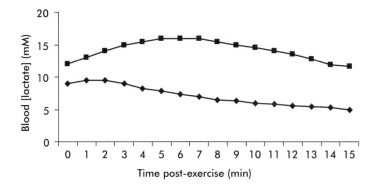

Figure 12.3 Schematic illustration of the response of blood [lactate] in the first 15 min of recovery from exhaustive high-intensity exercise in an endurance-trained athlete (closed diamonds) and a sprint-trained athlete (closed squares). Note that the peak blood [lactate] is higher and occurs later in recovery in the sprint-trained athlete

peak blood [lactate] measured in the recovery period following a bout or bouts of maximal-intensity exercise could be considered to provide a crude estimate of the extent to which energy has been supplied through anaerobic glycolysis. Strictly, it remains an upper bound figure, because a component of the lactate production remains aerobic as it is at work rates just above LT, but all the power output additional to that achieved at VO_{2max} has, of course, no alternative source of energy than anaerobic glycolysis, and this is likely to be the majority lactate source in a subject working at maximal intensity. In support of this general concept, sprint-trained athletes almost invariably demonstrate higher peak blood [lactate] values than their endurance-trained counterparts (Figure 12.3). Interestingly, the time at which the peak blood [lactate] is attained during the recovery period also differs between sprint and endurance athletes (being later in the sprint-trained) so that frequent blood samples are necessary if the peak value is to be accurately determined. Finally, whether one is considering maximal or sub-maximal exercise, it should be remembered that the blood [lactate] measured at any moment represents a conflation of the rate of lactate production in the active muscles, the rate of efflux of lactate from muscle to blood, and the rate at which lactate is cleared from the blood by muscle and other (chiefly visceral) organs (Brooks, 1991). Thus if subject A shows a lower blood [lactate] than subject B in a given test, A's muscles may be releasing less lactate in unit time than B's, *or* A's clearance mechanisms may be more active. In fact, both changes are likely consequences of aerobic training, but blood [lactate] measurements can provide no estimate of the balance between them.

REFERENCES

Brooks, G.A. (1991). Current concepts in lactate exchange. *Medicine and Science in Sports and Exercise*, 23: 895–906.

Connett, R.J., Honig, C.R., Gayeski, T.E.J. and Brooks, G.A. (1990). Defining hypoxia: a systems view of VO$_2$, glycolysis energetics and intracellular PO$_2$. *Journal of Applied Physiology*, 68: 833–842.

Gullstrand, L., Sjodin, B. and Svedenhag, J. (1994). Blood sampling during continuous running and 30-second intervals on a treadmill: effects on the lactate threshold results? *Scandinavian Journal of Medicine and Science in Sports*, 4: 239–242.

Holloszy, J.O. and Coyle, E.F. (1984). Adaptations of skeletal muscle to endurance exercise and their metabolic consequences. *Journal of Applied Physiology*, 56: 831–838.

Jones, A.M. and Carter, H. (2000). The effect of endurance training on parameters of aerobic fitness. *Sports Medicine*, 29: 373–386.

Jones, A.M. and Doust, J.H. (2001). Limitations to submaximal exercise performance. In R.G. Eston and T.P. Reilly (eds). *Exercise and Laboratory Test Manual*, 235–262, 2nd edn. E & FN Spon.

Pringle, J.S. and Jones, A.M. (2002). Maximal lactate steady state, critical power and EMG during cycling. *European Journal of Applied Physiology*, 88: 214–226.

Smith, C.G. and Jones, A.M. (2001). The relationship between critical velocity, maximal lactate steady-state velocity and lactate turnpoint velocity in runners. *European Journal of Applied Physiology*, 85: 19–26.

Spurway, N.C. (1992). Aerobic exercise, anaerobic exercise and the lactate threshold. *British Medical Bulletin*, 48: 569–591.

Tegtbur, U., Busse, M.W. and Braumann, K.M. (1993). Estimation of individual equilibrium between lactate production and catabolism during exercise. *Medicine and Science in Sports and Exercise*, 24: 620–627.

Wasserman, K., Hansen, J.E., Sue, D.Y., Whipp, B.J. and Casaburi, R. (1994). *Principles of Exercise Testing and Interpretation*, Philadelphia, PA: Lea & Febiger.

CHAPTER 13

RATINGS OF PERCEIVED EXERTION

John Buckley and Roger Eston

INTRODUCTION

Following two decades of research, Gunnar Borg's original rating of perceived exertion (RPE) scale was accepted in 1973 as a valid tool within the field of exercise science and sports medicine (Noble and Robertson, 1996). His seminal research provided the basic tool for numerous studies in which an individual's effort perception was of interest. It also provided the basis and incentive for the development of other scales, particularly those used with children. Borg's initial research validated the scale against heart rate and oxygen uptake. Later research focussed on the curvilinear growth of perceived exertion with lactate, ventilation and muscle pain responses, and led to the development of the category-ratio (CR-10) scale.

The general aim of using RPE is to quantify an individual's subjective perception of exertion as a means of determining the exercise intensity or regulating exercise intensity (Borg, 1998). In this way it acts as a surrogate or concurrent marker to key relative physiological responses including: percentage of maximal heart rate (%HRmax), percentage of maximal oxygen uptake (%VO_{2max}) and blood lactate. The strongest stimuli influencing an individual's RPE are breathing/ventilatory work and sensations of strain from the muscles (Cafarelli, 1977, 1982; Chen *et al.*, 2002). Other correlates include perceptions of limb speed, body temperature and joint strain (Robertson and Noble, 1997). A common misunderstanding is to assume that changes in heart rate, oxygen uptake and blood lactate, are factors, which influence RPE. However, one does not actually perceive heart rate, oxygen uptake or the accumulation of muscle and blood lactate. It is the sensations associated with increased ventilatory work and muscle and joint strains, which correspond with these physiological markers, that an individual perceives.

MODES OF USING THE RPE

Traditionally, RPE was developed as a dependent response variable to a given exercise intensity known as *estimation mode* (Noble and Robertson, 1996). Smutok *et al.* (1980) were one of the first to evaluate RPE as an independent exercise intensity regulator. They asked participants to adjust their treadmill running speeds to elicit a given RPE. This is known as *production mode*. This study also raised concern about the ability of some individuals to repeat the same heart rate and running speed for the same RPE, when RPE was used in production mode. From a practitioner's perspective, it is important to confirm that an individual can reliably elicit a given RPE for a given exercise intensity (heart rate or work rate) before being requested or directed to use RPE as a sole intensity regulator.

In this regard, one should not assume that exercise intensity measures derived from estimation–production paradigms are the same; they involve passive and active information processing procedures, respectively. In the *estimation–production* paradigm, objective intensity measures (*expected or derived*) from a previous estimation trial are compared to values produced during a subsequent exercise trial(s) in which the participant *actively* self-regulates exercise intensity levels using assigned RPEs. The memory of exercise experience is particularly relevant in the active paradigm. Following an exercise situation, memory will degrade and may impact upon future active productions. In comparison, the passive paradigm is based upon the interpretation of current stimulation. This information may then be used to compare responses between conditions after some form of intervention or to assist in the prescription of exercise intensity. These considerations are vital when RPE is used in clinical or older populations.

RPE AND RELATIVE MEASURES OF EXERCISE INTENSITY

Table 13.1 summarises the relationship between RPE scores and related physiological markers. During exercise testing or training, the robust relationship between RPE and objective physiological markers may allow the investigator to estimate the participant's relative exercise intensity. For example, once

Table 13.1   Summary of the relationship between the percentages of maximal aerobic power ($\%VO_{2max}$), maximal heart rate reserve ($\%HRR_{max}$), maximal heart rate ($\%HR_{max}$) and Borg's rating of perceived exertion (RPE)

$\%VO_{2max}$	<20	20–39	**40–59**	**60–84**	≥85	100
$\%HRR_{max}$	<20	20–39	**40–59**	**60–84**	≥85	100
$\%HR_{max}$	<35	**35–54**	**55–69**	**70–89**	≥90	100
RPE	<10	10–11	**12–13**	**14–16**	17–19	19–20

Source: adapted from ACSM, 2005; Noble and Robertson, 1996; Pollock *et al.*, 1978

an individual has given an RPE greater than 16 on the RPE scale, or 6–7 on the CR-10 scale, it is highly probable that he/she has surpassed the level where lactate levels may lead to muscular fatigue and accelerated ventilation. This allows the investigator to prepare for test termination. Eston *et al.* (2005) have demonstrated the ability to predict VO_{2max} from a perceptually–guided submaximal exercise test using RPE as the independent variable (production mode). They observed that VO_{2max} values predicted from a series of submaximal RPE: VO_2 values in the range RPE 9–15 and RPE 9–17 were remarkably similar, and within (bias $\pm$ 1.96 $\times$ SDdiff) 2 $\pm$ 8 and $-1. \pm 6$ ml·kg^{-1}·min^{-1}, respectively.

Inspection of the values within Table 13.1 indicates that there is a range of up to 20% of any relative physiological measure for a given RPE. This can be largely attributed to two factors: (1) the subjective nature of rating perceived levels of exertion, and (2) inter-individual differences in training status (Berry *et al.*, 1989; Boutcher *et al.*, 1989; Brisswalter and Delignierè, 1997). Thus, physical training is characterised by a reduction in RPE for a given percentage of maximal HR or VO_{2max}.

FACTORS INFLUENCING RPE

During exercise testing, the inter-trial agreement of either RPE or a concurrent physiological response at a given RPE, increases with each use of the RPE scale (Buckley *et al.*, 2000, 2004; Eston *et al.*, 2000, 2005). Typically, the agreement is shown to be acceptable within three trials when the participant is exposed to a variety of exercise intensities.

Psychosocial factors can influence up to 30% of the variability in an RPE score (Dishman and Landy, 1988; Williams and Eston, 1989). Furthermore the literature has identified numerous modulators of RPE including: the mode of exercise, age, audio-visual distractions, circadian rhythms, gender, haematological and nutritional status, medication, muscle mechanics and biochemical status, the physical environment, and the psycho-social status or competitive milieu of the testing and training environment. These factors are exemplified in Borg's effort continua proposed in 1973 (Borg, 1998). Beta-blocking medication exerts an influence during extended periods of exercise and at intensities greater than 65% VO_{2max} (Eston and Connolly, 1996; Head *et al.*, 1997).

In healthy or clinical populations that may be fearful of the exercise-testing environment (e.g. cardiac patients), it is likely that they will inflate RPE (Morgan, 1973, 1994; Rejeski, 1981; Kohl and Shea, 1988; Biddle and Mutrie, 2001). Such inflation of RPE relates to individuals who either lack self-efficacy or who are unfamiliar or inhibited by the social situation of the exercise training or testing environment.

RPE AND STRENGTH/POWER TESTING AND TRAINING

Up until the late 1990s, most of the evidence in RPE focussed on application and research with aerobic type exercise. There is now a growing body of evidence in the use of monitoring somatic responses to local muscle sensations during resistive or strength training exercise (Borg, 1998; Gearhart *et al.*, 2002; Pincivero *et al.*, 2003; Lagally and Costigan, 2004). The important aspect to consider is that during short-term high-intensity exercise for a localised muscle group, where 8 to 15 repetitions are performed, RPE will grow by one point on the RPE or CR-10 for every 3 to 4 repetitions. For example if after 12 repetitions, one wishes to end his/her last repetition at an RPE of 15 or a CR-10 scale rating of 5 (hard, heavy), then the first or second repetition should elicit an RPE of ~12 or a CR-10 rating of 2 (between light and somewhat hard).

Which scale should I use?

In both Borg's RPE and CR-10 scale, the semantic verbal anchors and their corresponding numbers have been aligned to accommodate for the curvilinear nature (a power function between 1.6 and 2.0) of human physiological responses (Borg, 1998). The CR-10 scale, with its ratio or semi-ratio properties was specifically designed with this in mind. The RPE 6–20 scale was originally designed for whole body aerobic type activity where perceived responses are pooled to concur with the linear increments in heart rate and oxygen uptake, as exercise intensity is increased. The CR-10 scale is best suited when there is an overriding sensation arising either from a specific area of the body, for example, muscle pain, ache or fatigue in the quadriceps or from pulmonary responses. Examples of this individualised or differentiated response have been applied in patients with McArdle's disease (Buckley *et al.*, 2003) and chronic obstructive pulmonary disease (O'Donnell *et al.*, 2004).

PERCEIVED EXERTION IN CHILDREN

Simplified numerical and pictorial scales

There have been important advances in the study of effort perception in children in the last 15 years. The topic has been the subject of several critical reviews with the most recent being (Eston and Lamb, 2000; Eston and Parfitt, 2006). The idea for a simplified perceived exertion scale, which would be more suitable for use with children emanated from the study by Williams *et al.* (1991). They first proposed the idea for a 1–10 scale anchored with more developmentally appropriate expressions of effort. This led to a significant development in the measurement of children's effort perception in 1994 with the publication of two papers (Eston *et al.*, 1994; Williams *et al.*, 1994), which proposed and validated an alternative child-specific rating scale – the Children's Effort Rating Table (CERT, Figure 13.1, Williams *et al.*, 1994).

Compared to the Borg Scale, the CERT has five fewer possible responses, a range of numbers (1–10) more familiar to children than the Borg 6–20 Scale and verbal expressions chosen by children as descriptors of exercise effort. This type of scale facilitates the child's perceptual understanding and therefore the

1 Very, very easy
2 Very easy
3 Easy
4 Just feeling a strain
5 Starting to get hard
6 Getting quite hard
7 Hard
8 Very hard
9 Very, very hard
10 So hard I'm going to stop

Figure 13.1   The Children's Effort Rating Table (CERT, Williams *et al.*, 1994)

ability to use it in either a passive or active paradigm with greater reliability. The CERT initiative for a simplified scale containing more 'developmentally appropriate' numerical and verbal expressions, led to the development of scales which combined numerical and pictorial ratings of perceived exertion scales. All of these scales depict four to five animated figures, portraying increased states of physical exertion. Like the CERT, the scales have embraced a similar, condensed numerical range and words or expressions which are either identical to the CERT (PCERT, Yelling *et al.*, 2002), abridged from the CERT (CALER, Eston *et al.*, 2000; Eston *et al.*, 2001) or similar in context to the CERT (OMNI, Robertson, 1997; Robertson *et al.*, 2000).

The Pictorial CERT (PCERT), initially described by Eston and Lamb (2000), has been validated for both effort estimation and effort production tasks during stepping exercise in adolescents (Yelling *et al.*, 2002). The scale depicts a child running up a 45° stepped grade at five stages of exertion, corresponding to CERT ratings of 2, 4, 6, 8 and 10. All the verbal descriptors from the original CERT are included in the scale.

The OMNI Scale has various pictorial forms. It has been validated for cycling (Robertson *et al.*, 2000), walking/running (Utter *et al.*, 2002) and stepping (Robertson *et al.*, 2005). Robertson and colleagues have also proposed 'adult' versions of the OMNI Scale for resistance exercise and cycling, although we are doubtful of the need to develop such pictorial scales for normal adults, given the well-established validity of the Borg 6–20 RPE and CR-10 Scales. The original idea behind the development of pictorial scales was to simplify the cognitive demands placed on the child. This does not seem necessary in normal adults.

Roemmich *et al.* (2006) have recently validated the OMNI and PCERT scales for submaximal exercise in children aged 11–12 years. They observed no difference in the slopes of the PCERT and OMNI scores when regressed against heart rate or VO_2. There was also no difference in the percentage of maximal PCERT and OMNI at each exercise stage. In effect, the results showed that the two scales could be used with equal validity. Although pictorially different, their results are not that surprising since the scales utilise basically the same limited number range. It perhaps questions the need for pictorial scales for children of this age range.

All the pictorial scales developed so far to assess the relationship between perceived exertion and exercise intensity in children have used either a horizontal line or one that has a linear slope. Eston and Parfitt (2006) have proposed a pic-torial 0–10 curvilinear scale which is founded on its inherently obvious face validity. As noted previously (Eston and Lamb, 2000), it is readily conceivable that a child will recognise from previous learning and experience that the steeper the hill, the harder it is to ascend.

FACTORS AFFECTING RPE IN CHILDREN

A discussion of the factors affecting RPE in children is provided in more detail by Eston and Parfitt (2006). The following identifies the key considerations in this group.

As indicated earlier, young children's ability to utilise traditional rating scales is affected by their numerical and verbal understanding. Pictorial scales with a narrower numerical range and fewer verbal references simplify the con-ceptual demands made on the child. An active paradigm places greater demands upon memory of exercise experience in order to generate a specific intensity in comparison to the passive paradigm that requires an instant response to the current exercise stimulation. Following an exercise situation, memory will degrade and be affected by a combination of factors associated with the three effort continua, particularly the interaction of perceptual and performance variables. This will impact upon future active productions and is an important consideration given the limited memory and range of experience in young children. As in adults, the accuracy of children's effort perception increases significantly with practice (Eston *et al.*, 2000).

The perceived effort response varies according to whether the exercise protocol is intermittent or continuous. The perceived exertion response appears to be higher in a continuous protocol. Intermittent protocols are therefore preferred with young children (Lamb *et al.*, 1997).

KEY POINTS FOR THE EFFECTIVE USE OF RPE IN ADULTS AND CHILDREN

In considering the factors described throughout this chapter, the following points for instructing participants, patients and athletes have been recommended (adapted from Maresh and Noble, 1984; Borg, 1998, 2004).

1   Make sure the participant understands what an RPE is. Before using the scale see if they can grasp the concept of sensing the exercise responses (breathing, muscle movement/strain, joint movement/speed).
2   Anchoring the perceptual range, which includes relating to the fact that no exertion at all is sitting still and maximal exertion is a theoretical con-cept of pushing the body to its absolute physical limits. Participants should then be exposed to differing levels of exercise intensity (as in an incremental test or during an exercise session) so as to understand to what

the various levels on the scale feel like. Just giving them one or two points on the scale to aim for will probably result in a great deal of variability.

3   Use the earlier points to explain the nature of the scale and that the participant should consider both the verbal descriptor and the numerical value. The participant should first concentrate on the sensations arising from the activity, look at the scale to see which verbal descriptor relates to the effort he/she is experiencing and then linking this to the corresponding numerical value.

4   Unless specifically directed, ensure that the participant focuses on all the different sensations arising from the exercise being performed. For aerobic exercise, the participant should pool all sensations to give one rating. If there is an overriding sensation then additionally make note of this differentiated rating. Differentiated ratings can be used during muscular strength activity or where exercise is limited more by breathlessness or leg pain, as in the case of pulmonary or peripheral vascular disease, respectively.

5   Confirm that there is no right or wrong answer and it is what the participant perceives. There are three important cases where the participant may give an incorrect rating:

(a)   When there is a preconceived idea about what exertion level is elicited by a specific activity (Borg, 1998).

(b)   When participants are asked to recall the exercise and give a rating. As with heart rate, RPEs should be taken while the participant is actually engaged in the movements; not after they have finished an activity.

(c)   When participants attempt to please the practitioner by stating what should be the appropriate level of RPE. This is typically the case when participants are advised ahead of time of the target RPE (e.g. in education sessions or during the warm-up). In the early stages of using RPE, the participant's exercise intensity should be set by heart rate or work rate (e.g. in METs) and participants need to reliably learn to match their RPE to this level in estimation mode. Once it has been established that the participant's rating concurs with the target heart rate or MET level reliably, then moving them on to production mode can be considered.

6   Keep RPE scales in full view at all times (e.g. on each machine or station or in fixed view in the exercise testing room) and keep reminding participants throughout their exercise session or test to think about what sort of sensations they have while making their judgement rating. Elite endurance athletes are known to be good perceivers, because in a race situation they work very hard mentally to concentrate (cognitively associate) on their sensations in order to regulate their pace effectively (Morgan, 2000).

REFERENCES

American College of Sports Medicine (ACSM) (2005). *Guidelines for Exercise Testing and Prescription*, 7th edn. Baltimore, MD: Lippincott, Williams and Wilkins.

Berry, M.J., Weyrich, A.S., Roberds, R.A., Krause, K.M. and Ingallis, C.P. (1989). Ratings of perceived exertion in individuals with varying fitness levels during walking and running. *European Journal of Applied Physiology and Occupational Physiology*, 58: 494–499.

Biddle, S.J.H. and Mutrie, N. (2001). *Psychology of Physical Activity; Determinants, Well-being and Interventions*. London: Routledge.

Borg, G. (1998). *Borg's Perceived Exertion and Pain Scales*. Champaign, IL: Human Kinetics.

Borg, G. (2004). *The Borg CR10 Folder. A Method for Measuring Intensity of Experience*. Stockholm, Sweden: Borg Perception.

Boutcher, S.H., Seip, R.L., Hetzler, R.K., Pierce, E.F., Snead, D. and Weltman, A. (1989). The effects of specificity of training on the rating of perceived exertion at the lactate threshold. *European Journal of Applied Physiology and Occupational Physiology*, 59: 365–369.

Brisswalter, J. and Delignierè, D. (1997). Influence of exercise duration on perceived exertion during controlled locomotion. *Perceptual and Motor Skills*, 85: 17–18.

Buckley, J.P., Eston, R.G. and Sim, J. (2000). Ratings of perceived exertion in Braille: validity and reliability in production mode. *British Journal of Sports Medicine*, 34: 297–302.

Buckley, J.P., Quinlivan, R.C.M., Sim, J. and Eston, R.G. (2003). Ratings of perceived pain and the second wind in McArdle's disease. *Medicine and Science in Sports and Exercise*, 35(Suppl. 5): 1604.

Buckley, J.P., Sim, J., Eston, R.G., Hession, R. and Fox, R. (2004). Reliability and validity of measures taken during the Chester step test to predict aerobic power and to prescribe aerobic exercise. *British Journal of Sports Medicine*, 38: 197–205.

Cafarelli, E. (1977). Peripheral and central inputs to the effort sense during cycling exercise. *European Journal of Applied Physiology and Occupational Physiology*, 37: 181–189.

Cafarelli, E. (1982). Peripheral contributions to the perception of effort. *Medicine and Science in Sports and Exercise*, 14: 382–389.

Chen, M.J., Fan, X. and Moe, S.T. (2002). Criterion-related validity of the Borg ratings of perceived exertion scale in healthy individuals: a meta-analysis. *Journal of Sports Sciences*, 20: 873–899.

Dishman, R.K. and Landy, F.J. (1988). Psychological factors and prolonged exercise. In D.R. Lamb and R. Murray (eds), *Perspectives in Exercise Science and Sports Medicine*, pp. 281–355. Indianapolis, IN: Benckmark Press.

Eston, R.G. and Connolly, D. (1996). The use of ratings of perceived exertion for exercise prescription in patients receiving β-blocker therapy. *Sports Medicine*, 21: 176–190.

Eston, R.G. and Lamb, K.L. (2000). Effort perception. In N. Armstrong and W. Van-Mechelen (eds), *Paediatric Exercise Science and Medicine*, pp. 85–91, Oxford, UK: Oxford University Press.

Eston, R.G. and Parfitt, G. (2006). Perceived exertion. In N. Armstrong (ed.), *Paediatric Exercise Physiology*. Elsevier, London (in Press).

Eston, R.G., Lamb, K.L., Bain, A., Williams, M. and Williams, J.G. (1994). Validity of a perceived exertion scale for children: a pilot study. *Perceptual and Motor Skills*, 78: 691–697.

Eston, R.G., Parfitt, G., Campbell, L. and Lamb, K.L. (2000). Reliability of effort perception for regulating exercise intensity in children using a Cart and Load Effort Rating (CALER) Scale. *Pediatric Exercise Science*, 12: 388–397.

Eston, R.G., Parfitt, G. and Shepherd, P. (2001). Effort perception in children: implications for validity and reliability. In A. Papaionnou, M. Goudas and Y. Theodorakis (eds), *Proceedings of 10th World Congress of Sport Psychology, Skiathos*, Greece, Volume 5, pp. 104–106.

Eston, R.G., Lamb, K.L., Parfitt, C.G. and King, N. (2005). The validity of predicting maximal oxygen uptake from a perceptually regulated graded exercise test. *European Journal of Applied Physiology*, 94: 221–227.

Gearhart, R.F. Jr, Goss, F.L., Lagally, K.M., Jakicic, J.M., Gallagher, J., Gallagher, K.I. and Robertson, R. (2002). Ratings of perceived exertion in active muscle during high-intensity and low-intensity resistance exercise. *Strength and Conditioning Research*, 16(1): 87–91.

Head, A., Maxwell, S. and Kendall, M.J. (1997). Exercise metabolism in healthy volunteers taking celiprolol, atenolol, and placebo. *British Journal of Sports Medicine*, 31: 120–125.

Kohl, R.M. and Shea, C.H. (1988). Perceived exertion: influences of locus of control and expected work intensity and duration. *Journal of Human Movement Studies*, 15: 225–272.

Lagally, K.M. and Costigan, E.M. (2004). Anchoring procedures in reliability of ratings of perceived exertion during resistance exercise. *Perceptual and Motor Skills*, 98(3 Pt 2): 1285–1295.

Lamb, K.L. and Eston, R.G. (1997). Effort perception in children. *Sports Medicine*, 23: 139–148.

Lamb, K.L., Trask, S. and Eston, R.G. (1997). Effort perception in children: a focus on testing methodology. In N. Armstrong, B.J. Kirby and J.R. Welsman (eds), *Children and Exercise XIX Promoting Health and Well Being*, pp. 258–266. London: E & FN Spon.

Maresh, C. and Noble, B.J. (1984). Utilization of perceived exertion ratings during exercise testing and training. In L.K. Hall, G.C. Meyer and H.K. Hellerstein (eds), *Cardiac Rehabilitation: Exercise Testing and Prescription*, pp. 155–173. Great Neck, NY: Spectrum.

Morgan, W.P. (1973). Psychological factors influencing perceived exertion. *Medicine and Science in Sports and Exercise*, 5: 97–103.

Morgan, W.P. (1994). Psychological components of effort sense. *Medicine and Science in Sports and Exercise*, 26: 1071–1077.

Morgan, W. (2000). Psychological factors associated with distance running and the marathon. In D. Tunstall-Pedoe (ed.), *Marathon Medicine*. London: Royal Society of Medicine Press.

Noble, B. and Robertson, R. (1996). *Perceived Exertion*. Champaign, IL: Human Kinetics.

O'Donnell, D.E., Fluge, T., Gerken, F., Hamilton, A., Webb, K., Make, B. and Magnussen, H. (2004). Effects of tiotropium on lung hyperinflation, dyspnoea and exercise tolerance in COPD. *European Respiratory Journal*, 23(6): 832–840.

Pincivero, D.M., Campy, R.M. and Coelho, A.J. (2003). Knee flexor torque and perceived exertion: a gender and reliability analysis. *Medicine and Science in Sports and Exercise*, 35(10): 1720–1726.

Pollock, M.L., Wilmore, J.H. and Fox, S.M. (1978). *Health and Fitness Through Physical Activity*. New York: Wiley: American College of Sports Medicine Series.

Rejeski, W.J. (1981). The perception of exertion: a social psychophysiological integration. *Journal of Sport Psychology*, 4: 305–320.

Robertson, R.J. (1997). Perceived exertion in young people: future directions of enquiry. In J. Welsman, N. Armstrong and B. Kirby (eds), *Children and Exercise XIX* Volume II, pp. 33–39. Exeter: Washington: Singer Press.

Robertson, R.J. and Noble, B.J. (1997). Perception of physical exertion: methods, mediators and applications. *Exercise and Sports Science Reviews*, 25: 407–452.

Robertson, R.J., Goss, F.L., Boer, N.F., Peoples J.A., Foreman A.J., Dabayebeh I.M., Millich N.B., Balasekaran G., Riechman S.E., Gallagher J.D. and Thompkins T. (2000). Children's OMNI Scale of perceived exertion: mixed gender and race validation. *Medicine and Science in Sports and Exercise*, 32: 452–458.

Robertson, R.J., Goss, J.L., Bell, F.A., Dixon, C.B., Gallagher K.I., Lagally K.M., Timmer J.M., Abt K.L., Gallagher J.D. and Thompkins T. (2002). Self-regulated cycling using the Children's OMNI Scale of Perceived Exertion. *Medicine and Science in Sports and Exercise*, 34: 1168–1175.

Robertson, R.J., Goss, J.L., Andreacci, J.L. Dube J.J., Rutkowski J.J., Snee B.M., Kowallis R.A., Crawford K., Aaron D.J. and Metz K.F. (2005). Validation of the Children's OMNI RPE Scale for stepping exercise. *Medicine and Science in Sports and Exercise*, 37: 290–298.

Roemmich, J.N., Barkley, J.E. and Epstein, L.H., Lobarinas, C.L., White T.M. and Foster J.H. Validity of PCERT and OMNI walk/run ratings of perceived exertion. (2006). Validity of the PCERT and OMNI-walk/run ratings of perceived exertion scales. *Medicine and Science in Sports and Exercise*, 38: 1014–1019.

Smutok, M.A., Skrinar, G.S. and Pandolf, K.B. (1980). Exercise intensity: subjective regulation by perceived exertion. *Archives of Physical Medicine and Rehabilitation*, 61: 569–574.

Utter, A.C., Robertson, R.J., Nieman, D.C. and Kang, J. (2002) Children's OMNI Scale of perceived exertion: walking/running evaluation. *Medicine and Science in Sports and Exercise*, 34: 139–144.

Williams, J.G. and Eston, R.G. (1989). Determination of the intensity dimension in vigorous exercise programmes with particular reference to the use of the rating of perceived exertion. *Sports Medicine*, 8: 177–189.

Williams, J.G., Eston, R.G. and Stretch, C. (1991). Use of rating of perceived exertion to control exercise intensity in children. *Pediatric Exercise Science*, 3: 21–27.

Williams, J.G., Eston, R.G. and Furlong, B. (1994). CERT: a perceived exertion scale for young children. *Perceptual and Motor Skills*, 79: 1451–1458.

Williams, J.G., Furlong, B., MacKintosh, C. and Hockley, T.J. (1993). Rating and regulation of exercise intensity in young children. *Medicine and Science in Sports and Exercise*, 1993, 25 (Suppl. S8) (Abstract).

Yelling, M., Lamb, K. and Swaine, I.L. (2002). Validity of a pictorial perceived exertion scale for effort estimation and effort production during stepping exercise in adolescent children. *European Physical Education Review*, 8: 157–175.

CHAPTER 14

STRENGTH TESTING

Anthony J. Blazevich and Dale Cannavan

INTRODUCTION

Maximum strength can be defined as the 'maximum force or torque a muscle or group of muscles can generate at a specified determined velocity' (Komi *et al.*, 1992: 90–102). Information regarding a person's strength is often sought in order to monitor longitudinal adaptations to training and rehabilitation, compare strength levels between individuals (or groups of individuals), determine the importance of strength to performance in other physical tasks, and to determine single limb or inter-limb strength inadequacies/imbalances.

The three main forms of strength testing are: isometric, isokinetic and isotonic (isoinertial). Importantly, each form of testing measures different qualities so the tests cannot be used interchangeably. This is largely due to the complex interaction of muscular, tendinous and neural factors impacting on strength expression. In order to determine the best possible battery of tests, it is important to consider issues of test specificity and reliability, the safety of subjects and the ease of test administration (and re-administration: for example, reproducibility of environment, subject motivation to re-perform, etc.). However, Abernethy and Wilson (2000: 149) ask five important questions to determine which form/s of strength assessment is/are most appropriate:

1   How reliable is the particular measurement procedure?
2   What is the correlation between the test score and either whole or part of the athletic performance under consideration? (If the performances are not related, are they specific enough to each other?)
3   Does the test item discriminate between the performances of members of heterogeneous and/or homogeneous groups?
4   Is the measurement procedure sensitive to the effects of training, rehabilitation and/or acute bouts of exercise?

5   Does the technique provide insights into the mechanisms underpinning strength and power performance and/or adaptations to training?

It is probably useful to examine each form of testing in relation to these questions.

ISOMETRIC TESTING

Isometric strength testing requires subjects to produce maximum force or torque against an immovable resistance. Force or torque can be measured by a force platform, cable tensiometer, strain gauge, or metal- or crystal-based load cell. Isometric tests can be easily standardised and have a high reproducibility (correlation (r) = 0.85–0.99; Abernethy $et\ al.$, 1995), require minimal familiarisation, are generally easy to administer and safe to perform, can be used to assess strength over various ranges of motion, and can be conducted with relatively inexpensive equipment. Both maximum force (or torque) and the maximum rate of force development (RFD) can be quantified. RFD can be quantified as: (1) the time to reach a certain level of force, (2) the time to attain a relative force level (e.g. 30% of maximum), (3) the slope of the force–time curve over a given time interval or (4) the force or impulse (force × time) value reached in a specified time.

Despite the many benefits of isometric testing, the relationship between maximum isometric strength and athletic performance is generally poor (correlation coefficients <0.50). Also, isometric tests tend to be insensitive to changes in athletic performance or changes in isotonic or isokinetic strength (Baker $et\ al.$, 1994; Fry $et\ al.$, 1994). Thus, while isometric testing might provide information regarding isometric strength and RFD, its use in practical terms is questionable.

The lack of a strong relationship between isometric strength and various dynamic measures might be attributable to: (1) the significant differences in the neural activation of muscles during isometric versus dynamic movements (Nakazawa $et\ al.$, 1993), or (2) the fact that many dynamic movements are performed with considerable extension and recoil of elastic structures in the muscle–tendon units. This is most notable in movements where the whole muscle–tendon unit is stretched rapidly before shortening, the so-called stretch–shorten cycle. Thus, isometric testing largely examines muscle function under a specific set of conditions, without accounting for the effects of the elastic elements.

Suggested protocol for isometric testing

1   Appropriate warm-up and the performance of several practice contractions should precede testing. While little practice is required for many isometric tests, appropriate muscle control strategies would be developed with consistent practice. Therefore, increases in force seen after several testing sessions might not be completely attributable to changes in the contractile component of the muscle, but indicate some 'learning' of the test.

2   Prolonged stretching performed prior to testing can reduce maximum force production (Fowles *et al.*, 2000; Behm *et al.*, 2001), so stretching during warm-up should be minimal, and repeated exactly in subsequent testing sessions.

3   Repeated testing should be conducted at the same time of day with the same environmental conditions (e.g. room temperature), and after the same pre-testing routine is performed (e.g. warm-up, food intake, training, stimulant use, sleep, etc.).

4   Participants should be highly motivated for every trial. Usually up to three trials should be performed with the best performance recorded.

ISOKINETIC TESTING

Isokinetic testing involves the measurement of force or torque during a movement in which the velocity is constant, and non-zero. Typically, isokinetic testing is performed on a specialised machine where a motor drives a lever or bar to move at a specified speed while force or torque is measured via a load cell or force platform. Isokinetic testing is commonly used to profile the force – velocity or torque – angle characteristics of a muscle group or limb, muscle fatigability and recovery, or joint range of motion. Both eccentric (muscle lengthening) and concentric (muscle shortening) strength can be tested, although it is not possible to test stretch–shorten actions with most standard isokinetic machines. Isokinetic testing has been largely thought to provide information about the capacity of muscle, rather than tendon. While this is largely true, since gravitational energy cannot be stored in elastic structures during isokinetic testing, recent research examining concentric actions has shown that there is significant tendon lengthening early in a movement with subsequent recoil of the tendon as the movement proceeds; this phenomenon is greater at higher movement speeds (Ichinose *et al.*, 2000).

The reproducibility of isokinetic force or torque depends on the type of movement and the speed at which it is performed. Subject force/torque reliability is generally good, or very good, provided the subject has had several familiarisation sessions and a strict testing protocol is followed (discussed later). A slight exaggeration of force is sometimes seen early in a movement – the so-called torque overshoot, which is small at slow speeds but larger at high speeds. This occurs as the limb gains momentum and impacts with the cuff or pad onto which the limb is moving. Modern systems use damping mechanisms or impose a controlled period of acceleration to reduce the overshoot, however it might be necessary to set the dynamometer to move through a larger range of motion than is required so that some data can be excluded from analysis. Isokinetic machines generally move within $1°·s^{-1}$ of the set speed, with a larger discrepancy (up to $2°·s^{-1}$) occurring in the period of overshoot, so speed measurements can be considered accurate and reliable. If necessary, the accuracy and reliability of movement speed can be assessed using motion analysis.

The validity of isokinetic testing is likely to decrease as the test movement pattern becomes less similar to the task movement pattern, particularly if the task involves a stretch–shorten cycle action or the complexity of the task increases above that of the isokinetic test. It is therefore necessary to examine the specificity of isokinetic testing before adopting it.

Protocol for testing on an isokinetic dynamometer

1   As per points 1–3 for isometric testing; although several familiarisation sessions may be required.
2   Participants should be highly motivated for every trial.
3   The subjects should be tightly secured to the seat or bench in order that extraneous movements do not significantly impact on force development (refer to manufacturer's guidelines). The limb to be tested should be tightly secured to the machine using the straps provided. Certain machines (e.g. Kin-Com; Chatanooga Inc., USA) require accurate recording of the positioning of the attachment so that torque (force × distance) can be reliably calculated.
4   The axis of rotation of the lever of the dynamometer should be adjacent to the centre of rotation of the joint being assessed. When large forces are produced, there will be unavoidable movement of the subject and flexion of the dynamometer mountings, so alignment will not be properly maintained. This is rarely problematic and is reasonably consistent between trials, however quantification of misalignment, and correction using mathematical means, can be performed by combining video analysis with force or torque measurement.
5   Gravity correction should be performed as per the manufacturer's guidelines. The error created when gravity correction is not performed is greater for fatigue tests than tests of maximum strength.
6   Ranges of motion and movement speeds need to be carefully considered.
7   Up to three trials should be performed with the best performance recorded, although it is often necessary to increase the number of repetitions when moving continuously at higher movement speeds (e.g. for knee extension, 4 and 5 trials should be performed at $180°$ and $300°·s^{-1}$, respectively) in order for the subject to become accustomed to that speed. Fatigue tests may vary in their repetition number, however 30 and 50 repetitions are commonly used.
8   Rest intervals should be greater than 30 s, although up to 4 min may be required when testing at slower speeds where perceived exertion and contraction time are greater.
9   Test order generally progresses from slower speeds to faster and should be the same at consecutive testing sessions; this test order shows high reliability (Wilhite *et al.*, 1992).

ISOTONIC (ISOINERTIAL) TESTING

Isotonic strength testing involves moving a fixed mass with constant acceleration and deceleration. Since acceleration changes with joint angle during a movement, these movements are probably more correctly described as isoinertial (Abernethy and Jürimäe, 1996). Common tests of isoinertial strength include the one-repetition maximum (1-RM) tests such as the maximal bench press or barbell squat tests, maximal concentric and eccentric strength tests, static and countermovement vertical and horizontal jumps (with and without additional load), throwing tests, cycle ergometer and sprint running/swimming tests. Performance can be measured via force platforms and load cells (with measures described as peak forces/torques, RFD, work/power, force decrements, etc.), by the maximum weight lifted, or by the distance/height thrown or jumped, etc.

Since many sports require the acceleration of a mass with constant inertia, such tests generally show higher task validity than isometric and isokinetic tests. Correlations with athletic task performance are generally high when the movement characteristics match those of the task, but are reduced as they differ more widely (see Table 14.1). Since the use of a variety of tests can provide a greater amount of information about the factors affecting strength (e.g. muscle recruitment potential, elastic energy storage and recovery, maximal muscle contraction force, work rates and fatigue indices, etc.), it might sometimes be necessary to use tests that do not correlate highly with task performance. Test performances are also very sensitive to change after periods of isoinertial strength, power or sprint training, although changes may not be seen after isometric or isokinetic training.

Reliability of isoinertial tests varies largely depending on the test performed and the experience of the subject. For traditional maximum strength tests such as the 1-RM bench press or squat, reliability is very high ($r = 0.92–0.98$ typically) when strict procedures are followed. When the 1-RM is predicted by mathematical equations from 3 to 10 RM lifting tests, reliability is slightly reduced ($r = 0.89–0.96$) and results may vary by up to 2.5 kg depending on which equation is used (see Table 14.2 for examples).

Table 14.1 Correlation between sprint running and selected test performances

Isoinertial test	Correlation coefficient	
	2.5 m sprint (ct ≈ 0.17–2.1 s)	Fastest 10 m time (ct ≈ 0.9–1.2 s)
F30 (t = 30 ms)	− 0.46	− 0.49
MAX RFD (t = 56 ms)	− 0.62	− 0.73
F100/WEIGHT (t = 100 ms)	− 0.73	− 0.80
MDS/WEIGHT (t = 121 ms)	− 0.86	− 0.69

Notes
The validity of isoinertial strength tests increases as the movement characteristics become more similar to the performance task. In the above example, correlations between sprint running performance (2.5 m time and 'fastest 10-m' times) and test performance are greatest when test duration is most similar to contact time (ct), for example, performance in the F100/weight test, which takes approximately 100 ms, correlates highest with 10 m time, where the foot-ground contact time is also approximately 100 ms

F30: force developed in the first 30 ms of a weighted (19 kg) jump squat from 120° knee angle; MAX RFD: maximum rate of force development in jump squat (which occurred [mean] 0.056 s after movement initiation); F100/WEIGHT: force applied 100 ms into jump squat; MDS/WEIGHT: maximum force developed during jump squat normalised for bodyweight (occurred [mean] 0.121 s after movement initiation). For more detail, see Young et al. (1995)

Table 14.2 Examples of equations used to calculate 1-RM lifting performances from multiple maximal repetitions

Test exercise	Equation	Correlation	Difference between achieved and predicted 1RM[d]	Cross validation reference
Bench press	100·repetition mass/ (52.2 + 41.9·exp[0.055·reps])[a]	$r = 0.992$	0.5 kg ± 3.6 kg	LeSuer *et al.*, 1997
Squat	100·repetition mass/ (48.8 + 53.8·exp[0.075·reps])[b]	$r = 0.969$	0.5 kg ± 3.5 kg	LeSuer *et al.*, 1997
Multiple exercises	100·repetition mass/ (102.78–2.78·reps)[c]	$r = 0.633$– 0.896	Not available	Knutzen *et al.*, 1999

Notes
a Formula from Mayhew *et al.* (1992)
b Formula from Wathan (1994)
c Formula from Brzycki (1993)
d Mean difference between predicted and actual 1RM from a cross validation of prediction equations (LeSuer *et al.*, 1997)

Also, while factors such as gender appear not to affect prediction accuracy, the reliability of estimates seems to be greater for some lifts (e.g. bench press and leg press) than others (e.g. barbell curl and knee extension) (Hoeger *et al.*, 1990). Reliability of weighted jumps measured on a force platform or contact mat are good, although it tends to be reduced as loads increase. Sprint running and cycling tests usually show very good reliability, although performance reliability of well-trained subjects is usually higher than that of lesser-trained subjects. Importantly, reliability of these tests should be determined in the test population before being used to assess performance.

Protocol for isotonic (isoinertial) testing

1   As per points 1–3 for isometric testing.
2   Subjects may require several familiarisation sessions before test reliability is acceptable; familiarisation of 1-RM lifts is usually more rapid than for higher-velocity tests.
3   Participants should be highly motivated for every trial.
4   Tests should be selected that are closely related to the athletic or rehabilitation task being trained for, and/or provide significant information about the functioning of a specific part of the neuromusculotendinous system.
5   Most tests can be performed with a wide variety of techniques. A technique should be chosen that has close specificity to the task being trained for, and should be performed identically on subsequent testing occasions (particular attention should be paid to the techniques adopted for weighted and drop jump tests).
6   For more detail regarding isoinertial strength testing, see Logan *et al.* (2000: 200–221).

OTHER CONSIDERATIONS IN TEST SELECTION

A range of tests should be selected so that as much information as possible is available to assess inter-individual differences, monitor training/rehabilitation progress, or examine a person's strengths and weaknesses. Consideration should be given to using a selection of isometric, isokinetic and isoinertial tests. For example, testing isokinetic knee extensor, knee flexor and ankle plantarflexor strength at a range of velocities will allow some determination of the capacity of the muscle groups to generate force over a range of contraction speeds and ranges of motion. Also, the ratio of squat (static) jump to counter-movement jump height has been shown to provide a useful indication of the compliance of tendon structures in the lower limb (Kubo *et al.*, 1999). Thus, this test battery provides the examiner with information about both muscle and tendon function and allows appropriate training plans to be developed for a specific purpose. It is clear then, that the design of optimum test batteries requires a good scientific knowledge, and some creative design.

REFERENCES

Abernethy, P. and Jürimäe, J. (1996). Cross-sectional and longitudinal uses of isoinertial, isometric, and isokinetic dynamometry. *Medicine and Science in Sports and Exercise*, 28: 1180–1187.

Abernethy, P. and Wilson, G. (2000). Introduction to the assessment of strength and power. In C.J. Gore (ed.), *Physiological Tests for Elite Athletes*. Champaign, IL: Human Kinetics.

Abernethy, P., Wilson, G. and Logan, P. (1995). Strength and power assessment. Issues, controversies, and isokinetic dynamometry. *Sports Medicine*, 19: 401–417.

Baker, D., Wilson, G. and Carlyon, B. (1994). Generality versus specificity: a comparison of dynamic and isometric measures of strength and speed-strength. *European Journal of Applied Physiology*, 68: 350–355.

Behm, D.G., Button, D.C. and Butt, J.C. (2001). Factors affecting force loss with prolonged stretching. *Canadian Journal of Applied Physiology*, 26: 261–272.

Brzycki, M. (1993). Strength testing – predicting a one-rep max from reps-to fatigue. *Journal of Health Physical Education Recreation and Dance*, 64: 88–90.

Fowles, J.R., Sale, D.G. and MacDougall, J.D. (2000). Reduced strength after passive stretch of the human plantarflexors. *Journal of Applied Physiology*, 89: 1179–1188.

Fry, A.C., Kraemer, W.J., van Borselen, F., Lynch, J.M., Marsit, J.L., Roy, E.P., Triplett, N.T. and Knuttgen, H.G. (1994). Performance decrements with high intensity resistance exercise overtraining. *Medicine and Science in Sports and Exercise*, 26: 1165–1173.

Hoeger, W.W.K., Hopkins, D.R. and Barette, S.L. (1990). Relationship between repetitions and selected percentages of one repetition maximum: a comparison between trained and untrained males and females. *Journal of Applied Sports Science Research*, 4: 47–54.

Ichinose, Y., Kawakami, Y., Ito, M., Kanehisa, H. and Fukunaga, T. (2000). In vivo estimation of contraction velocity of human vastus lateralis muscle during 'isokinetic' action. *Journal of Applied Physiology*, 88: 851–856.

Komi, P.V., Suominen, H., Keikkinen, E., Karlsson, J. and Tesch, P. (1992). Effects of heavy resistance training and explosive type strength training methods on mechanical, functional and metabolic aspects of performance. In P.V. Komi (ed.), *Exercise and Sports Biology*, Champaign, IL: Human Kinetics.

Kubo, K., Kawakami, Y. and Fukunaga, T. (1999). Influence of elastic properties of tendon structures on jump performance in humans. *Journal of Applied Physiology*, 87: 2090–2096.

LeSuer, D.A., McCormick, J.H., Mayhew, J.L., Wasserstein, R.L. and Arnold, M.D. (1997). The accuracy of prediction equations for estimating 1-RM performance in the bench press, squat, and deadlift. *Journal of Strength and Conditioning Research*, 11: 211–213.

Logan, P., Fornasiero, D., Abernethy, P. and Lynch, K. (2000). Protocols for the assessment of isoinertial strength. In C.J. Gore (ed.), *Physiological Tests for Elite Athletes*. Champaign, IL: Human Kinetics.

Mayhew, J.L., Ball, T.E., Arnold, M.D. and Bowen, J.C. (1992). Relative muscular endurance performance as a predictor of bench press strength in college men and women. *Journal of Applied Sports Science Research*, 6: 200–206.

Nakazawa, K., Kawakami, Y., Fukunaga, T., Yano, H. and Miyashita, M. (1993). Differences in activation patterns in elbow flexors during isometric, concentric and eccentric contractions. *European Journal of Applied Physiology*, 66: 214–220.

Wathan, D. (1994). Load assignment. In T.R. Baechle (ed.), *Essentials of Strength Training and Conditioning*. Champaign, IL: Human Kinetics.

Wilhite, M.R., Cohen, E.R. and Wilhite, S.C. (1992). Reliability of concentric and eccentric measurements of quadriceps performance using the KIN-COM dynamometer: the effect of testing order for three different speeds. *Journal of Orthopaedic and Sports Physical Therapy*, 15: 175–182.

Young, W., McLean, B. and Ardagna, J. (1995). Relationship between strength qualities and sprinting performance. *Journal of Sports Medicine and Physical Fitness*, 35: 13–19.

CHAPTER 15

UPPER-BODY EXERCISE

Paul M. Smith and Mike J.Price

PREAMBLE

Upper-body exercise testing holds important practical applications for many populations including specifically trained competitors who pursue events such as canoeing and kayaking, and individuals who do not have the habitual use of their legs. Furthermore, this mode of exercise can be useful in clinical rehabilitation.

Several testing rigs such as kayak and wheelchair ergometers and swim benches have been designed to mimic the movement patterns and physiological demands of specific upper-body sports. However, arm crank ergometry (ACE) provides the sport and exercise scientist with a generic means by which physiological responses and adaptations of individuals to upper-body exercise can practically be examined. Work with ACE has concentrated principally on the development of protocols used to examine individual aerobic and anaerobic exercise capability. Nevertheless, few recommendations for exercise testing exist in this area. While electrically braked arm ergometers are now increasingly available, most laboratories use less expensive, suitably adapted friction-braked cycle ergometers to perform ACE tests. In some instances the use of a friction-braked ergometer will make the implementation of some of the testing protocols (e.g. ramp testing) problematic. Where such issues arise alternative protocol designs have been recommended.

AEROBIC TESTING

Previous studies have concentrated on methodological aspects including the use of continuous or discontinuous protocols, effects of crank rate selection and pattern by which exercise intensity changes. An important point to note is that the continuation of exercise during incremental ACE protocols is predominantly constrained by peripheral as opposed to centrally limiting factors. Consequently, in assessments of maximum oxygen uptake the term VO_{2peak} is preferred (refer to Chapter 5 for general information on methodological aspects of aerobic testing).

BODY POSITION

While some studies have required subjects to stand, the majority have adopted unrestrained, seated positions. The crankshaft of the ergometer is usually horizontally aligned with the centre of the glenohumeral joint. The subject is required to sit at a distance from the ergometer so that with their back vertical the arms are slightly bent at the furthest horizontal point of the duty cycle.

Variations in procedures used to brace either the legs and/or torso have been reported. To reflect what the athlete might experience in the field bracing is not necessary. However, it is recommended that a standard and consistent procedure be adopted where subjects should keep their back vertical with their feet flat on the floor and their knees at 90°.

Discontinuous protocols can be used in an attempt to postpone peripheral fatigue, though similar sub-maximal and peak physiological responses have been reported compared to continuous tests. The use of discontinuous protocols can be advantageous if a supplementary measurement such as blood pressure is required.

CRANK MODE AND RATE

The majority of studies adopt asynchronous cranking, though direct comparisons of physiological responses to exercise are available for synchronous and asynchronous modalities. It has consistently been demonstrated that influences in crank rate effect submaximal and peak physiological responses during ACE even when differences in the internal work needed simply to move the limbs is considered. At any given work rate during incremental exercise mechanical efficiency is lower using a faster crank rate resulting in greater energy expenditure. Previous editions of the BASES testing guidelines published in 1986 and 1988 recommended that a crank rate of 60 rev.min^{-1} be used with ACE. However, more recent work has shown that the use of a faster crank rate (70 and 80 rev.min^{-1}) elicits a higher and therefore, more valid peak physiological responses (Price and Campbell, 1997; Smith et al., 2001). The principal reason for this is that a faster crank rate will postpone the onset of peripheral muscular fatigue ensuring higher exercise intensities are achieved during incremental exercise (Smith et al., 2001). Faster crank rates also lead to lower differentiated ratings of perceived exertion (RPE) associated with perceptions of localised fatigue and strain in the active musculature. Conversely higher central ratings have being reported at the point of volitional exhaustion using a faster crank rate (please refer to Chapter 13 for further information on the use of RPE scales). It should be noted that if the crank rate employed is too slow (50 rev.min^{-1}) or too fast (90 rev.min^{-1}) premature fatigue can occur.

INCREMENTS

The initial exercise intensity and subsequent increases crucially influence the duration of a test designed to assess peak aerobic capacity. Step or ramp tests can elicit peak physiological responses, though it is important to note that they should not be used interchangeably (Smith *et al.*, 2004). Typically the VO$_{2peak}$ test should last between 8 and 15 min and a standard graded exercise test can be adopted, as illustrated in Figure 15.1. It is important to note that following the initial 3 min warm-up period, the total amount of work completed during each successive 2 min stage is equivalent between tests.

In any test to volitional exhaustion there is a trade-off between the duration and number of exercise stages that can be completed. Usually 2 min exercise stages during stepwise ACE protocols: (1) permit a valid measurement of peak physiological responses, and (2) evaluate the influence of changes in exercise intensity on the evolution of physiological responses to the point of volitional exhaustion.

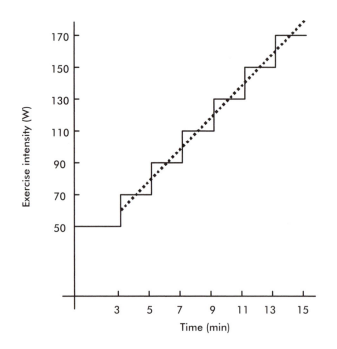

Figure 15.1   An illustration of step (solid lines) and ramp (broken line) patterns of increases in exercise intensity used to elicit peak physiological responses during a graded arm crank ergometry test

Table 15.1 Recommended starting and increments in exercise intensity (W) for graded arm crank ergometry tests

		Step test		Ramp test	
		Start (W)	Increment (W)	Start (W)	Increment (W)
Male	Trained	50	30 every 2 min	50	1 every 4 s
	Untrained	40	20 every 2 min	40	1 every 6 s
Female	Trained	30	15 every 2 min	30	1 every 8 s
	Untrained	20	10 every 2 min	20	1 every 10 s

PROTOCOL RECOMMENDATIONS

Table 15.1 summarises recommendations for trained and untrained, male and female subjects where step or ramp tests are used. Time permitting, we recommend an individualised approach to both starting and increments in exercise intensity. To this end, an initial incremental protocol should be conducted following the guidelines in Table 15.1 to establish the mean exercise intensity achieved during the final minute of the test or peak minute power (PMP). A test can then be designed with a starting (warm-up) intensity equivalent to 30% of PMP, with subsequent stepwise increments of 10% of PMP every 2 min. If a ramp test is used the same initial exercise intensity can be adopted for the warm-up with subsequent increments of 1% of PMP every 12 s.

TYPICAL VALUES AND REPRODUCIBILITY

Information relating to normative values and the reproducibility of the parameters associated with ACE testing is limited. In non-specifically trained groups of men, typical values of VO_{2peak} range from 2.5 to 3.2 $l \cdot min^{-1}$. In specifically trained men values in excess of 3.5 $l \cdot min^{-1}$ are frequently observed. Limited information is available for women however it is likely that non-specifically trained groups would typically achieve VO_{2peak} values from 1.5 to 2.0 $l.min^{-1}$. For trained women 1.7–2.6 $l \cdot min^{-1}$ could be anticipated. An acceptable typical error measurement for VO_{2peak} on a test–retest basis is $\pm 5\%$ for all groups.

The value of PMP achieved by a non-specifically trained group of men ranges from 110 to 160 W. Specifically trained men are able to achieve PMP values ranging from 170 to 270 W. For non-specifically trained women PMP values of 70–110 W can be achieved, while trained female groups may achieve values of 100–120 W. An acceptable typical error measurement for all PMP values for all groups on a test–retest basis is $\pm 3\%$.

MAXIMAL INTENSITY EXERCISE

Considerable variations in methodological procedures associated with all-out exercise tests are also evident. Differences include equipment employed, body position adopted, resistive load used, and methods of power measurement and reporting.

Adapted friction-braked ergometers are most frequently used, with a standard resistive load usually determined according to a percentage of body weight. Studies tend to use resistive loads equivalent to 2.0–8.0% body weight. Commercially available computer software programs now permit the simultaneous measurement of uncorrected and corrected power outputs. Uncorrected data relate to, and can be used to assess, the force–velocity relationship of muscle. Corrected data is more concerned with the relationship between instantaneous torque production, which in turn, is calculated using algorithms that take into consideration information relating to the inertial characteristics of the heavy flywheel, the resistive (braking) load applied and the instantaneous rate of flywheel de-/acceleration. Most recent studies have recorded and reported values of corrected peak power output (PPO) over 1 s.

It is unlikely that subjects will be accustomed to the requirements placed upon them during an all-out upper-body sprint effort. Therefore, it is highly recommended that several practise tests are performed. For the purpose of standardisation, a similar seated position to that described earlier for the VO_{2peak} testing should be adopted though we recommend that for sprint tests the legs and ankles should be firmly braced.

PROTOCOL DESIGN

Although the Wingate Anaerobic Test (WAnT) was originally designed to last 30 s we have tended to use a 20 s test for the purpose of measuring values of PPO and mean power output (MPO) due to the rapid onset of fatigue. This is of particular relevance when high resistive loads are used. The test should be preceded by a standardised 3–5 min warm-up using a crank rate of 70 rev·min^{-1}, and a resistive load of 9.81 N. It is also recommended that during the latter stages of the warm-up several practise starts should be made with the resistive load to be used during the test. Thereafter, subjects are required to perform an all-out sprint effort for the full duration of the test. A rolling start of 70 rev·min^{-1} is recommended though it is important to start logging of data after the resistive load has been applied and before the subject begins to accelerate the flywheel so as to avoid a flying start. Once the subject has completed the test the resistive load should be reduced to 9.81 N and the subject should complete a warm-down using a crank rate of their choice. If repeated 20- or 30-s tests are performed it is recommended that at least 60 min of passive re covery be allowed between tests.

RESISTIVE LOAD

Recommendations associated with resistive loads are presented here as percentages of body weight. It is clear that the force–velocity relationship applies to the upper-body as it does for the legs. Corrected values of PPO are greater than uncorrected PPO values, and typically occur within the first 5 s of the test. However, few differences exist between uncorrected and corrected values of MPO.

When uncorrected PPO data are considered loading strategy is influential. Generally, uncorrected PPO increases as the resistive load increases (Figure 15.2). In contrast, a considerable inter-subject variation exists for corrected PPO and the resistive load used to elicit an optimal value (Figure 15.2). With this in mind, and time permitting, we recommend that an individual approach be used with respect to identifying the 'optimised' resistive load required to elicit corrected PPO. To achieve this, repeated 10 s tests are required employing the full range of resistive loads presented in Table 15.2. At least 20 min of passive recovery is required between tests and the order in which the resistive loads are used should be randomised. The test that elicits the highest value of corrected PPO represents the optimised resistive load. It is important to note that while an optimised value of corrected PPO will be achieved, this approach is unlikely to permit the concomitant assessment of an optimised value of uncorrected PPO or un-/corrected values of MPO. To achieve such measurements separate optimisation procedures would have to be conducted with respect to the power output measurement of interest.

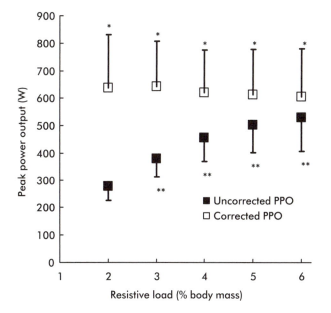

Figure 15.2 Mean (+/−SD) values of uncorrected and corrected PPO achieved using a range of resistive loads during an optimisation procedure conducted by 25 untrained men

Notes

* denotes corrected PPO greater ($P < 0.05$) than uncorrected PPO

** denotes the value of uncorrected PPO is greater ($P < 0.05$) compared to the value achieved using the previous resistive load

Table 15.2 Recommended ranges of resistive loads to be used in association with an optimisation procedure linked to corrected peak power output

Groups	Resistive load (% body weight)				
Trained males	4	5	**6**	7	8
Trained females	2	3	**4**	5	6
Untrained males	3	4	**5**	6	7
Untrained females	1	2	**3**	4	5

Note

Values in **bold and italicised** text represent the standard resistive loads that should be used by the respective subject populations if a single test is to be used

TYPICAL VALUES AND REPRODUCIBILITY

Typical values of uncorrected and corrected 1 s PPO for a non-specifically trained group of men range from 300 to 550 W and 400 to 700 W, respectively. For a specifically trained male group, respective values of 550–800 W and 600–1,100 W may be achieved. There is generally little difference between uncorrected and corrected values of MPO measured over 20 or 30 s. A non-specifically trained group of men would be able to achieve values ranging from 250 to 600 W, while a specifically trained group would achieve 400–700 W.

Typical values of uncorrected and corrected 1 s PPO for a group of non-specifically trained women range from 175 to 250 W and 200 to 300 W, respectively. For a specifically trained female group typical values would range from 200 to 300 W and 250 to 400 W, respectively. For 20 s MPO, a non-specifically trained group of women would be expected to achieve values from 175 to 250 W, while a specifically trained group can achieve values between 250 and 400 W. An acceptable level of typical error measurement for all power output values on a test–retest basis is ±5%.

REFERENCES

Price, M.J. and Campbell, I.G. (1997). Determination of peak oxygen uptake during upper body exercise. *Ergonomics*, 40, 491–499.

Smith, P.M., Price, M.J. and Doherty, M. (2001). The influence of crank rate on peak oxygen uptake during arm crank ergometry. *Journal of Sports Sciences*, 19, 955–960.

Smith, P.M., Doherty, M., Drake, D. and Price, M.J. (2004). The influence of step and ramp type protocols on the attainment of peak physiological responses during arm crank ergometry. *International Journal of Sports Medicine*, 25, 616–621.

PART 4

CLINICAL EXERCISE PHYSIOLOGY

CHAPTER 16

EXERCISE TESTING FOR PEOPLE WITH DIABETES

Pelagia Koufaki

INTRODUCTION

Diabetes is a metabolic disorder that results in elevated levels of blood glucose due to either pancreatic inability to produce insulin (type 1 diabetes) or cells' inability to effectively respond to circulating insulin (insulin resistance) (Diabetes UK, 2004). There are four diabetic categories. *Type 1 diabetes* is characterised by complete lack of insulin production and therefore regular supply of insulin is needed. *Type 2 diabetes* is mainly characterised by insulin resistance which may develop into insufficient insulin production. Common treatment approach involves administration of oral hypoglycaemic agents or insulin sensitising antihyperglycaemic agents. About 35–40% of patients with long-term type 2 diabetes may also require exogenous insulin administration. *Gestational diabetes* may develop during pregnancy but usually elevated levels of glucose return to normal after delivery. The fourth category is termed 'other specific types' which are strongly related to certain diseases or genetic predispositions (American Diabetes Association, 2004a). The general criteria for diagnosing diabetes are presented in Table 16.1.

Although symptoms of type 1 diabetes are well described (polyuria, polydipsia, unexplained weight loss) type 2 diabetes is not associated with specific symptoms and can go unnoticed for many years (Diabetes UK, 2004). However, individuals who present with problems of obesity, hypertension, hyperlipidaemia and physical inactivity are more likely to also present with impaired glucose metabolism that may progress into type 2 diabetes (Wilson *et al.*, 2005).

The prevalence of diabetes in the United Kingdom is ~3%, which means that 1.8 million people are affected. However, it is estimated that there are up to one million people in the UK population with undiagnosed type 2 diabetes. Worldwide figures show that 5% of the population is affected by diabetes with prevalence doubling with every generation (Diabetes UK, 2004).

Table 16.1 Plasma glucose levels for the diagnosis of diabetes and in impaired glucose tolerance state. Target range refers to glucose levels goal following usual medical treatment. Normal ranges refer to apparently healthy individuals

	Diabetes	*Impaired glucose tolerance*	*Target range*	*Normal ranges*
Random[a] glucose concentration (mmol·l⁻¹)	≥ 11.1		5.5–7.8	< 6.1
Fasting[b] plasma glucose (mmol·l⁻¹)	≥ 7	≥ 7.8	4.4–6.7	< 5
Plasma glucose after OGTT[c] (mmol·l⁻¹)	≥ 11.1	7.8–11.1	—	—
Hb_{A1C}[d] (%)	> 8	~7	< 7	< 6

Notes
a Random: at any time of the day without regard of last meal
b Fasting: at least 8 h since last meal
c OGTT: 2 h post-oral glucose tolerance test using a 75 g glucose load
d Glycosylated haemoglobin: index that reflects average glucose concentration over previous months 2–3

Diabetes is very strongly associated with cardiovascular disease morbidity and mortality (Diabetes UK, 2004; Wilson *et al.*, 2005) and therefore effective management of the condition could minimise the incidence of diabetic and cardiovascular complications. Currently there is no cure for diabetes. All available interventions and lifestyle guidelines aim to manage the condition by keeping glucose levels stable within normal limits. Recommendations for optimal management include a combination of pharmaceutical, diet and exercise interventions (American Diabetes Association, 2004b,c; Albright *et al.*, 2000).

DIABETIC COMPLICATIONS AND EXERCISE-RELATED PATHOPHYSIOLOGY

Chronically elevated levels of glucose (hyperglycaemia) can cause microvascular and/or macrovascular complications such as damage to peripheral nerves and the autonomic nervous system, retinopathy which may be accompanied by partial or complete loss of vision, renal failure, atherosclerotic cardiac and/or peripheral vascular disease and stroke (Albright *et al.*, 2000; Diabetes UK, 2004; American Diabetes Association, 2004b; Verity, 2005). Diabetic neuropathy and small vessel disease are also responsible for lower limb amputations. The 2004 report of Diabetes UK indicates that the rate of amputation in people with diabetes is 15 times higher than in people without diabetes. Moreover, elevated levels of blood glucose significantly alter lipid and protein metabolism with significant effects on weight management and muscle structure and function at rest and during physical activity (Horton, 1999; Ivy *et al.*, 1999; Sigal *et al.*, 2004). It is not surprising therefore that exercise tolerance is significantly impaired compared to apparently healthy individuals especially when other comorbidities are present (Regensteiner *et al.*, 1998; Wei *et al.*, 2000).

Metabolic adjustment to initiate and sustain exercise is a very finely tuned process that requires an integrated response from many physiological systems (cardiovascular, hormonal, neural) to ensure adequate oxygen delivery and fuel to active muscles. People with diabetes are characterised by diminished ability to effectively regulate all physiological processes during exercise. In brief, upon initiation of exercise, sympathetic nervous activity and catecholamine release is increased, whereas, with initiation of muscular activity blood glucose levels and circulating free fatty acids (FFA) start decreasing. Under normal conditions these responses suppress insulin secretion which in turn stimulates hepatic glucose production and adipose tissue lipolysis and therefore adequate FFA acids and glucose get delivered to insulin-sensitive working muscles. Glucose uptake by working muscles is enhanced and thus blood glucose levels stay within normal levels (Horton, 1999; Sigal *et al.*, 2004). On the other hand, in people with diabetes who take exogenous insulin or have insulin deficiency, the earlier mechanisms are altered. Resultantly, insulin response may not fully adjust to hormonal and metabolic changes and therefore the overall effect on glucose production is not optimal (Sigal *et al.*, 1994; Marliss and Vranic, 2002) (see Figure 16.1 (A)). Complications such as exercise-induced hypoglycaemia, post-exercise-induced hyperglycaemia, and exercise-induced ketosis can prove dangerous if necessary precautions and actions are not taken in advance to prevent them. The risk-to-benefit ratio also worsens with prolonged exercise at higher intensities during which metabolic demand is increased and good metabolic control becomes even more important.

Although exercise-associated complications become more prominent during sustained exercise conditions (exercise training) and even more so at higher intensities, it is important that personnel involved with physical function assessment in people with diabetes have a good knowledge and understanding of the disease-specific characteristics and their potential interactions with exercise metabolism.

THE ROLE OF PHYSICAL FUNCTION ASSESSMENT

Assessment of physical function in patients with diabetes is recommended when the patients express an interest in participating in moderate or high-intensity exercise training or when information of clinical significance is required by the care team (gas exchange indices, cardiac function, angina and peripheral arterial disease pain thresholds, exercise chronotropic response, peak HR and BP or derived indices, etc.). In both cases it is advised that a fully integrated graded exercise testing protocol is executed (12 lead ECG, gas exchange, BP monitoring and ratings of perceived exertion, angina and breathlessness on relevant scales). Autonomic and peripheral neuropathy and CV disease is prevalent amongst people with diabetes (Albright *et al.*, 2000; Diabetes UK, 2004; Wilson *et al.*, 2005). Manifestations of the earlier include evidence of silent cardiac ischaemia, other cardiac rhythm abnormalities and abnormal BP responses to metabolic stress (Albright *et al*, 2000; Diabetes UK, 2004; Wilson *et al.*, 2005). Therefore, proper evaluation of these factors is necessary to ensure safety of training and accurate risk factor profile development. Physical function testing is also useful in evaluating effectiveness of medical or dietary interventions.

The choice of exercise modality (treadmill or cycle ergometer) will be influenced by the presence of factors such as severe peripheral neuropathy with or without loss of sensation, foot ulcers or balance problems, peripheral arterial disease and other orthopaedic limitations. All the aforementioned conditions may limit the ability of patients to perform treadmill exercise and therefore cause early cessation of the test before meaningful physiological stress has been achieved. Cycle ergometry may be more suitable for people with a cluster of conditions. On the other hand, cycling exercise may be perceived as more physically stressful due to the more localised muscular effort and for some obese individuals it may be extremely uncomfortable to sustain.

A variety of standard and customised graded exercise protocols have been used to assess the exercise tolerance of patients with diabetes (Regensteiner *et al.*, 1998; Wei *et al.*, 2000; Maiorana *et al.*, 2002). However, it is generally recommended that, in people with chronic disease and impaired physical capacity, baseline exercise assessment should employ a ramp incremental protocol with increments of $10-15\,W{\cdot}min^{-1}$. If the physical function status of the patient is good at baseline and diabetes does not co-exist with other serious medical conditions, increments of $20-25\,W{\cdot}min^{-1}$ may be used in either a step or ramp fashion. For those individuals who do not produce insulin at all, or are insulin deficient, it is recommended that the total testing time does not exceed 20–30 min of continuous exercise including warm-up and cool-down times.

In terms of functional capacity testing modes and protocols, there are no disease-specific guidelines and therefore interested readers can choose any tests from those recommended for people with cardiovascular disease or other metabolic diseases (e.g. renal failure). As a rule all general guidelines for the conduct of physical function assessments and test termination in people with chronic disease also apply to diabetes. (Specific guidelines are provided in Tables 20.1 and 20.3 in Chapter 20. Currently, there is no available published information about the reproducibility or validity of physical function assessments in patients with diabetes. This lack of information constitutes a gap in the diabetic physical function literature. Given this lack of information, clinical exercise specialists are advised to use reproducibility information derived from studies performed in CV disease and renal failure. Disease-specific guidelines do, however, exist for pre- and post-exercise precautions and safety measures and it would be prudent to consider these when scheduling physical function assessments for this patient population. Failure to comply with these guidelines may result in adverse consequences which, at the extreme, can be life threatening.

PRE-PHYSICAL FUNCTION ASSESSMENT CONSIDERATIONS

1 *Take detailed medical history*. Identification of co-existing conditions is important to help make a decision about the appropriate type of testing modality

and exercise protocol. For example if retinopathy is present, sub-maximal exercise testing or simple functional capacity tests should be considered instead of peak exercise tolerance tests, in order to avoid excessive increases in BP responses. Near maximal isometric contractions and prolonged weight lifting tests are also best avoided. In cases of severe autonomic dysfunction, and in the presence of postural hypotension, physical function tests that require rapid changes in body position (climbing stairs, sit to stand tests) should be avoided.

2   *If available, consider blood biochemistry and in particular glucose and glycosylated haemoglobin (HbA$_{1C}$).* Diabetes rarely exists in isolation. Renal dysfunction or even failure, cardiomyopathies and heart failure co-exist in the vast majority of diabetic patients resulting in abnormal blood biochemistry values and fluid retention. Patients should be tested for glucose levels and only allowed to perform exercise if blood glucose is within a safe range (5.5–11.1 mmol·l^{-1} or 100–200 mg·dl^{-1}). If blood glucose is low patients should be advised to consume a high-carbohydrate beverage and blood glucose should be reassessed after 15–20 min. If blood glucose is more than 12–13 mmol·l^{-1} exercise testing should be abandoned. The physical function assessment team should be aware that especially long-standing diabetic patients may not present with any symptoms of hypoglycaemia or may not realise them early enough. Hypoglycaemic symptoms include hunger, weakness, dizziness, sweating, confusion, headaches and trembling.

3   *Obtain detailed information about dosage and timing of administration of medications (primary to glucose control and secondary to diabetic complications).* The main concern regarding timing of administration and dosage of insulin and all other oral glucose control agents, is that when taken so that the peak effect of their action coincides with exercise, the risk of hypoglycaemic episodes is significantly increased (Dube *et al.*, 2005). It is advisable, therefore, to avoid exercise testing and strenuous exercise participation at such times. Detailed information about the 'peak times' for several types of insulin and oral hypoglycaemic agents is provided by Hornsby and Albright (2003). To further minimise the hypoglycaemic effect of insulin, patients should be advised in advance to alter the dose of insulin depending on the exercise protocol (Dube *et al.*, 2005) or inject insulin into predominantly 'non-exercising' muscles. Although the risk of exercise-induced hypoglycaemia is associated primarily with type 1 diabetes, hypoglycaemic episodes are also observed in type 2 diabetes. The likelihood of such an episode is, however, minimal during most commonly used exercise testing protocols.

Secondary medications to control diabetic complications are also commonly prescribed. Such medications include antihypertensives, lipid lowering agents or medications to promote weight loss, medications for pain management and diuretics. In general, exercise testing should be performed with the patient taking their usual medication unless there are instructions and a particular reason for the opposite. Repeat testing should also be performed at the same time of day if possible, following exactly the same pattern and timing of medication uptake and food intake as the original test.

CONSIDERATIONS DURING PHYSICAL FUNCTION ASSESSMENT

1   It is essential when performing maximal exercise tests to monitor vital signs including blood pressure (BP), heart rate (HR) and preferably the electro-cardiogram (ECG) (either a 3–5 lead ECG for basic rhythm recognition or a full 12 lead ECG). Patients with severe cardiovascular autonomic disturbance quite often experience abnormal responses in BP and HR regulation during exercise, which can result in loss of consciousness. Pallor, failure to respond normally (either by eye contact or verbally) and/or a sudden inability to maintain pedal cadence/walking speed, are indications for immediate cessation of exercise and prompt initiation of treatment to restore cerebral perfusion and oxygenation (e.g. laying the patient down and raising the legs ± administration of high-flow oxygen).

2   Assessment of glucose level during testing procedures will be beneficial.

3   Patients should be instructed to avoid Valsalva manoeuvere especially during muscular assessment when there may be a tendency towards breath-holding. This is especially relevant in patients with retinopathy, hypertension and autonomic dysfunction.

POST-PHYSICAL FUNCTION TESTING CONSIDERATIONS

1   *Active recovery* of at least 5 min duration with minimal or no resistance (depending on the patient's fitness level) should be incorporated in the graded exercise testing protocol. After the active recovery period the patient should recover in the sitting position for at least 15–20 min or until cardiovascular values have returned to, or near to, pre-exercise levels. Blood glucose levels should also be monitored immediately after exercise and just before the patient leaves the assessment area to ensure that they are within safe limits for the patient.

2   *Late onset-hypoglycaemic episodes* are possible for up to 12–15 h following the cessation of exercise. Late onset post-exercise hypogly-caemia is related to increased glycogen store repletion in muscle and liver. Such episodes are associated mostly with intense and prolonged exercise but can also occur following physical function assessments, especially those that require patients to perform a battery of tests within a discrete time period. If such assessment days are scheduled, as is often the case in clinical trials, adequate recovery time should be programmed between tests. Sessions could be arranged in such a way as to ensure that more demanding tests are interspersed with less-strenuous assessments such as anthropometric measurement or questionnaires. Also, patients should be encouraged to have a light meal (depending on the type and intensity of assessments) and to continue self-monitoring of blood glucose levels once they return home.

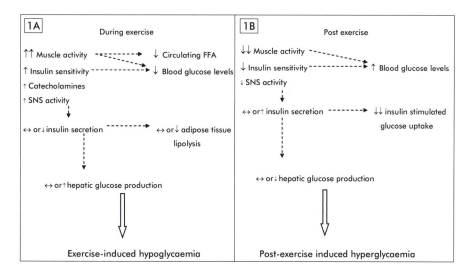

Figure 16.1 Simplified schematic representation of exercise-induced hypoglycaemia and post-exercise-induced hyperglycaemia in type 1 diabetes and in people with long-standing insulin deficiency. Broken arrows indicate causal relationships. In people with diabetes the hormonal and sympathetic nervous system response during exercise is impaired and therefore the overall effect on insulin levels adjustment is diminished (small arrows). This lack of coordinated response results is an imbalance between hepatic glucose production and glucose use

3   *Hyperglycaemic episodes* can also occur especially in people who suffer from type 1 diabetes. Immediately post-exercise glucose levels have been observed to be higher in people with diabetes compared to healthy individuals and remain higher for longer (Sigal *et al.*, 1994). A normal response to cessation of intense exercise (e.g. maximal exercise test) is an increase in insulin that inhibits the increased hepatic glucose production. The latter, combined with enhanced post-exercise muscle glucose uptake, result in regulation of glucose within normal limits. In diabetes on the other hand, due to a lack or absence of physiological insulin variability, this effect is minimised and glucose levels remain elevated (see Figure 16.1(B)) (Sigal *et al.*, 1994; Horton, 1999; Marliss and Vranic, 2002). In this case patients should be advised to self-monitor their glucose levels after they get home and avoid any carbohydrate-rich beverages or foods until glucose levels fall to within their usual range (usually within 2–3 h).

CONCLUSION

Exercise-related metabolism is a very finely tuned process that requires co-ordinated responses from many physiological systems. In diabetes the insulin-like effect of exercise can be beneficial as well as potentially dangerous. Although risks associated with physical function assessment under properly supervised and controlled conditions are minimal, health care professionals and exercise physiologists involved with physical function assessment need to have a good understanding of exercise-related pathophysiology and knowledge of specific techniques to prevent adverse side effects.

Prevention starts with educating and advising patients on how to best control glucose levels and to learn to identify symptoms indicative of poor diabetic control. The conduct of an effective and safe physical function assessment is built on the platform of the detailed clinical evaluation of the patient's health status in order to estimate the risk to benefit ratio of performing physical function testing. Subsequently, testing modalities and protocols should be chosen so as to best suit the patient's clinical picture, capabilities and fitness level. If all reasonable safety steps have been taken and explained to patients then they can feel reassured and able to give their best during physical function assessment.

REFERENCES

Albright, A., Franz, M., Hornsby, G., Kriska, A., Marrero, D., Ullrich, I. and Verity, L.S. (2000). American College of Sports Medicine. Position stand. Exercise and type 2 diabetes. *Medicine and Science in Sports and Exercice*, 32: 1345–1360.

American Diabetes Association. (2004a). Diagnosis and classification of diabetes mellitus. *Diabetes Care*, 27(S1): S5–S10.

American Diabetes Association. (2004b). Standards of medical care in diabetes. *Diabetes Care*, 27(S1): S58–S62.

American Diabetes Association. (2004c). Physical activity/exercise and diabetes. *Diabetes Care*, 27(S1): S58–S62.

Diabetes UK. A report From Diabetes UK 2004. Available from: http://www.diabetes. org.uk/catalogue/reports.htm.

Dube, M.C., Weisnagel, S.J., Prud'homme, D. and Lavoie, C. (2005). Exercise and new insulins. How much to avoid hypoglycaemia? *Medicine and Science in Sports and Exercise*, 37(8): 1276–1282.

Hornsby, W.G. and Albright, A.L. (2003). Diabetes. In J.L. Durstine and G.E. Moore, (eds), *ACSM's Exercise Management for Persons with Chronic Diseases and Disabilities*, 2nd edn. Champaign, IL: Human Kinetics.

Horton, E.S. (1999). Diabetes mellitus. In W.R. Frontera, D.M. Dawson and D.M. Slovik, (ed.), *Exercise in Rehabilitation Medicine*. Champaign, IL: Human Kinetics.

Ivy, J.L., Zderic, T.W. and Fogt, D.L. (1999). Prevention and treatment of non-insulin dependent diabetes mellitus. *Exercise and Sports Sciences Reviews*, 27: 2–35.

Marliss, E.B. and Vranic, M. (2002). Intense exercise has unique effects on both insulin release and its roles in glucoregulation implications for diabetes. *Diabetes*, 51: S271–S283.

Maiorana, A., O'Driscoll, G., Goodman, C., Taylor, R. and Green, D. (2002). Combined aerobic and resistance exercise improves glycemic control and fitness in type 2 diabetes. *Diabetes Research and Clinical Practice*, 56: 115–123.

Regensteiner J.G., Bauer, T.A., Reusch, J.E.B., Brandenburg, S.L., Sippel, J.M., Vogelsong, A.M., Smith S., Wolfel, E.E, Eckel, R.H. and Hiatt, W.R. (1998). Abnormal oxygen uptake kinetic responses in women with type 2 diabetes mellitus. *Journal of Applied Physiology*, 85: 310–317.

Sigal, R.J., Purdon, C., Fisher, S.J., Halter, J.B., Vranic, M. and Marliss, E.B. (1994). Hyperinsulinemia prevents prolonged hyperglycemia after intense exercise in insulin-dependent diabetic subjects. *Journal of Clinical Endocrinology and Metabolism*, 79: 1049–1057.

Sigal, R.J., Kenny, G.P., Wasserman, D.H. and Castaneda-Sceppa, C. (2004). Physical activity/exercise and type 2 Diabetes. *Diabetes Care*, 27(10): 2518–2539.

Verity, L.S. (2005). Diabetes mellitus and exercise. In L.A. Cminsky, K.A. Bonzheim, C.E. Garber, S.C. Glass, L.F. Hamm, H.W and Kohl, A.Mikesky (ed.) G.E. Garber *et al.* (ed.), *ACSM's Resource Manual for Guidelines and Exercise Testing and Prescription*. Baltimore, MD: Lippincott Williams & Wilkins.

Wei, M., Gibbons, L.W., Kambert, J.B., Nichaman, M.Z. and Blair S.N. (2000). Low cardiorespiratory fitness and physical inactivity as predictors of mortality in men with type 2 diabetes. *Annals of Internal Medicine*, 132: 605–611.

Wilson, P.W., D'Agostino, R.B., Parise, H., Sullivan, L. and Meigs, J.B. (2005). Metabolic syndrome as a precursor of cardiovascular disease and type 2 diabetes mellitus. *Circulation*, 112(20): 3066–3072.

CHAPTER 17

CARDIAC DISORDERS

*Keith George, Paul D. Bromley and
Gregory P. Whyte*

INTRODUCTION

Cardiac, or more broadly cardiovascular (CV), disease provides one of the biggest challenges to exercise and health professionals in the United Kingdom and worldwide. This is primarily due to the scale of the problem as well as the diversity and complexity of the diseases. It is well known that CV diseases are the most common pathology in 'Western' societies accounting for 238,000 deaths in 2002 in the United Kingdom. About 50% of these deaths were due to coronary heart disease (British Heart Foundation, 2004). CV diseases constitute a huge medical burden to the NHS as most diseases are progressive and impose a life-long burden of intervention and treatment that require the investment of time, labour, drug therapy and other broader cost implications.

The umbrella term of CV disease is an oversimplification of an exceptionally diverse set of pathologies that is often simply represented by coronary heart disease. It should be recognised that any disease of the central or peripheral circulation is covered in such a term (e.g. coronary artery disease, chronic heart failure, as well as a host of congenital diseases). All CV diseases are complex and this chapter cannot do all of them full justice. In the current chapter we have chosen to present some basic information related to central CV diseases with the next chapter providing some insight on peripheral CV diseases.

One increasingly common intervention to aid prevention and improve treatment of CV diseases is the promotion of physical activity (Thomas *et al.*, 2003). A structured approach when attempting to increase levels of physical activity generally begins with the assessment of aspects of CV health (structure and function) as well as the determination of an individual's maximal or symptom limited CV performance capacity via an exercise test. The knowledge of CV health and physical performance capabilities are then used as a source of information that will shape a host of processes including risk stratification and exercise prescription. This, and the next, chapter cannot cover all variables and tests associated with CV disease patients, therefore the current chapter will cover two aspects of the assessment of CV health and performance capacity. First, we will detail and briefly discuss various methods that can be used in the assessment of a variety of CV variables (e.g. heart rate, cardiac output). Second, a range of exercise tests that have been employed to assess or estimate CV performance capacity will be reviewed. In this section we wish to move on from just a standard graded exercise tolerance test (e.g. Corra *et al.*, 2004) and detail other methods of assessment of CV performance capacity that may include tests that are sub-maximal in nature and/or may be functionally relevant (e.g. Olsson *et al.*, 2005). The next chapter will follow this general organisation with specific respect to peripheral CV diseases.

CARDIOVASCULAR VARIABLE ASSESSMENT

Heart rate and electrical conduction

One of the simplest CV parameters to assess is heart rate; normally recorded as the number of complete cardiac cycles (or beats) per minute. We often assess resting heart as well as exercise heart rates. Care, of course, must be taken with heart rate interpretation in CV disease patients who may be taking medications with a chronotropic effect (e.g. beta blockers).

Heart rate is normally assessed by palpation, short-range telemetry or an electrocardiogram (ECG). Heart rate assessment via palpation can occur at any superficial artery but is commonly measured at the carotid or radial arteries. This is a simple method that is invaluable in the field or laboratory setting. Care must be taken to avoid palpating with the thumb as it often has its own strong pulse that can be mistaken for the pulse of the subject at rest. Care must also be taken not to apply too much pressure when palpating the carotid artery because of the proximity of the carotid bodies. Only one carotid artery should be palpated at a time as there is a risk of collapse if both carotid arteries are simultaneously occluded. Second, heart rate can be displayed via short-range telemetry involving an electrical sensing system on the chest wall and a receiving/display unit often worn as a wristwatch. The system detects electrical peaks (R wave of the ECG) and then displays a heart rate that is normally averaged over a few seconds. Such devices are quite flexible and can often store data for downloading after exercise. These systems are considered to be very accurate and are in common use in exercise physiology laboratories, gymnasiums, sports clubs and rehabilitation units.

The most common method of heart rate assessment in clinical practice is the ECG (see Figure 17.1). An ECG requires a number of electrodes to be placed at specific sites on the chest wall that can generate a range of electrical traces that represent different 'views' of the overall electrical activity of all the cardiomyocytes.

A basic understanding of ECG nomenclature and waveforms is crucial even to the assessment of something as simple as heart rate. It is essential to manually check the heart rate display on ECG machines (check paper speed and count squares between adjacent R waves). This is especially important if the

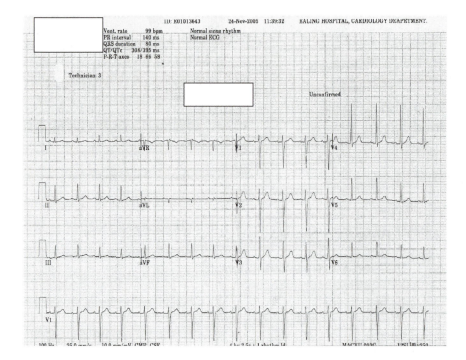

Figure 17.1   An exemplar '12-lead' ECG

rhythm is irregular. The PQRST nomenclature of the standard ECG represents the normal pattern of electrical conduction through the heart as viewed from lead II in a standard 12-lead configuration. This conduction pathway begins at the Sino-Atrial (SA) node, passes across the atria (which produces the P wave) to the Atrio-Ventricular (AV) node (junction) where the signal passes through specialised fibres that slow the signal conduction (bundle of His; and results in the delay between P and R waves) on through the left and right bundle branches and ending at the Purkinje fibres (which produce the QRS complex). The T wave represents ventricular repolarisation with atrial repolarisation occurring within the QRS complex. The passage of electrical depolarisation along this pathway results in sinus rhythm and normal cardiac function.

The cardiac cycle at rest lasts ~0.8 s reflecting a normal resting heart rate of c.70 beats·min^{-1}. During exercise, heart rate rises in parallel with exercise intensity associated with a number of neural and hormonal changes. Maximal heart rate in normally healthy individuals is commonly associated with age (max HR ≈220-age) although the exact equation is still debated and contains significant individual variability.

Arrhythmias (sometimes termed dysrhythmias) are abnormal heart rhythms associated with abnormalities in the electrical conduction system and are common in a range of CV diseases. Arrhythmias often result in sub-optimal cardiac function and can, of course, significantly impact upon the assessment of heart rate. Extensive ECG interpretation is beyond the scope of this text and lies within clinical boundaries. We would urge those with a real and strong interest in this area to consult appropriate texts (e.g. Wagner, 2001) and seek out appropriate clinically supervised training.

Stroke volume and cardiac output

Cardiac output is defined as the volume of blood ejected from the ventricle, per unit time. In adult humans, cardiac output ranges from 4 to 7 $l \cdot min^{-1}$ at rest and can achieve a three-to six-fold increase during intense exercise. A more restricted range of outputs is seen in the diseased heart, making the assessment of cardiac output a useful diagnostic indicator. Cardiac output can be simply described by:

$$\dot{Q}T = SV \cdot f_c$$

where SV = stroke volume in ml·beat and f_c = the frequency of cardiac cycles, or heart rate, in beats·min^{-1}.

Measurement of cardiac output during exercise presents a difficult challenge to exercise scientists. Measurements need to be applied rapidly and with ease if accurate measurements are to be taken. The method used should be capable of detecting beat-to-beat changes in cardiac output.

Invasive methods

Generally considered the standard for the determination of cardiac output, the direct Fick method requires the estimation of whole body oxygen uptake from expired air measurements and the sampling of arterial and mixed venous blood, via catheterisation, for oxygen concentration. The risks associated with catheterisation as well as the slow response (only valid in steady-state exercise) make it generally unsuitable for use during heavy exercise.

Indicator dilution techniques use an indirect Fick method where the substance to be measured, a metabolically inert dye or radioiodine labelled albumin, is injected as a bolus into the systemic circulation. The bolus becomes diluted in the returning venous blood and by taking arterial blood samples at frequent intervals the concentration of injectate in the arterial plasma can be plotted against time and cardiac output can be estimated as the area under the concentration–time curve.

It is now more common to use a thermodilution method, whereby a fixed volume of cold solution (e.g. NaCl, D5 W or autologous blood) is injected into the right atrium and the change in blood temperature (dilution) is measured continuously by a thermistor mounted on a pulmonary artery catheter. Cardiac output is determined from the area under the temperature–time curve. Both indicator dilution and thermal dilution methods can be used with acceptable accuracy during exercise, with error reported to be less than ±5%.

Non-invasive methods

Blood flow velocity can be computed from either continuous-wave or pulsed-wave Doppler echocardiography. Measurements are taken in the left ventricular outflow tract (apical position) or the ascending aorta (suprasternal position). Evaluation of the flow–velocity time curve for each cardiac cycle provides a measure of blood flow, which when allied to an M-mode estimation of aortic cross-sectional area is equivalent to stroke volume and hence can be used to estimate cardiac output. Stroke volume is calculated as:

$$SV = CSA \cdot FVI$$

where CSA = aortic cross-sectional area at the site of velocity measurement in cm^2 and FVI = flow – velocity integral or stroke distance in cm.

The non-invasive nature and speed of this method provide advantages over other methods but it does suffer from limitations of calibration and noise. The major limitation of the use of Doppler in the accurate assessment of cardiac output is that of aliasing which is of particular concern when measuring cardiac output during or immediately following vigorous exercise. Accuracy of the method during exercise may be as low as $\pm 44\%$ (Coats, 1990). Thus, Doppler methods offer a safe but only moderately reproducible and accurate method for measuring cardiac output.

Impedance cardiography relies on a direct correlation between blood flow through a body segment and the changes in bioimpedance across that segment to estimate SV and thus cardiac output. Simply stated, the increase in blood volume and velocity in the aorta during ventricular systole causes a decrease in bioimpedance that can be detected by electrodes placed at either end of the thoracic cavity. In this way SV can be estimated from the Sramek equation (Sramek *et al.*, 1983):

$$SV = VEPT \cdot VET \cdot [EVI/TFI]$$

where VEPT = physical volume of electrically participating tissue in ml, VET = the ventricular ejection time in s, EVI = ejection velocity index in $\Omega \cdot s^{-1}$ and TFI = thoracic fluid index [the total bioimpedance between the sensing electrodes] in Ω.

Belardinelli *et al.* (1996) found no significant differences in cardiac output values determined by impedance cardiography, thermodilution, and direct Fick methods at rest and over a wide range of exercise workloads. Agreement between the methods was between 0.01 and 0.04 $l \cdot min^{-1}$ at rest and between 0.2 and 0.5 $l \cdot min^{-1}$ at peak exercise (≈ 80–$140\,W$). The method may become less reliable at higher intensities ($\sim 180\,W$) of exercise (Moore *et al.*, 1992).

Gas exchange methods are a common non-invasive technique for the estimation of cardiac output. The rate of uptake or excretion of physiological gasses (e.g. O_2, CO_2) or inert soluble gasses (e.g. acetylene, nitrous oxide, Freon), determined from analysis of alveolar gas exchange, can be used to estimate pulmonary capillary blood flow ($\dot{Q}_c$) without the need for blood sampling. The most commonly used gas exchange technique is the CO_2 rebreathing method. Rebreathing a gas mixture containing CO_2 is well tolerated by both trained and untrained subjects. The rebreathing method employs an indirect Fick principle such that:

$$\dot{Q}_c = \frac{\dot{V}_{CO_2}}{C\,\bar{V}_{CO_2} - Ca_{CO_2}}$$

Instead of measuring the concentrations of CO_2 in arterial blood, Ca_{CO_2} is estimated by measuring the partial pressure of CO_2 (P_{CO_2}) in alveolar gas and converting it to the equivalent arterial gas concentration with the use of a CO_2 dissociation curve. PCO_2 can be easily converted to C_{CO_2} provided pH and oxyhaemoglobin concentration are known or are unchanged during the measurement (McHardy, 1967). Modern metabolic analysis systems perform this computation automatically. Estimation of $C\bar{V}_{CO_2}$ is somewhat more challenging and is achieved by measuring the PCO_2 of expired air during a rebreathing manoeuvre.

The two methods of the CO_2 rebreathing technique commonly employed use either an equilibrium technique (Collier, 1956) or an exponential technique (Defares, 1958). In the equilibrium method, rebreathing a CO_2 mixture reverses the normal $P\bar{V}_{CO_2} - Pa_{CO_2}$ concentration gradient bringing the expired CO_2 measurement into equilibrium with that in the blood passing through the pulmonary circulation. In the exponential method, the subject rebreathes a gas mixture with an initial CO_2 concentration of 5% and a volume at least equal to the subject's tidal volume (V_T). Estimation of $P\bar{V}_{CO_2}$ is achieved by plotting a best-fit line through a series of end-tidal CO_2 (PET_{CO_2}) data points.

Carbon dioxide rebreathing procedures have been shown to provide acceptable levels of accuracy and precision in the estimation of $\dot{Q}T$ during steady-state exercise (Reybrouk et al., 1978). Indeed, both accuracy (Mahler et al., 1985) and reliability (Nugent et al., 1994) appear to improve during exercise. Measurements during non-steady-state exercise have, however, produced mixed results and further investigation of the technique is necessary before its accuracy can be confirmed.

Cardiovascular structures

A vast number of cardiac structures have been assessed in clinical practice using a broad array of techniques. In this chapter we limit our discussion primarily to left ventricular assessment. Likewise, we have limited the brief description of techniques to the most common clinical imaging technique: ultrasound (echocardiography) as well as providing some reference to radionuclide angiography and magnetic resonance imaging (MRI).

Clinical assessment of cardiac structures advanced significantly with the practical application of ultrasound imaging that became widespread in the 1970s. Initially with M-mode (see Figure 17.2) and subsequently with 2-D and 3-D sector echocardiography, clinicians were able to differentiate and measure

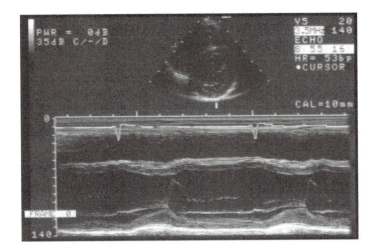

Figure 17.2   An example of an M-mode echocardiogram across the left ventricle

parameters such as LV volume at end-diastole and end-systole, LV wall thickness and LV mass. From these measurements came the ability to estimate some functional variables such as stroke volume and ejection fraction. Other structural variables that can be assessed include some aspects of the major vessels leading to and from the chambers of the heart. In newer machines, with better resolution, portions of the cardiac arterial tree can be imaged. There are a number of studies that have demonstrated good validity for ultrasound measures (e.g. Devereux and Reichek, 1977) when compared with autopsy studies and both intra- and inter-tester reliability is acceptable in the hands of a skilled technician (Stefadouros and Canedo, 1977) working with standard imaging and measurement guidelines (e.g. Schiller *et al.*, 1989).

Radionuclide techniques (e.g. radionuclide angiography) include a range of tests/procedures that utilise radioactive 'agents' that are injected into the subject, as a contrast medium for viewing cardiac chambers and arterial lumens when scanning. A common use of radionuclide testing is to examine the coronary arteries in suspected coronary artery disease. Other uses have included the assessment of global left ventricular function in health, exercise and sporting contexts (e.g. Spina *et al.*, 1993). Whilst highly accurate (e.g. Borges-Neto *et al.*, 1997) it has some limitations with the most accurate data for LV function gathered from 'multiple-pass' scanning that restricts its use within exercise interventions to steady-state (often in the supine position). MRI is a powerful tool for assessing CV structures and function. The combination of a magnetic field with radiofrequency energy produces images of cardiovascular tissues that reflect their different hydrogen (mainly water content), thus providing clear tissue differentiation. The resolution and clarity of images are better than other techniques (Bottini *et al.*, 1995) and no harmful effects of the testing have been documented. Cost, technical and clinical requirements are such that both radionuclide techniques and MRI are likely to remain a clinical and/or research tool.

EXERCISE TESTING IN CARDIAC DISORDERS

Congenital, inherited and acquired heart disease

Heart disease can be broadly categorised into three main groups: congenital, inherited and acquired. The term 'congenital' refers to an inborn (existing at birth) defect affecting the heart and proximal blood vessels. A list of common congenital cardiovascular defects can be found in Table 17.1. Congenital cardiovascular defects are present in about 1% of live births and represent the most common congenital malformations in newborns. The majority of congenital cardiovascular diseases obstruct blood flow in the heart or proximal vessels, or cause an abnormal pattern of blood flow through the heart. The natural history of congenital CV defects is not fully understood. Amongst the possible candidates for causative factors are heredity, viral infections (e.g. rubella), certain conditions affecting multiple organs (e.g. Down's syndrome), some prescription drugs and over-the-counter medicines, as well as alcohol and 'street' drugs.

The term 'inherited' refers to diseases that have a genetic origin and are often familial (i.e. diseases that run in families). The inherited heart diseases are disorders of the DNA code (known as 'mutations') of specific genes.

Table 17.1   Common congenital cardiovascular defects

Aortic Stenosis (AS)

Atrial Septal Defect (ASD)

Atrioventricular (AV) Canal Defect

Bicuspid Aortic Valve

Coarctation of the Aorta

Ebstein's Anomaly

Eisenmenger's Complex

Hypoplastic Left Heart Syndrome

Patent Ductus Arteriosus (PDA)

Anomalous Coronary Arteries

Pulmonary Stenosis

Pulmonary Atresia

Subaortic Stenosis

Tetralogy of Fallot

Total anomalous pulmonary venous (P-V) Connection

Transposition of the Great Vessels

Tricupsid Atresia

Truncus Arteriosus

Ventricular Septal Defect (VSD)

Table 17.2 Common inherited cardiovascular diseases

Hypertrophic Cardiomyopathy (HCM)
Arrhythmogenic Right Ventricular Cardiomyopathy (ARVC)
Dilated Cardiomyopathy (DCM)
The ionchannelopathies (Long QT, Brugadas)
Marfans Syndrome (not strictly a cardiac disease but does have cardiac/cardiovascular implications)

The process of inheritance depends upon whether the gene is dominant or recessive and the number of affected siblings in a family will depend upon the penetrance and the chromosome within which the abnormal gene resides. Inherited heart diseases are present at birth, however, the genotype is not always expressed in the phenotype, and thus some inherited heart diseases may not be termed 'congenital'. A list of common inherited cardiovascular diseases can be found in Table 17.2.

Acquired heart disease covers a broad spectrum of CV diseases that can be attributable to lifestyle and environment (although some genetic component may be present) and develop over a more prolonged period of time. Specifically these diseases, such as coronary artery disease, are not present at birth and normally manifest themselves in mid-to later-life. We now possess a degree of knowledge related to the development of acquired heart disease as well as some of the key risk factors including hypertension, hyperlipidaemia, physical inactivity, obesity, smoking and excess alcohol consumption. Because of their prevalence and their impact upon lifestyle, socio-economics and morbidity/mortality statistics, such diseases are at the core of the health-related roles now fulfilled by appropriately trained sport and exercise scientists.

Exercise testing in congenital, genetic and acquired heart disease

Careful consideration regarding the nature of the underlying disease is crucial in the safe management of exercise testing and exercise prescription in all patients with heart disease. Specific concerns in congenital and genetic heart disease are related to the variety of structural and/or functional alterations of the heart or proximal vessels and an abnormal cardiovascular response to exercise is expected. The abnormalities associated with congenital and genetic heart diseases, as well as the problems related to acquired heart diseases, affect the electrical conduction through the heart, the functional capacity of the heart and the function of the peripheral vasculature. In all patients with cardiac disease the impact of drug therapy on exercise tolerance and physiological response to exercise should be considered; particularly those associated with chronotropic and inotropic function. Further, exercise stress testing in morbidly sedentary patients may not yield maximum values for various physiological parameters. The use of gas exchange response during testing in these patients may be a valuable addition in the diagnosis of the condition, evaluation of exercise capacity and prescription of exercise (Graham *et al.*, 1994; Whyte *et al.*, 1999; Lainchbury and Richards, 2002). Contraindications to exercise should be carefully evaluated and, given the increased potential for adverse outcome, particularly during maximal exercise testing, appropriate steps should be taken to avoid incidents including modification of protocols and availability of appropriately trained personnel. Because of the range of observed abnormalities, integrated cardiopulmonary stress testing including simultaneous 12-Lead ECG, blood pressure and gas exchange during and post-exercise is recommended in most cases for hospital-based clinical assessment.

The normal exercise test employed in the clinical environment in patients with, or suspected of having, CV disease is the integrated cardiopulmonary stress test. The importance of such a test in both determining the presence of significant heart disease, and specifically coronary artery disease, is not in doubt (Whaley *et al.*, 2005). Further, in patients with known heart disease such tests are useful for assessing functional tolerance (e.g. anginal thresholds), progress of rehabilitation, influence of drug administration and other important issues. It is normal for the GXT test to be treadmill-based, for the greatest cardiovascular work, and be continuous with exercise intensity progression achieved by staged changes in speed, incline or both. Other clinical laboratory-based tests may use stepping protocols or cycling protocols but the treadmill test remains the 'gold standard'.

Tests of exercise capacity or tolerance are often determined outside of the clinical laboratory (e.g. phase III and IV cardiac rehabilitation in gyms, exercise physiology laboratories) and thus come more within the direct remit of sport and exercise scientists. Over the last 10 years significant interest has arisen in tests of functional capacity that more closely reflect activities of daily living. Most interest and activity has surrounded the use of a variety of walking tests and these have been used to assess functional capacity or to predict clinical outcomes and events (e.g. Girish *et al.*, 2001) and have included protocols such as walks for time, walks for distance and shuttle walks. Walking tests have been used in a variety of heart disease populations including patients with pacemakers (Payne and Skehan, 1996), heart failure (Delahaye *et al.*, 1997) and coronary artery disease (Gayda *et al.*, 2003). The research evidence generally points to the utility of walking-based exercise tests. For example, in heart failure patients a shuttle walk test accurately predicted event free survival at one year (Morales *et al.*, 2000) as well as predicting $\dot{V}O_{2peak}$ (Morales *et al.*, 1999). Payne and Skehan (1996) concluded that 'the shuttle walk is easy to administer, requiring little equipment...that produces a symptom limited maximal performance'. Green *et al.* (2001) provided evidence to support the reliability of the shuttle walk test as well as describing a closer relationship between treadmill $\dot{V}O_{2peak}$ and distance ambulated in the shuttle walk test than with the 6-min walk test. More recent research has validated the 20-m shuttle walk test in patients with coronary artery disease where maximal walking pace was not to different maximal treadmill speed (Gayda *et al.*, 2003). There are now a number of valid and reliable exercise test alternatives to a maximal treadmill test that may be used, with appropriate considerations for the patient and the disease, in a broader range of exercise settings.

SUMMARY OF KNOWLEDGE AND FUTURE DIRECTIONS

When working with clinical populations it is always important to know where the boundaries of our roles and competencies lie with respect to the patient, the disease and the tests employed. It is likely that our work in these scenarios will broaden alongside important developments in our understanding of CV diseases and their prevention, detection and treatment. It is incumbent on the sport and exercise scientist to be familiar with an ever-changing literature base related to CV disease. Specifically, we should also endeavour to keep abreast of new literature related to new methods of assessment as well as data pertaining to the accuracy and quality of any estimated or measured variables.

REFERENCES

Belardinelli, R., Ciampani, N., Costantini, C., Blandini, A. and Purcaro, A. (1996). Comparison of impedance cardiography with thermodilution and direct Fick methods for non-invasive measurement of stroke volume and cardiac output during incremental exercise in patients with ischemic cardiomyopathy. *American Journal of Cardiology*, 77: 1293–1301.

Borges-Neto, S., Shaw, L.J., Kesler, K., Sell, T., Peterson, E.D., Coleman, R.E. and Jones, R.H. (1997). Usefulness of serial radionuclide angiography in predicting cardiac death after coronary artery bypass grafting and comparison with clinical and cardiac catheterization data. *American Journal of Cardiology*, 79: 851–855.

Bottini, P., Carr, A., Prisant, L., Flickinger, F., Allison, J. and Gottdiener, J. (1995). Magnetic resonance imaging compared to echocardiography to assess left ventricular mass in the hypertensive patient. *American Journal of Hypertension*, 8: 221–228.

British Heart Foundation (2004). *Coronary Heart Disease Statistics: Factsheet*. Oxford, UK: British Heart Foundation.

Coats, A.J. (1990). Doppler ultrasonic measurement of cardiac output: reproducibility and validation. *European Heart Journal*, 11 (Suppl. I): 49–61.

Collier, C.R. (1956). Determination of mixed venous CO_2 tensions by rebreathing. *Journal of Applied Physiology*, 9: 25–29.

Corra, U., Mezzani, A., Bosimini, E. and Giannuzzi, P. (2004). Cardiopulmonary exercise testing and prognosis in chronic heart failure: a prognosticating algorithm for the individual patient. *Chest*, 126: 942–950.

Defares, J.G. (1958). Determination of $PvCO_2$ from the exponential CO_2 rise during rebreathing. *Journal of Applied Physiology*, 13: 159–164.

Delahaye, N., Cohen-Solal, A., Faraggi, M., Czitrom, D., Foult, J.M., Doau, D., Peker, C., Gourgou, R. and Le Guludec, D. (1997). Comparison of the left ventricular responses to the six minute walk test, stair climbing and maximal upright bicycle exercise in patients with congestive heart failure due to idiopathic dilated cardiomyopathy. *American Journal of Cardiology*, 80: 65–70.

Dent, J. (2003). Congenital heart disease and exercise. *Clinics in Sports Medicine*, 22: 81–99.

Devereux, R.B. and Reichek, N. (1977). Echocardiographic determination of left ventricular mass in man: anatomic validation of the method. *Circulation*, 55: 613.

Gayda, M., Choquet, D., Temfemo, A. and Ahmaidi, S. (2003). Cardiorespiratory fitness and functional capacity assessed by the 20-meter shuttle walking test in patients with coronary artery disease. *Archives in Physical Medicine and Rehabilitation*, 84: 1012–1016.

Girish, M., Trayner, E. Jr., Dammann, O., Pinto-Plata, V. and Celli, B. (2001). Symptom-limited stair climbing as a predictor of postoperative cardiopulmonary complications after high risk surgery. *Chest*, 120: 1147–1151.

Graham, T. Jr, Bricker, J., James, F. and Strong, W. (1994). 26th Bethesda conference: recommendations for determining eligibility for competition in athletes with cardiovascular abnormalities. Task Force 1: congenital heart disease. *Journal of the American College Cardiology*, 24: 867–873.

Green, D.J., Watts, K., Rankin, S., Wong, P. and O'Driscoll, J.G. (2001). A comparison of the shuttle and 6 minute walking tests with measured peak oxygen consumption in patients with heart failure. *Journal of Science and Medicine in Sports*, 4: 292–300.

Jones, N.L., McHardy, G.J., Naimark, A. and Campbell, E.J. (1966). Physiological dead space and alveolar-arterial gas pressure differences during exercise. *Clinical Science*, 34: 19–29.

Lainchbury, J. and Richards, A. (2002). Exercise testing in the assessment of chronic congestive heart failure. *Heart*, 88: 538–543.

Mahler, D.A., Matthay, R.A., Snyder, P.E., Neff, R.K. and Loke, J. (1985). Determination of cardiac output at rest and during exercise by carbon dioxide rebreathing method in obstructive airway disease. *American Review of Respiratory Disease*, 131: 73–78.

Maron, B., Mitchell, J., Isner, J. and McKenna, W. (1994). 26th Bethesda conference: recommendations for determining eligibility for competition in athletes with cardiovascular abnormalities. *Journal of the American College Cardiology*, 24: 880–885.

McHardy, G.J.R. (1967). The relationship between the differences in pressure and content of carbon dioxide in arterial and venous blood. *Clinical Science*, 32: 299–309.

Moore, R., Sansores, R., Guimond, V. and Abboud, R. (1992). Evaluation of cardiac output by thoracic electrical bioimpedance during exercise in normal subjects. *Chest*, 102: 448–455.

Morales, F.J., Martinez, A., Mendez, M., Agarrado, A., Ortega, F., Fernandez-Guerra, J., Montemayor, T. and Burgos, J. (1999). A shuttle walk test for the assessment of functional capacity in chronic heart failure. *American Heart Journal*, 138: 291–298.

Morales, F.J., Montemayor, T. and Martinez, A. (2000). Shuttle vs. six-minute walk test in the prediction of outcome in chronic heart failure. *International Journal of Cardiology*, 76: 101–105.

Nugent, A.M., McParland, J., McEneaney, D.J., Steele, I., Campbell, N.P., Stanford, C.F. and Nicholls, D.P. (1994). Non-invasive measurement of cardiac output by a carbon dioxide rebreathing method at rest and during exercise. *European Heart Journal*, 15: 361–368.

Olsson, L.G., Swedberg, K., Clark, A.L., Witte, K.K. and Cleland, J.G. (2005). Six minute corridor walk test as an outcome measure for the assessment of treatment in randomized, blinded, intervention trials of chronic heart failure: a systematic review. *European Heart Journal*, 26: 778–793.

Payne, G.E. and Skehan, J.D. (1996). Shuttle walking test: a new approach for evaluating patients with pacemakers. *Heart*, 75: 414–418.

Reybrouck, T., Amery, A., Billiet, L., Fagard, R. and Stijns, H. (1978). Comparison of cardiac output determined by a carbon dioxide-rebreathing and direct Fick method at rest and during exercise. *Clinical Science and Molecular Medicine*, 55: 445–452.

Schiller, N.B., Shah, P.M., Crawford, M., DeMaria, A., Devereux, R., Feigenbaum, H., Gutgesell, H., Reichek, N., Sahn, D. and Schnittger, I. (1989). Recommendations for quantitation of the left ventricle by two-dimensional echocardiography. American Society of Echocardiography Committee on Standards, Subcommittee on

Quantitation of Two-Dimensional Echocardiograms. *Journal of American Society of Echocardiography*, 2: 358–367.

Spina, R.J., Ogawa, T., Kohrt, W.M., Martin, W.H. III, Holloszy, J.O. and Ehsani, A.A. (1993). Differences in cardiovascular adaptations to endurance exercise training between older men and women. *Journal of Applied Physiology*, 75: 849–855.

Sramek, B.B., Rose, D.M. and Miyamoto, A. (1983). Stroke volume equation with a linear base impedance model and its accuracy, as compared to thermodilution and electromagnetic flow meter techniques in animals and humans. *Proceedings of the Sixth International Conference on Electrical Bioimpedance*, Zadar, Yugoslavia.

Stefadouros, M.A. and Canedo, M.I. (1977). Reproducibility of echocardiographic estimates of left ventricular dimensions. *British Heart Journal*, 39: 390–398.

Thaulow, E. and Fredriksen, P. (2004). Exercise and training in adults with congenital heart disease. *International Journal of Cardiology*, 97 (Suppl. 1): 35–38.

Thomas, N.E., Baker, J.S. and Davies, B. (2003). Established and recently identified coronary heart disease risk factors in young people: the influence of physical activity and physical fitness. *Sports Medicine*, 33: 633–650.

Wagner, G.S. (2001). *Marriott's Practical Electrocardiography*, 10th edn. Philadelphia, PA: Lippincott Williams and Wilkins.

Whaley, M.H., Brubaker, P.H and Otto, R.M. (2005). ACSM's Guidelines for Exercise Testing and Prescription, 7th edn. Philadelphi, PA: Lippincott Williams and Wilkins.

Whyte, G., George, K., Sharma, S. and McKenna, W.J. (1999). Exercise gas exchange response in the differentiation of physiologic and pathologic left ventricular hypertrophy. *Medicine and Science in Sports and Exercise*, 31: 1237–1241.

CHAPTER 18

PERIPHERAL CIRCULATORY DISORDERS

John M. Saxton and Nigel T. Cable

INTRODUCTION

Impaired functioning of the vascular endothelium and decreased peripheral vasodilatory capacity are observed in many age-related cardiovascular conditions, including hypertension (Panza *et al.*, 1990), coronary artery disease (Thanyasiri *et al.*, 2005), congestive heart failure (Zelis *et al.*, 1968) and peripheral arterial disease (PAD) (Sanada *et al.*, 2005), as well as in individuals with increased risk of cardiovascular disease (Creager *et al.*, 1990; Celermajer *et al.*, 1994; Al Suwaidi *et al.*, 2001). In the United Kingdom, the number of people aged 65 and over is expected to increase at 10 times the overall rate of population growth in the next 40 years (Dean, 2003), which means that the prevalence of age-related cardiovascular disorders and their sequelae can be expected to increase. Techniques which can detect impairment of peripheral blood flow, and monitor the progression of impairment in disease states or underpinning mechanisms of symptomatic improvement following interventions in patient groups or 'at-risk' populations, are useful tools for exercise scientists working in health-related areas or clinical settings.

This chapter begins with a section on blood pressure measurement, which is normally measured in the brachial artery, though in patients with PAD it is also measured at sites in the lower limb. Given that mean arterial pressure (MAP) is the product of cardiac output ($\dot{Q}_T$) and total peripheral resistance (TPR) (MAP = $\dot{Q}_T \times$ TPR), the assessment of arterial pressure provides an overall index of cardiovascular function and a linkage between the measurement of central (cardiac output) and peripheral circulations (peripheral blood flow). The chapter then provides an overview of useful physiological techniques for assessing peripheral blood flow and skeletal muscle oxygenation, before concluding with a section on assessment of exercise capacity in patients with impaired lower-limb arterial function.

ARTERIAL BLOOD PRESSURE MEASUREMENT

Arterial blood pressure (systolic and diastolic) is most accurately measured in the major arteries using rapidly responding pressure transducers. Fortunately, values measured using this invasive technique can be estimated with acceptable accuracy using the indirect technique of auscultation. This technique requires the use of a sphygmomanometer and stethoscope, and is dependent upon the observer detecting the characteristic Korotkoff sounds that are produced following occlusion of the circulation to the forearm (Cable, 2001). When resting environmental conditions and measurement protocol are standardised, this indirect method gives reliable estimations of blood pressures, particularly when used by experienced personnel. In addition, this technique can be used during static and dynamic exercise in steady-state conditions. Indeed, when used to predict mean arterial pressure (diastolic pressure + 1/3 (systolic − diastolic pressure)), this technique has been shown to provide a good estimation of blood pressure measured directly in the brachial artery during exercise (MacDougall *et al.*, 1999). Under resting or recovery conditions, blood pressure can also be indirectly measured using various automated systems (e.g. Dinamap Vital Signs Monitor, Criticom).

More advanced beat to beat indirect assessment of arterial pressure is achieved with photoplethysmographic techniques using systems such as FINAPRES (Ohmeda, USA) or PORTAPRES (TNO, Netherlands). These systems estimate systolic, diastolic and mean arterial pressures in the digital artery of the finger and have been shown to accurately measure (weighted accuracy, -1.6 ± 8.5 mmHg (see Imholz *et al.*, 1998)) changes in blood pressure in response to various interventions (such as psychological stress or orthostasis). In addition, the latter system, through the use of mathematical modelling of the pressure waveform, can estimate stroke volume and hence give a measurement of $\dot{Q}_T$ and TPR. This assessment has been compared with echocardiographic assessment of $\dot{Q}_T$ and found to accurately determine the degree of change in $\dot{Q}_T$ during orthostasis, and the technique is reliable during submaximal exercise.

Lower-limb arterial blood pressure measurement in peripheral arterial disease

Overview of peripheral arterial disease

The PAD mainly affects the arteries of the lower limbs. Although the condition is usually caused by atherosclerotic occlusion, it can also reflect the presence of other diseases such as arteritis, aneurysm and embolism. The disease can be unilateral or bilateral and is characterised by lesions within the aorto-iliac and/or femoropopliteal arterial segments. Intermittent claudication is the most common symptomatic manifestation of mild to moderate PAD, with an annual incidence of 2% in people over 65 years of age (Kannel and McGee, 1985). This is the cramp-like pain felt in the calf, thigh or buttock regions during walking, when the arterial oxygen supply is insufficient to meet an increased metabolic demand of the active skeletal muscles (Regensteiner and Hiatt, 1995).

Diagnosis of PAD is established through the patient's history, physical examination and confirmed by Doppler assessment of the ankle to brachial pressure index (ABPI). This is defined as the ratio of systolic blood pressure measured in the ankle region to that measured at the level of the brachial artery. In the vascular laboratory, analyses of Doppler spectra can provide further information about disease severity, where non-invasive pressure measurements alone are insensitive (Evans *et al.*, 1989). Other techniques such as duplex scanning, magnetic resonance imaging, computer tomography and digital subtraction angiography are also useful for the collection of anatomical and functional data, but tend to be used for the anatomical localisation of arterial disease before surgical intervention, rather than for initial diagnosis (Norman *et al.*, 2004).

Assessment of the ankle to brachial pressure index

Patients should rest for 10 min in the testing position (supine or recumbent, but with consistency of body position between repeated assessments). Measurement sites need to be prepared by the application of electro-conductive gel. In the arm, a hand-held 5-MHZ Doppler probe is placed over the brachial artery and at the ankle, over the posterior tibial and dorsalis pedis artery. The posterior tibial artery can be palpated behind the medial malleolus and the dorsalis pedis artery can be palpated between the first and second metatarsal bones, approximately half way down the dorsum of the foot. Appropriately sized blood pressure cuffs are positioned over the brachial artery and above each malleolus. For measurement, the cuff is quickly inflated to 20 mmHg above estimated systolic blood pressure, before being deflated at a rate of 2–3 mm·s^{-1} and the first audible systolic blood pressure at each site recorded.

The ABPI is determined for each leg by dividing the averaged systolic pressures from the posterior tibial and dorsalis pedis arteries by the averaged

Table 18.1 Interpretation of ABPI results

ABPI	Interpretation
1.0–1.1	Normal ABPI
0.9–0.99	Borderline PAD, requires an exercise test/ further investigation for confirmation
<0.9	Characteristic of PAD
Severity of disease	
0.7–0.89	Mild to moderate PAD (asymptomatic or intermittent claudication)
0.4–0.69	Moderate to severe PAD (intermittent claudication or rest pain)
<0.4	Severe PAD (intermittent claudication and rest pain more likely)

systolic pressure measured at the level of the brachial artery (left and right). There is evidence of a stronger association between ABPI and lower-extremity function when ABPI is calculated using averaged values in this way (McDermott *et al.*, 2000; McDermott *et al.*, 2002). However, if the brachial pressure between the left and right arms differs by at least 10 mmHg, upper extremity arterial stenosis is suspected and the higher of the two values is used to calculate ABPI. Furthermore, a pulse may not be detectable at both ankle sites in some patients with more severe disease pathology, and in such cases, a single measure of posterior tibial or dorsalis pedis pressure is acceptable (Table 18.1).

PERIPHERAL BLOOD FLOW AND SKELETAL MUSCLE OXYGENATION

Peripheral blood flow measurement

Blood flow in the peripheral circulation (usually the forearm or calf) can be measured non-invasively using the techniques of venous occlusion plethysmography and laser Doppler flowmetry. Venous occlusion plethysmography impedes venous outflow from the limb (using a pressure cuff inflated to 50 mmHg) for a period of 10 s (repeated over a number of cycles). Arterial inflow into the limb is not impeded, hence expanding the volume of the limb, which is detected as a change in limb circumference by a strain gauge located about the widest part of the limb. The change in circumference is directly proportional to arterial blood flow. This technique measures whole limb blood flow, which is a product of both muscle and skin blood flow. Blood flow through the skin can be directly measured using laser Doppler flowmetry. This technique uses a beam of laser-generated monochromatic light to measure the movement of red blood cells 2–3 mm under the skin surface and operates on the principle that the frequency shift of laser light reflected from the skin is linearly related to red blood cell flux and thus, tissue blood flow. The laser probes are small and therefore skin blood flow can be measured at any site.

Both techniques can be used to measure baseline (or resting) blood flow in the limb or skin, or more importantly maximum limb and skin blood flow. Maximum flow in both circulations can be induced by arterial occlusion (for 10 min) and local heating to 42°C respectively, and these manoeuvres give a direct indication of the structural capacity (i.e. the size and number of vessels in the circulation) for vasodilatation. Both these techniques can also be used to assess the integrity of the endothelium and smooth muscle to release and respond to vasoactive substances, respectively using invasive techniques of intra-brachial infusions or microdialysis or the non-invasive introduction of vasoactive substances using iontophoresis. Such techniques provide a valuable insight into the effects of various pathologies on decreases in peripheral blood flow due to an increase in resistance to flow or conversely, how exercise interventions can be used to improve flow to these circulations. When peripheral flow is measured in conjunction with blood pressure and reported as limb and skin vascular resistance (Resistance = Pressure/Flow) or limb and skin vascular conductance (Conductance = Flow/Pressure), further powerful indices of peripheral vascular function are provided.

Skeletal muscle oxygenation during exercise

Near infrared spectroscopy (NIRS) is a technique that has been developed in recent years that can be used to assess skeletal muscle oxygenation during exercise. A major advantage of this technique is the continuous and fast signals (real time) and the fact that it is non-invasive and easy to use. NIRS is based on the relative tissue transparency for light in the near infrared region and on the existence of five chromophores in biological tissues whose light absorbing properties vary with the level of oxygenation. These chromophores are oxy- and deoxyhaemoglobin, oxy- and deoxymyoglobin, and cytochrome oxidase. However, studies have shown that more than 90% of the signal is derived from haemoglobin (Seiyama et al., 1988). Furthermore, most of the haemoglobin signal is considered to come from the small tissue vessels because larger vessels (>1 mm in diameter) have high haem concentrations that absorb all the light (McCully et al., 2003), making changes in oxygen saturation undetectable.

A number of research studies have now used NIRS to assess changes in skeletal muscle oxygenation in clinical populations during walking (Komiyama et al., 1997; Kooijman et al., 1997; Egun et al., 2002; McCully et al., 2003) and other forms of exercise (McCully et al., 1997; Casavola et al., 1999). In patients with PAD, a relationship has been reported between the severity of claudication pain and the decline in calf muscle oxygen saturation during walking exercise (Komiyama et al., 2002). Other studies have shown that NIRS can be a reproducible and effective non-invasive method for assessing skeletal muscle oxygenation during exercise. In patients with PAD, Komiyama et al. (2000) reported an intraclass correlation coefficient (ICC) of 0.92 for time to recovery of muscle oxygenation after an incremental treadmill test (which is mainly dependent upon blood flow). In another study, an ICC of 0.99 was reported for an NIRS-derived measure of leg vessel conductance in cardiac patients, which was validated using a thermodilution technique (Watanabe et al., 2005). Thus, NIRS can be used to complement other techniques in the investigation of changes in peripheral circulation and skeletal muscle oxygenation after physical activity interventions or programmes of exercise rehabilitation.

TESTS OF EXERCISE CAPACITY IN PATIENTS WITH IMPAIRED LOWER-LIMB ARTERIAL FUNCTION

Treadmill walking protocols for patients with PAD

Resting ABPI is frequently a poor predictor of walking performance in patients with symptomatic PAD (Regensteiner and Hiatt, 1995), which means that monitoring ABPI alone is inadequate for assessing the impact of the disease on functional impairment. For this reason, walking performance is usually assessed using a standardised treadmill test. A variety of different testing protocols have been used, including constant-pace tests (e.g. slow constant speed of 2.4–3.2 km·h^{-1} and fixed grade of 8–12%) and graded or incremental protocols (e.g. slow constant speed of 3.2 km·h^{-1}, with gradient increasing 2% every 2 min). Treadmill testing is also used in the clinical setting to exceed the capacity of lower-limb collateral circulation in 5% of patients with PAD who have a normal resting ABPI, thereby helping to establish the diagnosis of exercise-induced leg pain (McDermott et al., 2002). After treadmill exercise, ABPI characteristically decreases in patients with PAD due to a decrease in systolic pressure at the ankle, relative to an increase in pressure proximal to the site of stenosis.

Following a Transatlantic conference on clinical trial guidelines in PAD (Labs et al., 1999), two internationally accepted treadmill protocols were recommended:

Constant-pace treadmill protocol   Constant walking speed of 3.2 km·h^{-1} at 12% gradient.

Graded (incremental) treadmill protocol   Starting horizontally at constant walking speed, but with the gradient increasing in pre-defined steps (e.g. 2%) at pre-defined time intervals (e.g. every 2 min).

Measured variables

The main measured variables in tests of walking performance are (1) distance or time to the onset of claudication pain (claudication distance, CD), and (2) maximum walking distance or time (MWD), at which point patients can no longer tolerate the claudication pain. Patients must report the onset of claudication pain verbally and CD is considered a less reliable walking performance measure than MWD, particularly in incremental treadmill tests (Hiatt et al., 1988; Gardner et al., 1991; Hiatt et al., 1995; Labs et al., 1999). To reduce measurement error, it is good practice to ensure that patients are fully accustomed to the testing procedures before assessment, as many elderly people are not familiar with treadmill walking. In addition, it is important to confirm that patients terminated the test due to intolerable claudication pain and not due to some other reason, for example, breathlessness or unrelated exercise pain due to co-morbidities that are common in this patient group.

Constant-pace vs. graded (incremental) treadmill protocols

Constant-pace tests are generally easier to administer and do not require a programmable treadmill. In addition, there is a larger historical database derived from constant-pace tests, as many of the earlier published studies used such protocols. However, incremental (graded) protocols have the advantage that they can be used to assess walking performance in more heterogeneous patient populations with wide-ranging walking abilities (Hiatt et al., 1995; Regensteiner and Hiatt, 1995). In addition, incremental protocols are likely to be more useful for re-assessing patients after a treatment intervention (in which an improvement is expected), as they do not exhibit the 'ceiling' effects which are more characteristic of constant-pace protocols. Incremental treadmill protocols are also considered to have higher test–retest reproducibility for MWD in comparison to constant-pace treadmill protocols (Hiatt *et al.*, 1995; Regensteiner and Hiatt, 1995; Labs *et al.*, 1999). Coefficients of variation (CVs) in the range of 30–45% for CD and MWD have been reported for constant-pace tests, in comparison to CVs of 15–25% for CD and 12–13% for MWD on incremental tests (Hiatt *et al.*, 1995).

Incremental shuttle-walk test

An alternative or complementary exercise testing modality to treadmill walking for assessing the effect of the disease or treatment intervention on functional capacity is the incremental shuttle-walk test (Zwierska *et al.*, 2004). Patients walk back and forth between two cones placed 10 m apart on a flat floor, at a pace that is controlled by audio tape bleeps. The initial walking speed for the incremental shuttle walk is 3 km·h^{-1} and at the end of each minute, the time interval between audible bleeps is decreased, resulting in a step-increase in walking speed of 0.5 km·h^{-1}. The accuracy of the timed bleep can be assured by inclusion of a 1 min calibration period at the beginning of the audio tape. This test has been shown to have similar test–retest reproducibility to standardised treadmill testing (Zwierska *et al.*, 2004) and performance is highly correlated with community-based measures of physical activity and physical function (Zwierska *et al.*, 2002). An intra-class correlation coefficient of 0.87 has been reported for MWD between repeated incremental shuttle-walk tests in patients with symptomatic PAD, which was similar to that observed for repeated standardised treadmill testing in the same patient group (Zwierska *et al.*, 2004).

Summary

Exercise rehabilitation can be a relatively inexpensive alternative or adjunctive treatment approach to pharmacological (or surgical) interventions in many cardiovascular conditions that affect peripheral vascular function and can have a clinically important impact on functional capacity and quality of life. Physiological adaptations resulting from exercise rehabilitation that can underpin improvements in physical function include peripheral blood flow adaptations, changes in blood rheology, altered nitric oxide metabolism and improved systemic endothelial vasoreactivity, which can all enhance blood flow to exercising skeletal muscles. With appropriate training, the techniques described in this chapter can be used to indirectly monitor changes in peripheral vascular function following exercise and/or lifestyle interventions in individuals at increased risk of developing cardiovascular disease or in patient groups. The techniques can also be used to assess the relative efficacy of different exercise training regimens for promoting positive changes in peripheral blood flow and skeletal muscle oxygenation.

REFERENCES

Al Suwaidi, J., Higano, S.T., Holmes, D.R. Jr, Lennon, R. and Lerman, A. (2001). Obesity is independently associated with coronary endothelial dysfunction in patients with normal or mildly diseased coronary arteries. *Journal of the American College of Cardiology*, 37: 1523–1528.

Cable, N.T. (2001). Cardiovascular function: In R. Eston and T. Reilly (eds), *Kinathropometry and Exercise Physiology Laboratory Manual: Tests, Procedures and Data*. London: Routledge.

Casavola, C., Paunescu, L.A., Fantini, S., Franceschini, M.A., Lugara, P.M. and Gratton, E. (1999). Application of near-infrared tissue oxymetry to the diagnosis of peripheral vascular disease. *Clinical Hemorheology and Microcirculation*, 21: 389–393.

Celermajer, D.S., Sorensen, K.E., Bull, C., Robinson, J. and Deanfield, J.E. (1994). Endothelium-dependent dilation in the systemic arteries of asymptomatic subjects relates to coronary risk factors and their interaction. *Journal of the American College of Cardiology*, 24: 1468–1474.

Creager, M.A., Cooke, J.P., Mendelsohn, M.E., Gallagher, S.J., Coleman, S.M., Loscalzo, J. and Dzau, V.J. (1990). Impaired vasodilation of forearm resistance vessels in hypercholesterolemic humans. *Journal of Clinical Investigation*, 86: 228–234.

Dean, M. (2003). Growing older in the 21st century: an ESRC research programme on extending quality of life. Economic and Social Research Council.

Egun, A., Farooq, V., Torella, F., Cowley, R., Thorniley, M.S. and McCollum, C.N. (2002). The severity of muscle ischemia during intermittent claudication. *Journal of Vascular Surgery*, 36: 89–93.

Evans, D.H., McDicken, W.N., Skidmore, R. and Woodcock, J.P. (1989). Doppler applications in the lower limb. In Evans, D.H. (ed.), *Doppler Ultrasound: Physics, Instrumentation, and Clinical Applications*, pp. 233–242. Chichester: John Wiley & Sons Ltd.

Gardner, A.W., Skinner, J.S., Cantwell, B.W. and Smith, L.K. (1991). Progressive vs single-stage treadmill tests for evaluation of claudication. *Medicine and Science in Sports and Exercise*, 23: 402–408.

Hiatt, W.R., Nawaz, S., Regensteiner, J.G. and Hossack, K.F. (1988). The evaluation of exercise performance in patients with peripheral vascular disease. *Journal of Cardiopulmonary Rehabilitation*, 12: 525–532.

Hiatt, W.R., Hirsch, A.T., Regensteiner, J.G. and Brass, E.P. (1995). Clinical trials for claudication: assessment of exercise performance, functional status and clinical end points. *Circulation*, 92: 614–621.

Imholz, B.P.M., Wieling, W., Langewouters, G.J. and van Montfrans, G.A. (1998). Continuous finger arterial pressure: utility in the cardiovascular laboratory. *Clinical Autonomic Research*, 1: 43–53.

Kannel, W.B. and McGee, D.L. (1985). Update on some epidemiologic features of intermittent claudication: the Framingham Study. *Journal of the American Geriatric Society*, 33: 13–18.

Komiyama, T., Shigematsu, H., Yasuhara, H. and Muto, T. (2000). Near-infrared spectroscopy grades and the severity of intermittent claudication in diabetics more accurately than ankle pressure measurement. *British Journal of Surgery*, 87: 459–466.

Komiyama, T., Onozuka, A., Miyata, T. and Shigematsu H. (2002). Oxygen saturation measurement of calf muscle during exercise in intermittent claudication. *European Journal of Vascular and Endovascular Surgery*, 23: 388–392.

Kooijman, H.M., Hopman, M.T., Colier, W.N., van der Vliet, J.A. and Oeseburg, B. (1997). Near infrared spectroscopy for noninvasive assessment of claudication. *Journal of Surgical Research*, 72: 1–7.

Labs, K.H., Dormandy, J.A., Jaeger, K.A., Stuerzebecher, C.S. and Hiatt, W.R. (1999). Transatlantic conference on clinical trial guidelines in peripheral arterial disease: clinical trial methodology. Basel PAD Clinical Trial Methodology Group. *Circulation*, 100: 75–81.

McCully, K.K. and Hamaoka, T. (2003). Near-infrared spectroscopy: what can it tell us about oxygen saturation in skeletal muscle? *Exercise and Sports Sciences Reviews*, 28: 123–127.

McCully, K.K., Halber, C. and Posner, J.D. (1994). Exercise-induced changes in oxygen saturation in the calf muscles of elderly subjects with peripheral vascular disease. *Journal of Gerontology*, 49: B128–B134.

McCully, K.K., Landsberg, L., Suarez, M., Hofmann, M. and Posner, J.D. (1997). Identification of peripheral vascular disease in elderly subjects using optical spectroscopy. *Journal of Gerontology Series A: Biological Sciences and Medical Sciences*, 52: B159–B165.

McDermott, M.M., Criqui, M.H., Liu, K., Guralnik, J.M., Greenland, P., Martin, G.J. and Pearce, W. (2000). Lower ankle/brachial index, as calculated by averaging the dorsalis pedis and posterior tibial arterial pressures, and association with leg functioning in peripheral arterial disease. *Journal of Vascular Surgery*, 32: 1164–1171.

McDermott, M.M., Greenland, P., Liu, K., Guralnik, J.M., Celic, L., Criqui, M.H., Chan, C., Martin, G.J., Schneider, J., Pearce, W.H., Taylor, L.M., and Clark, E. (2002). The ankle brachial index is associated with leg function and physical activity: the Walking and Leg Circulation Study. *Annals of Internal Medicine*, 136: 873–883.

MacDougall, J.D., Brittain, M., MacDonald, J.R., McKelvie, R.S., Moroz, D.E., Tarnopolosky, M.A. and Moroz, J.S. (1999). Validity of predicting mean arterial blood pressure during exercise. *Medicine and Science in Sports and Exercise*, 31: 1876–1879.

Norman, P.E., Eikelboom, J.W. and Hankey, G.J. (2004). Peripheral arterial disease: prognostic significance and prevention of atherothrombotic complications. *Medical Journal of Australia*, 181: 150–154.

Panza, J.A., Quyyumi, A.A., Brush, J.E. and Epstein, S.E. (1990). Abnormal endothelium-dependent vascular relaxation in patients with essential hypertension. *New England Journal of Medicine*, 323: 22–27.

Regensteiner, J.G. and Hiatt, W.R. (1995). Exercise rehabilitation for patients with peripheral arterial disease. *Exercise and Sport Science Reviews*, 23: 1–24.

Sanada, H., Higashi, Y., Goto, C., Chayama, K., Yoshizumi, M. and Sueda, T. (2005). Vascular function in patients with lower extremity peripheral arterial disease: a comparison of functions in upper and lower extremities. *Atherosclerosis*, 178: 179–185.

Seiyama, A., Hazeki, O. and Tamura, M. (1988). Noninvasive quantitative analysis of blood oxygenation in rat skeletal muscle. *Journal of Biochemistry (Tokyo)*, 103: 419–424.

Thanyasiri, P., Celermajer, D.S. and Adams, M.R. (2005). Endothelial dysfunction occurs in peripheral circulation patients with acute and stable coronary artery disease. *American Journal of Physiology*, 289: H513–H517.

Watanabe. S., Ishii, C., Takeyasu, N., Ajisaka, R., Nishina, H., Morimoto, T., Sakamoto, K., Eda, K., Ishiyama, M., Saito, T., Aihara, H., Arai, E., Toyama, M., Shintomi, Y. and Yamaguchi, I. (2005). Assessing muscle vasodilation using near-infrared spectroscopy in cardiac patients. *Circulation Journal*, 69: 802–814.

Zelis, R., Mason, D.T. and Braunwald, E. (1968). A comparison of the effects of vasodilator stimuli on peripheral resistance vessels in normal subjects and patients with congestive heart failure. *Journal of Clinical Investigation*, 47: 960–970.

Zwierska, I., Saxton, J.M., Male, J.S., Pockley, A.G. and Wood, R.F.M. (2002). Relationship between incremental shuttle-walk performance and community-based walking ability in elderly patients with peripheral arterial disease (abstract). *Journal of Sport Sciences*, 21: 339–340.

Zwierska, I., Nawaz, S., Walker, R.D., Wood, R.F., Pockley, A.G. and Saxton, J.M. (2004). Treadmill versus shuttle walk tests of walking ability in intermittent claudication. *Medicine and Science in Sports and Exercise*, 36: 1835–1840.

CHAPTER 19

CARDIOPULMONARY EXERCISE TESTING IN PATIENTS WITH VENTILATORY DISORDERS

Lee M. Romer

INTRODUCTION

Exercise intolerance in patients with chronic ventilatory disorders has important implications for quality of life (Ferrer *et al.*, 1997; Jones, 2001), morbidity (Kessler *et al.*, 1999; Garcia-Aymerich *et al.*, 2003) and mortality (Hiraga *et al.*, 2003; Oga *et al.*, 2003). Consequently, cardiopulmonary exercise testing is considered an essential component in the routine clinical assessment of these patients' functional status. The primary aims of this chapter are to describe the indications for cardiopulmonary exercise testing and to provide recommendations concerning methodology (e.g. exercise modality, protocols and measurements). An in-depth discussion of data interpretation is beyond the scope of this chapter, but the interested reader is directed towards a recent joint statement on cardiopulmonary exercise testing by the American Thoracic Society and the American College of Chest Physicians (ATS/ACCP, 2003). The following sections describe the general categories of ventilatory dysfunction and the health and economic burden of respiratory disease.

DEFINITIONS

There are two broad categories of ventilatory dysfunction: obstructive and restrictive. Obstructive ventilatory disorders include bronchial asthma and chronic obstructive pulmonary disease (COPD), which is the term used to describe patients with emphysema, chronic bronchitis or a mixture of the two. Obstructive disorders are characterised by low expiratory flow (e.g. forced expiratory volume in 1 s (FEV_1)) relative to age, sex and height predicted values. In COPD, the airway obstruction is due to airway and parenchymal damage, which results from chronic inflammation that differs from that seen in asthma and which is usually the result of tobacco smoke. In contrast to asthma, COPD is usually progressive, not fully reversible and does not change markedly over several months. Restrictive ventilatory disorders are those in which the expansion of the lung is restricted either because of alterations in the lung parenchyma (e.g. pulmonary fibrosis) or pleura (pneumothorax), or because of disorders of the respiratory pump (e.g. muscle weakness, chest deformities, rigidity of the thoracic cage, muscle and motor nerve disorders, and extreme obesity). Restrictive disorders are characterised by a reduced vital capacity, but the airway resistance is not increased. Although restrictive ventilatory disorders are different from the obstructive diseases in their pure form, mixed conditions can occur.

CLINICAL CONTEXT

Respiratory disease kills one in four people in the United Kingdom (British Thoracic Society (BTS), 2000). COPD is the third biggest cause of respiratory related death, and accounts for more than 5% of all deaths and 20% of all respiratory related deaths (pneumonia and cancers of the respiratory system account for ~43% and 23%, respectively) (BTS, 2000). The morbidity from respiratory disease is high: almost one-third (31%) of the population of England and Wales consult their GP for a respiratory condition at least once during the year (BTS, 2000) and up to 1 in 8 emergency hospital admissions is due to COPD (National Collaborating Centre for Chronic Conditions, 2004). The economic impact of ventilatory disorders is also substantial: ~28 million working days are lost each year and the total estimated annual cost to the National Health Service is £2,576 million (BTS, 2000).

INDICATIONS FOR CARDIOPULMONARY EXERCISE TESTING

The most important reasons for the exercise testing of pulmonary patients are to determine whether exercise tolerance is limited and to identify the source of the limitation. Occasionally, exercise tests can be diagnostic, for example, in exercise-induced asthma (see section on 'Constant Load Exercise Protocols' and chapter on 'Pulmonary Function Testing'). In general, however, the diagnostic value of exercise testing for pulmonary disease is not significantly better than other more traditional clinical assessments such as spirometry. Nevertheless, the results from an integrated exercise test can serve to define the specific organ system limiting exercise. Exercise testing can be helpful in predicting survival, guiding therapeutic strategy, determining appropriate exercise intensity domains for pulmonary rehabilitation, and evaluating the effectiveness of therapeutic interventions (e.g. mechanical ventilation, exercise training, respiratory muscle training, bronchodilators, etc.) on overall functional capacity and components of the exercise response (ATS/ACCP, 2003). Exercise testing is also useful in the pre-operative evaluation of risk for patients about to undergo lung cancer resectional surgery (Bolliger *et al.*, 1995), lung transplant surgery (Howard *et al.*, 1994) and lung volume reduction surgery (Fishman *et al.*, 2003). In practice, exercise testing in patients with pulmonary disease is usually considered when specific questions remain unanswered after an appropriate assessment of the patient by medical history, physical examination, chest radiograph, resting pulmonary function testing and electrocardiograph (ECG).

METHODS

The following sections describe the characteristics of several different exercise protocols. In general, the clinical question to be addressed and the resources available will dictate both the mode of exercise and the type of protocol to be used, as well as the variables to be considered in the interpretation of the test.

Exercise modality

A major aim of exercise testing is to assess the effect of intense physical stress on the various organ systems. Therefore, it is necessary to recruit large muscle groups, such as the lower extremities used during pedalling a cycle ergometer or walking/running on a motorised treadmill. Depending on the reasons for the exercise test and equipment availability, cycle ergometry is usually the preferred mode of exercise for patients with pulmonary disease (ATS/ACCP, 2003; European Respiratory Society (ERS), 1997). The main advantage of the cycle ergometer is that it provides a more accurate measure of the external work rate of the subject compared with treadmill exercise. Furthermore, the cycle ergometer is generally less expensive than the treadmill, less intimidating, safer, more easily mastered, less prone to movement or noise artefacts, and requires less space. However, the results from treadmill exercise are better applied to activities of daily living and there is a greater stress on the various organ systems, which may be important in the detection of coexisting disease (e.g. myocardial ischaemia). If the test results are used to prescribe subsequent exercise training it may be advantageous to use the same exercise modality in testing as for training. In general, arm ergometry should not be used in patients with COPD because the arm cranking interferes with the use of the inspiratory accessory muscles, which could result in significant symptoms and distress for the patient (Celli *et al.*, 1986).

Exercise protocols

Maximal incremental cycle ergometry

Maximal, symptom-limited incremental exercise tests are usually used to assess the physiological response of the patient to the entire range of exercise intensities in a short period of time. The exercise should last ~8–12 min, although durations outside this range produce only small differences in maximal physiological function (Buchfuhrer et al., 1983). Tests that are too short may not allow a sufficient quantity of data to be collected whereas tests that are too long might be terminated because of boredom or discomfort. Additional data should be collected during 3 min of rest, during 3 min of unloaded exercise (0 W) and during at least 2 min of active recovery. The work rate can be applied either in steps (e.g. every minute) or as a continuous ramp (see Figure 19.1). Similar metabolic and cardiopulmonary values are obtained from step and ramp protocols (Zhang et al., 1991). To achieve an exercise time of 8–12 min the incremental rate should be adjusted on an individual basis (typically between 5 and 25 W·min⁻¹). To determine the incremental rate (W·min⁻¹) necessary to elicit an individual's estimated $\dot{V}O_{2max}$ in ~10 min, the following equation is used:

$$\frac{\text{Estimated } \dot{V}O_{2max} - \text{Estimated } \dot{V}O_2 \text{ during unloaded cycling}}{100}$$

where estimated $\dot{V}O_{2max}$ in ml·min⁻¹ = (stature in cm − age in years) × 20 for sedentary men and × 14 for sedentary women; and estimated $\dot{V}O_2$ during unloaded cycling in ml·min⁻¹ = 150 + (6 × body mass in kg) (Wasserman et al., 2004). In practise, the incremental rate is selected after considering the patient's history, physical examination and pulmonary function. For example, if the patient has a forced expired volume in 1 s, a maximal voluntary ventilation or a lung diffusion capacity less than 80% of predicted, the estimated $\dot{V}O_{2max}$ would be reduced proportionally. If in doubt, it is better to overestimate the incremental rate, thereby if retesting is necessary the patient will recover quicker after a shorter test.

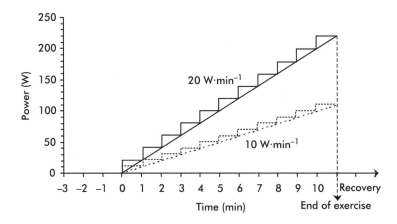

Figure 19.1 Graphical representation of standard incremental exercise protocols. Equivalent results are obtained when work rate is either increased continuously (ramp test) or by a uniform amount each minute (1-min incremental test) until the patient is limited by symptoms (he/she cannot cycle >40 rpm) or is unable to continue safely. The incremental rate of 10–20 W·min⁻¹ is set according to the characteristics of the patient in order to obtain ~10 min duration of the incremental part of the protocol
Source: Adapted from European Respiratory Society (1997)

In an attempt to enable a single test to be used for subjects with a range of fitness several exercise protocols have been developed (Northridge *et al.*, 1990; Riley *et al.*, 1992). In these protocols, which are suitable for either cycle ergometry or treadmill exercise, the work rate is increased exponentially by 15% of the previous workload every minute, resulting in a test that lasts less than about 15 min in fitter individuals and only a few minutes less in severely debilitated subjects. No clear advantage has been shown in the use of these exponential protocols over more conventional incremental protocols.

Maximal incremental treadmill exercise

Although cycle ergometry is the preferred modality for exercising patients with pulmonary disease (discussed earlier), treadmill exercise protocols have been used widely to assess the physiological responses to exercise in patients with ventilatory disorders. The modified Balke protocol is considered the most appropriate for use in patients with moderate to severe pulmonary disease (ERS, 1997; ATS/ACCP, 2003). With this protocol, treadmill gradient is increased progressively ($1–2\%\cdot\text{min}^{-1}$) while speed is kept constant ($5–6\text{ km}\cdot\text{h}^{-1}$). As mentioned previously, the standardised exponential exercise protocol can also be used with treadmills (Northridge *et al.*, 1990; Riley *et al.*, 1992).

Termination of maximal incremental exercise tests

The exercise intensity is reduced if the patient becomes distressed, if systolic or mean blood pressure fall by more than 10 mmHg from the highest value during the test, if a significant arrhythmia develops, if there is a 3 mm or greater ST segment depression, if the patient becomes limited by symptoms (e.g. loss of coordination, mental confusion, dizziness or faintness), or if the exercise cannot be continued safely. Where cycle ergometry is used, exercise is terminated if the patient is unable to maintain a pedal cadence above 40 rpm.

Constant-load exercise protocols

Constant-load tests are sometimes used to monitor physiological responses to a range of therapeutic interventions because the exercise intensity is usually selected to coincide with levels approximating the subject's usual daily activities. These constant-load protocols have been used to determine the dynamic behaviour of ventilatory and gas exchange indices. However, the utility of quantifying the dynamic responses to constant-load exercise in patients with respiratory disease remains to be established, primarily because there is limited information regarding normative values and reproducibility, and the predictive value of the derived parameters in specific patient populations is unclear (Roca and Rabinovich, 2005). Nevertheless, the extent of any increase of O_2 uptake between 3 and 6 min of constant-load exercise has been used to verify the workload associated with the lactate threshold (Casaburi *et al.*, 1989). Furthermore,

6 min of near-maximal, constant-load exercise with pre- and post-exercise measurements of FEV_1 and related parameters have been used to diagnose exercise-induced asthma, although alternative procedures may be more diagnostic (Anderson *et al.*, 2003; see also chapter on Pulmonary Function Testing).

Field exercise tests

In addition to laboratory exercise tests, complementary information regarding the functional capacity of a patient can be provided by incremental shuttle-walk tests (Revill *et al.*, 1999) and timed walk tests (Butland *et al.*, 1982). Timed walk tests provide information that is useful in predicting morbidity and mortality (Kessler *et al.*, 1999; Celli *et al.*, 2004) and they have an advantage over laboratory tests in that they better reflect the functional exercise level for daily physical activities. Furthermore, timed walk tests are sensitive to interventions such as supplemental O_2, inhaled bronchodilators, lung transplantation, lung resection, lung volume reduction surgery, whole-body exercise training and specific inspiratory muscle training (ATS, 2002).

The most widely validated and used field test in patients with pulmonary disease is the 6-min walk test (ATS, 2002). The aim of this test is for patients to walk as far as possible in 6 min over a 30 m course set up along a corridor or other flat terrain. Observations are made of distance covered, heart rate and, if available, arterial O_2 saturation via pulse oximetry. The distance covered during the 6-min walk test is reasonably reliable between-visits (coefficient of variation ~8%; ATS, 2002), although reliability may be improved further with at least one prior practise test (Sciurba *et al.*, 2003). For individual patients with COPD, an improvement of more than 70 m is required to be 95% confident of a clinically significant change (Redelmeier *et al.*, 1997; Sciurba *et al.*, 2003).

Measured variables

Primary measurements during laboratory exercise testing should include breath-by-breath ventilatory and pulmonary gas exchange, external work, heart rate and systemic arterial pressure. Arterial O_2 saturation (via pulse oximetry) and ECG should also be monitored continuously throughout the test. Perceptual ratings of dyspnoea (breathlessness) and limb discomfort should be assessed during the exercise and at the point when the patient discontinues exercise using standardised procedures (e.g. Borg's category ratio 10 scale or a visual analogue scale). After at least 2 min of recovery, the mouthpiece should be removed and the patient questioned about what symptoms caused them to stop exercise and whether the symptoms are the same as those experienced by the patient outside the laboratory.

The source and degree of ventilatory constraint can be determined by plotting exercise tidal flow-volume loops within the maximal flow-volume loop assessed immediately after exercise. Inspiratory capacity (IC) manoeuvres performed during exercise are used to place the spontaneous flow-volume loops within the maximal post-exercise loop. This procedure can also be used to calculate dynamic lung volumes (i.e. end-expiratory lung volume and end-inspiratory lung volume), which can be used to indicate the degree of dynamic lung hyperinflation that occurs with expiratory flow limitation (Johnson *et al.*, 1999). Assessment of dynamic hyperinflation is important in the context of obstructive ventilatory disorders because the associated change in end-expiratory lung volume correlates significantly with intensity of dyspnoea (O'Donnell and Webb, 1993).

Where pulmonary gas exchange abnormalities are suspected it is often necessary to evaluate directly the adequacy of gas exchange via arterial blood gases (ATS/ACCP, 2003). This procedure requires an arterial catheter to be placed, preferably into the radial artery because of the collateral circulation to the hand afforded by the ulnar artery in the event that the radial artery is blocked. For incremental exercise protocols, blood samples are taken at rest,

Table 19.1 Discriminating measurements during exercise in patients with obstructive and restrictive ventilatory disorders

Obstructive ventilatory disorders

Low peak $\dot{V}O_2$

Low breathing reserve

High heart rate reserve

High V_D/V_T

Increased $P(a - ET)CO_2$ during exercise

Usually high $P(A - a)O_2$

Increased O_2 cost of exercise

Failure to develop respiratory compensation for exercise metabolic acidosis

Decreased IC with exercise (air trapping)

Abnormal expiratory flow pattern

Restrictive ventilatory disorders

Low peak $\dot{V}O_2$

High V_T/IC

Breathing frequency >50 at max WR

Low breathing reserve

High V_D/V_T

High $P(a - ET)CO_2$

High $\dot{V}_E/\dot{V}CO_2$ @ LT

PaO_2 decreased and $P(A - a)O_2$ increases as WR is increased

$\Delta\dot{V}O_2/\Delta WR$ is reduced

Notes

V_D/V_T, physiological dead space/tidal volume ration; $P(a - ET)CO_2$, arterial-end tidal PCO_2 difference; $P(A - a)O_2$, alveolar-arterial PO_2 difference; IC, inspiratory capacity; V_T/IC, ratio between tidal volume and inspiratory capacity; WR, work rate; $\dot{V}_E/\dot{V}CO_2$ @ LT, ventilatory equivalent for CO_2 at lactate threshold; $\Delta\dot{V}O_2/\Delta WR$, increase in $\dot{V}O_2$ relative to increase in work rate

Source: Adapted from Wasserman *et al.* (2004)

at the end of unloaded pedalling, every 2 min during incremental exercise and at 2 min of recovery, for subsequent determination of PaO_2 and $PaCO_2$ and calculation of the alveolar-arterial difference for oxygen pressure $[P(A - a)O_2]$. The arterial catheter also enables data to be collected on acid–base status (i.e. pH, lactate concentration and base excess), arterial O_2 saturation (via co-oximetry) and intra-arterial blood pressure. Resting arterial blood samples should be obtained with the subject seated and off the mouthpiece to avoid breathing pattern effects induced by the mouthpiece. Although valid measurements of $PaCO_2$ and pH can be achieved using arterialised venous blood (e.g. from a heated dorsal hand vein), this is not the case for PaO_2 (Forster *et al.*, 1972). Pulse oximeters with optodes attached to an extremity (e.g. fingertip, earlobe or forehead) provide a reasonable estimate of arterial O_2 saturation during exercise, although the accuracy of these devices tends to decrease at levels below ~75% (Clark *et al.*, 1992). However, measurement of PaO_2 is usually more relevant in assessing the effects of lung disease on pulmonary gas exchange because the oxyhaemoglobin dissociation curve dictates that O_2 saturation is relatively insensitive to small changes in PaO_2. The discriminating measurements during exercise in patients with obstructive and restrictive ventilatory disorders are presented in Table 19.1.

REFERENCES

American Thoracic Society (ATS). (2002). ATS Statement: Guidelines for the six-minute walk test. *American Journal of Respiratory and Critical Care Medicine*, 166: 111–117.

American Thoracic Society/American College of Chest Physicians. (2003). ATS/ACCP statement on cardiopulmonary exercise testing. *American Journal of Respiratory and Critical Care Medicine*, 167: 211–277.

Anderson, S.D. and Brannan, J.D. (2003). Methods for 'indirect' challenge tests including exercise, eucapnic voluntary hyperpnea, and hypertonic aerosols. *Clinical Review of Allergy Immunology*, 24: 27–54.

Bolliger, C.T., Jordan, P., Soler, M., Stulz, P., Gradel, E., Skarvan, K., Elsasser, S., Gonon, M., Wyser, C. and Tamm, M. (1995). Exercise capacity as a predictor of postoperative complications in lung resection candidates. *American Journal of Respiratory and Critical Care Medicine*, 151: 1472–1480.

British Thoracic Society. (2000). The burden of lung disease. A statistics report from the British Thoracic Society. London, UK: Munro & Forster Communications.

Buchfuhrer, M.J., Hansen, J.E., Robinson, T.E., Sue, D.Y., Wasserman, K. and Whip B.J. (1983). Optimizing the exercise protocol for cardiopulmonary assessment. *Journal of Applied Physiology*, 55: 1558–1564.

Butland, R.J.A., Pang, J., Gross, E.R., Woodcock, A.A. and Geddes, D.M. (1982). Two-, six-, and 12-minute walking tests in respiratory disease. *British Medical Journal*, 284: 1607–1608.

Casburi, R., Wasserman, K., Patessio, A., Ioli, F., Zanaboni, S. and Donner, C.F. (1989). A new perspective in pulmonary rehabilitation; anaerobic threshold as a discriminant in training. *European Journal of Respiratory Disease*, 2: 618–623.

Celli, B.R., Rassulo, J. and Make, B.J. (1986). Dyssynchronous breathing during arm but not leg exercise in patients with chronic airflow obstruction. *New England Journal Medicine*, 314: 1485–1490.

Celli, B.R., Cote, C.G., Marin, J.M., Casanova, C., Montes de Oca, M., Mendez, R.A., Pinto Plata, V. and Cabral, H.J. (2004). The body-mass index, airflow obstruction, dyspnea, and exercise capacity index in chronic obstructive pulmonary disease. *New England Journal of Medicine*, 350: 1005–1012.

Clark, J.S., Votteri, B., Arriagno, R.L., Cheung, P., Eichhorn, J.H., Fallat, R.J., Lee, S.E., Newth, C.J.L. and Sue, D.Y. (1992). Noninvasive assessment of blood gases. *American Review of Respiratory Disease*, 145: 220–232.

European Respiratory Society. (1997). Clinical exercise testing with reference to lung diseases: indications, standardization and interpretation strategies. ERS task force on standardisation of clinical exercise testing. *European Respiratory Journal*, 10: 2662–2689.

Ferrer, M., Alonso, A., Morera, J., Morera, J., Marrades, R.M., Khalaf, A., Aguar, M.C., Plaza, V., Prieto, L. and Anto, J.M. (1997). Chronic obstructive pulmonary disease stage and health-related quality of life. The quality of life of chronic obstructive pulmonary disease study group. *Annals of Internal Medicine*, 127: 1072–1079.

Fishman, A., Martinez, F., Naunheim, K., Pianadosi, S., Wise, R., Ries, A., Weinmann Wood, D.E., National Emphysema Treatment Trial Research Group. 2003). A randomized trial comparing lung-volume-reduction surgery with medical therapy for severe emphysema. *New England Journal of Medicine*, 348: 2059–2073.

Forster, H.V., Dempsey, J.A., Thomson, J.A., Vidruk E. and DoPico, G.A. (1972). Estimation of arterial PO2, PCO2, pH, and lactate from arterialized venous blood. *Journal of Applied Physiology*, 32(1): 134–137.

Garcia-Aymerich, J., Farrero, E., Felez, M.A., Izquierdo, J., Marrades, R.M. and Anto, J.M. (2003). Risk factors of readmission to hospital for a COPD exacerbation: a prospective study. *Thorax*, 58: 100–105.

Hiraga, T., Maekura, R., Okuda, Y., Okamoto, T., Hirotani, A., Kitada, S., Yoshimura, K., Yokota, S., Ito, M. and Ogura, T. (2003). Prognostic predictors for survival in patients with COPD using cardiopulmonary exercise testing. *Clinical Physiology and Functional Imaging*, 23: 324–331.

Howard, D.K. Iademarco, E.J. and Trulock, E.P. (1994). The role of cardiopulmonary exercise testing in lung and heart-transplantation. *Clinical Chest Medicine*, 15: 405–420.

Johnson, B.D., Weisman, I.M., Zeballos, R.J. and Beck, K.C. (1999). Emerging concepts in the evaluation of ventilatory limitation during exercise: the exercise tidal flow-volume loop. *Chest*, 116: 488–503.

Jones, P.W. (2001). Health status measurement in chronic obstructive pulmonary disease. *Thorax*, 56: 880–997.

Kessler, R., Faller, M., Fourgaut, G., Mennecier, B. and Weitzenblum, E. (1999). Predictive factors of hospitalization for acute exacerbation in a series of 64 patients with chronic obstructive pulmonary disease. *American Journal of Respiratory and Critical Care Medicine*, 159: 158–164.

National Collaborating Centre for Chronic Conditions (2004). Chronic obstructive pulmonary disease. National clinical guideline on management of chronic obstructive pulmonary disease in adults in primary and secondary care. *Thorax*, 59(S1): 1–232.

Northridge, D.B., Grant, S., Ford, I., Christie, J., McLenachan, J., Connelly, D., McMurray, J., Ray, S., Henderson, E. and Dargie, H.J. (1990). Novel exercise protocol suitable for use on a treadmill or a bicycle ergometer. *British Heart Journal*, 64: 313–316.

O'Donnell, D.E. and Webb, K.A. (1993). Exertional breathlessness in patients with chronic airflow limitation. The role of lung hyperinflation. *American Review of Respiratory Disease*, 148: 1351–1357.

Oga, T., Nishimura, K., Tsukino, M., Sato, S. and Hajiro, T. (2003). Analysis of the factors related to mortality in chronic obstructive pulmonary disease. *American Journal of Respiratory and Critical Care Medicine*, 167: 544–549.

Redelmeier, D.A., Bayoumi, A.M., Goldstein, R.S. and Guyatt, G.H. (1997). Interpreting small differences in functional status: the six minute walk test in chronic lung disease patients. *American Journal of Respiratory and Critical Care Medicine*, 155: 1278–1282.

Revill, S.M., Morgan, M.D.L., Scott, S., Walters, D. and Hardman, A.E. (1999). The endurance shuttle walk: a new field test for the assessment of endurance capacity in chronic obstructive pulmonary disease. *Thorax*, 54: 213–222.

Riley, M., Northridge, D.B., Henderson, E., Stanford, C.F., Nicholls, D.P. and Dargie, H.J. (1992). The use of an exponential protocol for bicycle and treadmill exercise testing in patients with chronic cardiac failure. *European Heart Journal*, 13: 1363–1367.

Rocca, J. and Rabinovich, R. (2005). Clinical exercise testing. In E.F.M. Wouters (ed.), *Lung Function Testing, European Respiratory Mon*, 31: 146–165.

Sciurba, F., Criner, G.J., Lee, S.M., Mohsenifar, Z., Shade, D., Slivka, W., Wise, R.A; National Emphysema Treatment Trial Research Group. (2003). Six-minute walk distance in chronic obstructive pulmonary disease: reproducibility and effect of walking course layout and length. *American Journal of Respiratory and Critical Care Medicine*, 167: 1522–1527.

Wasserman, K., Hansen, J.E., Sue, D.Y., Stringer, W.W. and Whipp, B.J. (2004). Principles of exercise testing and interpretation (4th edn.), Media, PA: Lippincott, Williams and Wilkins.

Zhang, Y.Y., Johnson, M.C., Chow, N. and Wasserman, K. (1991). Effect of exercise testing protocol on parameters of aerobic function. *Medicine and Science in Sports and Exercise*, 23: 625–630.

CHAPTER 20

EXERCISE ASSESSMENT FOR PEOPLE WITH END-STAGE RENAL FAILURE

Pelagia Koufaki and Thomas H. Mercer

INTRODUCTION

Progressive loss of kidney function is often described as chronic kidney disease (CKD). CKD may progress to end-stage renal failure (ESRF), at which point the kidneys are not able to perform their regulatory and excretory functions. The transition into end-stage renal failure, with the concomitant derangement of normal biochemical, metabolic and endocrine functions, is almost always accompanied by the clinical syndrome of uraemia. Symptoms such as anorexia, generalised lethargy and fatigue, sleep disorder, neurological dysfunction, nausea and vomiting are frequently evident. The appearance of these symptoms is remarkably consistent and appears to coincide with abnormal plasma levels of many substances including urea, creatinine, phosphate and parathyroid hormone, which have been identified as potential uraemic toxins. Accompanying clinical signs of ESRF include fluid retention (peripheral and pulmonary oedema), raised blood pressure, diminishing haemoglobin levels and abnormal biochemistry (creatinine, serum urea and potassium) (Bommer, 1992; Moore, 2000).

The partial or complete loss of kidney function requires that some form of renal replacement therapy be initiated to maintain life. Renal replacement therapy refers to treatments that aim to remove excess fluid and waste products from the body (dialysis or kidney transplantation) and administration of drugs to supplement residual kidney functions, or manage the effects of lack of kidney functions (UK Renal Registry, 2002). Haemodialysis (HD) and continuous ambulatory peritoneal dialysis (PD) are the principal dialysis techniques commonly used. The former involves the removal of excess fluid and toxic solutes from the blood through a dialysis machine (artificial kidney). Peritoneal dialysis utilises the peritoneal cavity, and a permanently implanted catheter, as the means by which the exchange of toxic metabolic by-products and removal of excess waste is achieved. For details on the differences between dialysis techniques the interested reader may refer to the *Oxford Handbook of Dialysis*

(Levy *et al.*, 2004). The guidelines discussed in this chapter refer only to patients undergoing dialysis therapy.

PATHOPHYSIOLOGY AND PHYSICAL DYSFUNCTION IN END-STAGE RENAL FAILURE

Kidney disease is associated with multi-systemic dysfunction including abnormalities of the cardiovascular, endocrine-metabolic and musculoskeletal systems, electrolyte and acid–base imbalances, neurological, haematological and psychosocial disorders (Moore, 2000). Renal failure may result as a consequence of underlying and/or pre-existing conditions such as diabetes, arteriosclerotic renovascular disease, genetic defects or kidney infections. Conversely, established renal failure itself may precipitate the development of co-existing conditions including ischaemic heart disease, peripheral vascular disease and heart failure. This produces a complex pathophysiology for each individual patient with ESRF that will influence the choice of dialysis mode, may reduce the effectiveness of dialysis therapy and ultimately will dictate clinical outcome.

In addition to the restrictions imposed by the multi-systemic dysfunction and the dialysis treatment itself, patients with ESRF are commonly physically inactive and characterised by limited levels of physical functioning (Deligiannis *et al.*, 1999; Johansen *et al.*, 2000). As a result, patients with ESRF have significantly reduced levels of exercise capacity. Typically, mean VO_{2peak} is around $19\,ml\cdot kg^{-1}\cdot min^{-1}$ and ranges from 13 to $28\,ml\cdot kg^{-1}\cdot min^{-1}$. This corresponds to ~65% of values reported for age, gender and physical activity-matched healthy controls (Moore *et al.*, 1993; Kouidi *et al.*, 1998; Deligiannis *et al.*, 1999; Koufaki *et al.*, 2002). Objective measurement of functional capacity, using reliable and validated tests, reveals an even greater degree of impairment of ESRF patients in relation to activities of daily living. Deficits ranging from 20% to 120% have been observed, especially in the older dialysis population, indicating that the extent of functional impairment may be greatly underestimated if one relies only on physiological measures of peak exercise capacity (Naish *et al.*, 2000; Painter *et al.*, 2000).

Correlates and 'predictors' of physical function in ESRF include: sedentary life style, cardiovascular comorbidity, number of additional comorbidities, age, serum albumin, serum creatinine, dialysis dose, nutritional status, muscle atrophy, muscle strength, dialysis age, functional capacity, systemic inflammation (Moore *et al.*, 1993; Johansen *et al.*, 2001; Sietesema *et al.*, 2002; Johansen *et al.*, 2003). Whilst these observations confirm the multi-systemic effects of renal disease they also highlight the difficulties of establishing a single best approach to characterise physical dysfunction in these patients. Nonetheless, it is imperative that any safe and accurate assessment of physical function must be conducted within the context of appropriate risk factor stratification. This must take into account the patient's medical history, the prevailing clinical picture and their life style. The choice of the most informative and feasible method of functional assessment should then be reviewed on an individual

Table 20.1 Absolute and relative contraindications to exercise testing in patients with ESRF

Absolute	Relative
• Hyper/hypokalaemia	• History of angina
• Excess inter-dialytic weight gain	• Resting BP >180/100 or <100/60 mmHg
• Unstable on dialysis treatment and medication regime	• Sustained tachyarrhythmias or bradyarrhythmias
• Unstable BP	• Orthostatic BP drop of >20 mmHg with symptoms
• Pulmonary congestion	• Resting blood glucose of <5 or >10 mmol·l^{-1}
• Peripheral oedema	
• Unstable cardiac condition	
• Suspected or known aneurysm	
• Uncontrolled diabetes	
• Recent cerebrovascular event	
• Acute infections	

> Patients that present with relative contraindications may be exercise-tested only after the risk/benefit ratio has been evaluated and close monitoring of vital signs is in place

> The presence of qualified clinical staff is also required

basis, bearing in mind that for some patients exercise assessment will be contraindicated (see Table 20.1).

EXERCISE TOLERANCE ASSESSMENT

The specific choice and type of protocol for physical function assessment will mainly depend on the primary purpose of the assessment (diagnostic, exercise training prescription, risk stratification, etc.). The execution of comprehensive physiological exercise testing that includes measures of gas exchange, cardiac function, systemic blood pressure monitoring, and patients' subjective responses to general and specific discomfort (ratings of perceived exertion, angina and breathlessness scales) is considered to be the 'gold standard' of exercise capacity assessment for ambulatory patients on dialysis. Measures of VO_{2peak} and VO_2 at lactate threshold (LT) obtained during this type of test can be used to:

- establish physiological impairment and determine prognosis;
- categorise patients to different risk factor groups;
- evaluate the presence and severity of symptoms;
- identify potential life-threatening situations;
- determine safe and effective exercise rehabilitation intensities;
- evaluate responses to interventions.

Table 20.2   Special considerations for exercise testing of patients with ESRF

- Assessments are recommended to be performed on non-dialysis days and preferably not immediately after a weekend for haemodialysis patients, as this will be the longest interval without dialysis

- Peritoneal dialysis patients may find it easier to perform tests with their abdominal cavity empty of the dialysing fluid, as this may increase pressure on the diaphragm and result in more symptoms of breathlessness and chest discomfort

- The arm with the arterio-venous fistula should not be used for BP monitoring or strength assessment, as that will give erroneous readings, and may possibly damage the fistula

- A complete list of medication regime and doses should be obtained and reviewed before each test to ensure informed decisions in case of adverse medication–exercise interaction effects

It is vital that patients fully understand the procedures, reasons and possible 'side effects' associated with all tests and agree to execute them. It is also essential that patients are given adequate opportunity to be habituated to all protocols and equipment. Although all conventional guidelines for the conduct of graded exercise testing of people with chronic disease need to be applied some additional ESRF condition-specific pre-testing considerations are highlighted in Table 20.2. In particular, patients should always be tested 'on' their usual regime of medication unless indicated otherwise by their physician.

Peak exercise capacity

The most commonly reported measures of integrated cardiorespiratory exercise capacity in patients with ESRF are peak VO_2, peak heart rate, peak power output and time to exhaustion, obtained during incremental treadmill or cycle ergometer protocols (Moore *et al.*, 1993; Deligiannis *et al.*, 1999; Koufaki *et al.*, 2001). The clinical value of peak exercise capacity assessment for patients with ESRF is underscored by a recent report indicating that VO_{2peak} ($>17.5\,\text{ml·kg}^{-1}\text{·min}^{-1}$) was in fact a stronger predictor of survival than many traditional prognostic variables, some of which are subject to ceiling effects (Sietsema *et al.*, 2004).

Exercise test mode

Cycle ergometers are the most frequently used mode of exercise testing in patients with ESRF. The main advantage of cycle ergometry is that the monitoring of ECG and BP responses are more easily achieved. Moreover, patients with orthopaedic limitations and impaired balance or orthostatic intolerance may feel more confident exercising in a seated position. On the other hand, treadmill-walking protocols more closely mimic activities of daily living that are familiar to patients and may also prevent earlier termination of the

Table 20.3 Reasons to terminate the exercise test

- Sustained cardiac arrhythmias
- No increases in BP with increasing workload
- Evidence of cardiac ischaemia
- When BP exceeds 220/110 mmHg
- When there is a sudden drop in BP by more than 20 mmHg
- Symptoms such as angina, dizziness, severe breathlessness, lack of responsiveness or cooperation to oral and/or visual signs
- Equipment failure
- Patient's request

test because of localised leg fatigue, a frequently reported cause of patient discomfort and test termination.

Typically, a period of at least 2–3 min of unloaded exercise is required as a warm-up, after which small increments of about 10–15 W·min^{-1} should be applied to ensure that peak performance capacity is reached after a total of 12–15 min of exercise. The increase in exercise intensity (or power output) can be applied either in a step or ramp fashion. In contrast, Kouidi (2001) advocates a longer duration protocol for the assessment of peak exercise capacity and has described a peak exercise capacity treadmill assessment protocol (*Nephron* – a modification of the Bruce treadmill protocol) that they have developed successfully and used for over 10 years with patients with ESRF. Regardless of the protocol employed, careful and continuous monitoring of all physiological responses is essential in order that adverse events be avoided and/or minimised during exercise assessment. Table 20.3 outlines abnormal responses that would indicate termination of the exercise test. Following the cessation of the peak exercise test patients should be encouraged to complete a gradual, active return to the non-exercising state (of at least 3 min duration), during which monitoring of all assessed variables is continued. Patients should remain supervised in the assessment area until all indices of cardiovascular function have stabilised to pre-exercise or resting levels.

Reproducibility information on exercise tolerance assessment and outcome measures in patients with ESRF is scarce in the literature. The only published study (Koufaki *et al.*, 2001) that has evaluated the reproducibility of peak exercise parameters during incremental cycle ergometry, on a representative sample of contemporary dialysis patients, reported coefficients of variation of 4.7% for VO_{2peak}, 9% for peak power output, 5.9% for peak HR and 13% for exercise test duration. These observations were based on repeated assessments, on non-dialysis days, for a group of maintenance dialysis patients characterised by stable fluid status and resting haemodynamics. There is no published information available regarding the estimation of VO_{2peak} values from incremental exercise tests where gas exchange data has not been recorded.

Submaximal exercise capacity

Peak exercise capacity measures provide valuable information on the upper limits of integrated cardio-respiratory physiology. However, that information may not necessarily reflect the ability of patients to perform activities of daily living. Functional independence is also associated with the ability to sustain tasks without experiencing fatigue and this information may be more easily and safely derived from sub-maximal exercise tests (Basset and Howley, 2000).

Measurement and/or estimation of lactate threshold (LT) using gas exchange data (GET/VT) during the execution of an incremental test is feasible and exhibits good reproducibility in patients undergoing dialysis. An important pre-test requirement for accurate and reliable measurement of these parameters is that standard clinical chemistry values are within the normal range for dialysis patients (for normal ranges see *Oxford Handbook of Dialysis*, 2004). Indicative CV% for VO_2 at VT, time at VT, power output at VT and HR at VT are 6.6%, 11.7%, 9.7% and 4.9%, respectively (Koufaki *et al.*, 2001). The use of sub-maximal indices associated with physiological anchor points, such as GET or LT are also less likely to be influenced by discomfort, tolerance and motivation and therefore may reflect more meaningful physiological changes in follow-up studies.

An additional sub-maximal index of exercise capacity/tolerance that has been described in patients with ESRF is the rate of adjustment of VO_2 (VO_2 – on kinetics) in response to constant load exercise (Koufaki *et al.*, 2002a). The rate at which VO_2 reaches steady state is believed to reflect an integrated physiological ability to meet sudden increased demands of energy production. If the oxygen supply at the beginning of a task is insufficient to meet O_2 demand then there is a delay in reaching steady state and the development of early fatigue is more prominent (Grassi, 2000).

In the clinical context constant load exercise tests are usually designed to allow patients to reach a steady state for VO_2 and as a result most tests are conducted at an exercise intensity level below the directly determined LT or GET (VT). The test typically comprises a 2–min period of 'loadless' cycling followed by a 'loaded' exercise period of ~6 min with a subsequent 'loadless' pedalling recovery period of a further 2 min. Reproducibility data on VO_2 kinetics for patients with ESRF indicate that there is a substantial variability/error associated with this measure based on the average values from two transitions performed twice within a week. The reported CV% associated with the mean response time kinetics for exercise intensity corresponding to 90% of GET (VT) was 19.8% (Koufaki *et al.*, 2002b). Non-clinical approaches to this type of assessment advocate the use of several 'rest-to-work' transitions (at least 4) to reduce problems with 'signal to noise ratio' (and thus intra-subject variability). However, in our experience this is rather impractical with ESRF patients as their fatigue tolerance threshold is very low and in most cases they can only tolerate a maximum of 2–3 transitions in a single assessment day.

Neuromuscular exercise function

Muscle mass and muscle function related measures have also been implicated in predicting disease progress and survival in patients on dialysis (Diesel *et al.*, 1990;

Beddhu *et al.*, 2003; Johansen *et al.*, 2003, Sietsema *et al.*, 2004). Accurate and reliable assessment of these parameters is essential therefore for the clinically meaningful interpretation of results.

Muscle function in the dialysis population has been assessed by means of measuring absolute dynamic muscle strength (1, 5 or 10 repetition maximums), peak force, rate of force development, rate of muscle relaxation, during both isokinetic and isometric contractions with or without superimposed electrical stimulation, of nearly all main muscle groups (leg extensors, hamstrings, leg abductors and adductors, dorsiflexors, forearm muscles, back extensors) (Diesel *et al.*, 1990; Kouidi *et al.*, 1998; Gleeson *et al.*, 2002; Johansen *et al.*, 2003). Investigators have used a wide variety of assessment protocols involving a range of joint angles and/or limb movement speeds. However, published information regarding the reliability of muscle performance assessment protocols in patients with ESRF is only provided by one research group (Gleeson *et al.*, 2002). Day-to-day variability expressed as CV% for peak force and rate of force development indices during maximal voluntary isometric force production of the knee extensor ($45°$ knee flexion angle ($0° = $ full knee extension)) was found to be 6.6% and 20.3%, respectively. Although it is evident from the literature that the application of many muscle performance assessment protocols is feasible in patients with renal failure, extra caution still needs to be applied as these people are more prone to muscle and tendon ruptures in response to sudden changes in forces. As a result, extensive whole body and muscle group-specific warm-up exercise and stretches are mandated before the execution of any strength assessment protocols.

FUNCTIONAL CAPACITY ASSESSMENT

Performance-based functional capacity assessment is an alternative and/or complementary way to fully describe physical function in patients with ESRF. Recent reports have stressed the observation that functional impairment of patients on dialysis is often underestimated by measures of physiological exercise capacity alone (Naish *et al.*, 2000). Moreover, it has recently been suggested that the utility of established clinical assessments of the nutritional status of patients on dialysis may be enhanced by the inclusion of simple and inexpensive measures of functional capacity, that reflect muscle mass and muscle function (Mercer *et al.*, 2004).

Several investigators have reported patients' functional capacity using the 6-min walk test, gait speed tests, stair climb and descent, sit-to-stand tests (STS), and sit-and-reach test (Mercer *et al.*, 1998; Painter *et al.*, 2000, Johansen *et al.*, 2001; Koufaki *et al.*, 2002a). Although many of these tests have been fully validated in the general rehabilitation and exercise gerontology literature (refer to Ageing chapter in this book), information about the validity and reproducibility of these tests in the ESRF population is available only for STS tests and stair climb and descent (Mercer *et al.*, 1998; Koufaki, 2001). Therefore, subsequent discussion will be restricted to those functional capacity tests that have been evaluated in the dialysis population.

North Staffordshire Royal Infirmary Walk (NSRI walk)

This test is composed of four distinctive parts. A walk of 50 m on flat ground, a stair climb (2 flights; 22 stairs of 15 cm height; total elevation 3.3 m), a stair descent, and another 50 m walk back to the start point. Total time and split time for constituent elements should be recorded. The patients should be instructed to perform the test as fast as they can. This test has been shown to significantly correlate with VO_{2peak} ($r = -0.83$) with a prediction error of 11% (Mercer *et al.*, 1998). Therefore, it seems to be a very useful overall assessment of functional capacity and in particular the ability to complete ambulatory tasks often required in daily living. Reproducibility analysis has shown that the overall CV% for the NSRI walk is 8.2% and the CV% separately for the stair climb and stair descent is 11.1% and 11.4%, respectively (Koufaki, 2001).

Sit-to-stands

These tests involve rising unassisted from a standard height chair (0.42–0.46 m) and sitting back on the chair as fast as possible. The patients should be instructed to keep their hands crossed over their chest so they do not use them to push themselves up and feet should remain on the ground at all times. The patients should also be instructed to squat over and touch the chair on the sitting down phase and fully extend their knees on the standing up phase. Several variations of the test exist such as STS−5 and STS−10 which is the fastest time (in seconds) at which patients can complete 5 or 10 STS cycles (Johansen, 2001; Painter, 2000). These tests have been interpreted as indicators of muscle power. The reported CV% for STS−5 based on contemporary dialysis patients is 15%. STS−60, on the other hand, has been used as an indicator of muscular endurance and fatiguability as it requires patients to perform as many STS as they can in 60 s. The CV% for this version of STS has been reported to be 12.8% (Koufaki, 2001). It is not unusual that some of the patients may need to take resting breaks especially during the STS-60 test. The number of STS-cycles at the exact time of break should be recorded, without stopping the timer. Also the time at which the patients resume the test should be noted.

SUMMARY

Measures of peak exercise tolerance and/or functional capacity have been shown to be related to clinically important outcomes (survival, morbidity and quality of life) in patients receiving dialysis-based renal replacement therapy. Given the prognostic potential of these factors it is recommended that their measurement should form part of the routine assessment (and management) of patients receiving maintenance dialysis therapy. If good practice is followed the available literature suggests that exercise tolerance and functional capacity assessment of the patient with ESRF is both safe and feasible.

REFERENCES

Basset D.R. and Howley, E.T. (2000). Limiting factors for maximum oxygen uptake and determinants of endurance performance. *Medicine and Science in Sports and Exercise*, 32(1): 70–84.

Beddhu, S., Pappas, L.M., Ramkumar, N. and Samore, M. (2003). Effects of body size and body composition on survival in hemodialysis patients. *Journal of the American Society of Nephrology*, 14(9): 2366–2372.

Bommer, J. (1992). Medical complications of the long term dialysis patient: In S. Cameron, A. Davidson, J.P. Grufeld, D. Kerr and E. Ritz (eds), *Oxford Textbook of Clinical Nephrology*. New York: Oxford.

Deligiannis, A., Kouidi E., Tassoulas, E., Gigis, P., Tourkantonis, A. and Coats, A. (1999). Cardiac effects of exercise rehabilitation in hemodialysis patients. *International Journal of Cardiology*, 70: 253–266.

Diesel, W., Noakes, T., Swanepoel, C. and Lambert, M. (1990). Isokinetic muscle strength predicts maximum exercise tolerance in renal patients on chronic haemodialysis. *American Journal of Kidney Disease*, 16: 109–114.

Gleeson, N.P., Naish, P.F., Wilcock, J.E. and Mercer, T.H. (2002). Reliability of indices of neuromuscular leg performance in end-stage renal disease. *Journal of Rehabilitation Medicine*, 34(6): 273–277.

Grassi, B. (2000). Skeletal muscle VO_2 − on kinetics. Set by O_2 delivery or by O_2 utilization? New insights into an old issue. *Medicine and Science in Sports and Exercise*, 32(1): 108–116.

Johansen, K.L., Chertow, G.M., Alexander, V.N.G., Mulligan, K., Carey, S., Schoenfeld, P. and Kent-Braun, J.A. (2000). Physical activity levels in patients on hemodialysis and healthy sedentary controls. *Kidney International*, 57: 2564–2570.

Johansen, K.L., Chertow, G.M., DaSilva, M., Carey, S. and Painter, P. (2001). Determinants of physical performance in ambulatory patients on hemodialysis. *Kidney International*, 60: 1586–1591.

Johansen, K.L., Schubert, T., Doyle, J., Soher, B., Sakkas, G.K. and Kent-Braun, J.A. (2003). Muscle atrophy in patients receiving haemodialysis: effects on muscle strength, muscle quality and physical function. *Kidney International*, 63: 291–297.

Koufaki, P. (2001). The effect of erythopoietin therapy and exercise rehabilitation on the cardiorespiratory performance of patients with end stage renal disease. Unpublished PhD thesis. The Manchester Metropolitan University.

Koufaki, P., Naish, P.F. and Mercer, T.H. (2001). Reproducibility of exercise tolerance in patients with end stage renal disease. *Archives of Physical Medicine and Rehabilitation*, 82: 1421–1424.

Koufaki, P., Mercer, T.H. and Naish, P.F. (2002a). Effects of exercise training on aerobic and functional capacity of end stage renal disease patients. *Clinical Physiology and Functional Imaging*, 22: 115–124.

Koufaki, P., Mercer T.H. and Naish P.F. (2002b). Evaluation of efficacy of exercise training in patients with chronic disease. *Medicine and Science in Sports and Exercise*, 34(8): 1234–1241.

Kouidi, E., Albanis, M., Natsis, K., Megalopoulos, A., Gigis, P., Tziampiri, O., Tourkantonis, A. and Deligiannis, A. (1998). The effects of exercise training on muscle atrophy in haemodialysis patients. *Nephrology Dialysis Transplantation*, 13: 685–699.

Kouidi, E.J. (2001). Central and peripheral adaptations to physical training in patients with end-stage renal disease. *Sports Medicine*, 31(9): 651–665.

Levy, J., Morgan, J. and Brown, E. (2004). *Oxford Handbook of Dialysis*. Oxford, UK: Oxford University Press.

Mercer, T.H., Naish, P.F., Gleeson, N.P., Wilcock, J.E. and Crawford, C. (1998). Development of a walking test for the assessment of functional capacity in non-anaemic maintenance dialysis patients. *Nephrology Dialysis Transplantation*, 13: 2023–2026.

Mercer, T.H., Koufaki, P. and Naish, P.F. (2004). Nutritional status, functional capacity and exercise rehabilitation in end stage renal disease. *Clinical Nephrology*, S1 61(1): S54-S59.

Moore, G.E. (2000). Integrated gas exchange response: chronic renal failure. In J. Roca, R. Rodriguez-Roisin and P.D. Wagner (eds), *Pulmonary and Peripheral Gas Exchange in Health and Disease*, pp. 649–684. New York: Marcel Dekker.

Moore, G.E., Parsons, D.B., Gundersen, J.S., Painter, P.L., Brinker, K.R. and Mitchell, J.H. (1993). Uraemic myopathy limits aerobic capacity in haemodialysis patients. *American Journal of Kidney Disease*, 22(2): 277–287.

Naish, P.F., Mercer, T.H., Koufaki, P. and Wilcock, J.E. (2000). VO_{2peak} underestimates physical dysfunction in elderly dialysis patients. *Medicine and Science in Sports and Exercise*, 32(5): S160.

Painter, P., Carlson, L., Carey, S., Paul, S.P. and Myll, J. (2000). Physical functioning and health related quality of life changes with exercise training in haemodialysis patients. *American Journal of Kidney Disease*, 35(3): 482–492.

Sietsema, K.E., Hiatt, E.R., Esler, A. and Adler, S.G., Amato, A. and Brass, E.P. (2002). Clinical and demographic predictors of exercise capacity in end stage renal disease. *American Journal of Kidney Disease*, 39(1): 76–85.

Sietsema, K.E., Amato, A., Adler, S.G. and Brass, E.P. (2004). Exercise capacity as a predictor of survival among ambulatory patients with end stage renal disease. *Kidney International*, 65: 719–724.

UK Renal Registry Report (2002). *UK Renal Registry, Fourth Annual Report*, D. Ansell, T. Feest and C. Byrne (eds), Bristol, UK.

CHAPTER 21

PHYSIOLOGICAL TESTING FOR NEUROMUSCULAR DISORDERS

David A. Jones and Joan M. Round

Weakness and fatigue are two of the most common complaints of patients with a wide range of diseases and they are also common concerns of athletes who are training or recovering from injury. Muscle function testing is often an important aid to diagnosis and can also play a valuable role in assessing the extent of a problem and, in many cases, the progress of recovery and return to full function. For a more extensive introduction to muscle physiology and pathology see, Jones *et al.* (2004) and McComas (1996).

MUSCLE WEAKNESS

Normal muscle function depends on the correct working of the chain of command that extends from motivation to the interaction of actin and myosin within the muscle fibre and there are diseases and conditions that can disrupt the chain at almost any point and lead to a loss of function. The chain of command is often simplified into *central* and *peripheral* elements that can be separated on the basis of electrical stimulation of the motor nerve or its branches. If the problem is central in origin, voluntary force can be improved by superimposing electrical stimulation while this has no effect on peripheral causes of weakness.

The major diseases and their main features are summarised in Table 21.1. Muscle weakness is a feature of a wide range of disorders ranging from immobilisation and disuse, where the muscle fibres atrophy (mainly the slower type 1 fibres) as a consequence of the loss of the stimuli that promote and maintain protein synthesis, to the secondary atrophic myopathies where fibre atrophy is a response to an endocrine disturbance and the faster type 2 fibres are preferentially affected. In severe cases, the loss of the fast contractile material can lead to a slowing of the muscle. Type 2 fibre atrophy can be a consequence of an

Table 21.1 Summary of the main disorders and diseases affecting skeletal muscle, arranged according to their main presenting symptom

Weakness

Secondary atrophic myopathies	Hypothyroidism
	Malnutrition
	Cachexia
	Cushings
	Prolonged steroid therapy
	Alcohol
	Injury to muscle, joint or tendon
	Immobilisation
	Peripheral vascular disease
Neuropathies	Motor neuron disease
	Spinal muscular atrophy
	Multiple sclerosis
	Alcoholic neuropathy
	Diabetic neuropathy
Muscular dystrophies	Duchenne
	Becker
	Limb girdle
Inflammatory myopathies	Polymyositis
	Dermatomyositis

Abnormal function

	Malignant hyperthermia
	Hypokalaemic periodic paralysis
	Hyperkalaemic periodic paralysis
	Myotonia

Excessive fatiguability

Glycolytic enzyme deficiencies	Myophosphorylase (McArdle's)
	Phosphofructokinase (Tauri')
Mitochondrial enzyme deficiencies	Pyruvate dehydrogenase
	Cytochromes
	Carnitine palmitoyl transferase

Myasthenia gravis

Peripheral vascular disease

Chronic fatigue syndrome

Post-viral states

Overtraining

Hypothyroidism

Depression

Most serious diseases; trauma and/or surgery

endocrine disorder or have some external cause such as malnutrition, alcohol abuse or prolonged glucocorticoid therapy for asthma or inflammatory conditions. Although weakness can be severe in these conditions, muscle fibre size and strength can fully recover if the underlying disease is recognised and successfully treated.

Central limitation is rarely a major factor in muscle weakness, the exception being where there is damage or inflammation of a joint, tendon or ligament that can provide a powerful inhibitory input to the alpha motoneuron.

Fibre atrophy, muscle wasting and weakness are also features of a range of neuropathies where the problems arise either because of degeneration of the motoneurons or damage to peripheral motor nerves. Motor neuron disease is relentless and fatal but in some of the peripheral neuropathies muscle can, at least partially, recover if healthy motor axons branch out and reinnervate motor units that have been deprived of neural input. This process gives rise to the characteristic fibre type grouping seen in muscle biopsy preparations and the giant action potentials recorded with EMG.

In contrast to these disorders where the cause of weakness is atrophy of individual fibres without them ever totally disappearing, there are several diseases classified as 'destructive' myopathies in which fibres are destroyed and often replaced with fat and/or connective tissue. In polymyositis and dermatomyositis which are probably variants of the same disease, there is destruction of muscle fibres as a result of an inflammatory autoimmune process. Characteristically muscle fibres are surrounded and invaded by inflammatory cells. In the early stages these are mainly lymphocytes but later macrophages predominate. These conditions can lead to profound weakness. Treatment is with immunosuppressant drugs. Responses to treatment vary and in the best cases substantial muscle regeneration occurs leading to slow recovery of normal function but, in other cases, the condition can not be fully controlled and relapses can occur.

The muscular dystrophies are a large group of diseases in which the skeletal muscle degenerates relentlessly over a period of years due to a genetic defect in one of the structural proteins of the fibres. The different types of dystrophy vary in the distribution of affected muscles, time course and severity. In Duchenne and Becker dystrophies the defect has been identified in the protein *dystrophin* while in the limb girdle dystrophies it is in *laminin*. The dystrophies usually become apparent in childhood and muscle strength steadily deteriorates with the loss of muscle fibres and replacement with fat and connective tissue. In the more severe forms death occurs in the third decade mainly as a result of respiratory muscles weakness.

Although the atrophic and destructive myopathies both give rise to weakness the two can generally be distinguished by measurement of circulating levels of creatine kinase. This enzyme (along with other soluble proteins) is released from damaged muscle fibres and is characteristically high in the destructive myopathies. Normal levels are around $200 \ \mathrm{IU \cdot l^{-1}}$ and pathological levels are in the order of $1,000–10,000 \ \mathrm{IU \cdot l^{-1}}$ or more. However, care needs to be taken because very high CK levels can occur in normal subjects following unaccustomed exercise (especially involving muscle stretching) but these values will return to normal within 7 days whilst pathological values are persistently elevated.

ABNORMAL FUNCTION

There are several diseases where the muscles are of relatively normal strength but have some disturbance of function, usually associated with an abnormality in one of the various ion channels in the surface membrane. While being of great interest to the electrophysiologist, they are extremely rare and will not be discussed here (see Table 21.1).

EXCESSIVE FATIGUE

What constitutes excessive fatigue in everyday and sporting life can be a matter of debate, the answer depending very much on expectations and state of training. However, there is little doubt that some disorders lead to fatigue that can only be described as pathological, severely limiting the activities of the sufferers.

Since muscular contraction is one of the major energy consuming process within the body and fatigue inevitably occurs when the supply of substrate or oxygen is interrupted, it is natural to look for a metabolic cause in any complaint of fatigue. Peripheral vascular disease limits physical activity with severe ischaemic pain being the main feature. There are also several genetic defects affecting the glycolytic and aerobic pathways in muscle. Patients with these disorders are of relatively normal strength but fatigue rapidly during moderate activity. In the case of glycolytic disorders (e.g. myophosphorylase and phosphofructokinase deficiency) there is a tendency for the active muscle to go into a painful contracture that resolves slowly. Characteristically these patients fatigue in the absence of any lactate production or acidosis.

Deficiencies of the electron transport chain limit aerobic activity and, in these cases, activity is accompanied by a massive acidosis and hyperventilation. Deficiencies of the fatty acid transporting enzyme carnitine palmitoyl transferase have only a limited effect on fatiguability, probably because fat is not an indispensable source of energy for muscle. However, these patients suffer from occasional muscle fibre breakdown (rhabdomyolysis), often after unusual physical activity which is probably due to an accumulation of free fatty acid in the muscle that dissolves cell membranes.

In myasthenia gravis there is an autoimmune attack on the acetyl choline receptors in the neuromuscular junction. The rested muscle is of relatively normal strength but fatigues rapidly as the quantity of acetyl choline released decreases and fails to compete adequately with the antibody to its receptors. Treatment is with immunosuppressant drugs to control the autoimmune process and anti-choline esterase agents to counteract the inhibition at the post-synaptic membrane.

It must be stressed that peripheral causes of fatigue such as glycolytic and mitochondrial deficiencies are very rare and most unlikely to be encountered in an exercise or sports science laboratory. The vast majority of patients complaining of fatigue have complicated conditions in which central factors probably play an important role.

Patients with muscle weakness due to loss of contractile material tend to fatigue more rapidly than normal when performing every-day activities simply because their muscles are having to work closer to their maximum capacity when, for instance, walking upstairs. Individuals who are overweight have a similar problem in as much as their muscles are subject to greater loads than normal and consequently fatigue more rapidly. It is notable that obese subjects do not seem to develop muscle hypertrophy to compensate for the additional load on their muscles, possibly because they tend to reduce their level of activity, thus sparing their relatively weak muscles.

Objective tests of muscle fatiguability often show surprisingly little abnormality even in patients complaining of the most severe fatigue. Hypothyroid patients, for whom fatigue is a prime symptom, prove to have muscles that are less fatiguable than normal. Chronic fatigue syndrome (CFS) patients have also been found to be somewhat better at sustaining a series of isometric contractions than normal subjects. Objective measurements of fatiguability tend to focus on a single muscle group and it is notable that what CFS patients find difficult is not such single tasks but the more complex business of whole body exercise. A little reflection indicates that this is not so unusual since most normal people frequently feel tired and fatigued at the end of the day or after walking slowly around the shops, tasks that are not at all demanding in terms of muscle contraction or energy consumption. It is likely that in a wide variety of disorders these same feelings are intensified until they become detrimental to mobility and the quality of life. Chronic fatigue syndrome, where muscle function has been extensively studied without finding any peripheral cause for the symptoms, typifies this type of condition. Research in this area is at an early stage but it appears that patients have a heightened perception of exertion, possibly being more sensitive than most to the sensations of exercise than most. Current interest centres on possible changes in the sensitivity of hypothalamic pathways but there are several other possible central pathways that could decrease motor output in response to the afferent input occurring during exercise. The overtraining syndrome, that is of concern for many elite athletes, probably falls into the same category as chronic fatigue syndrome, although the degree of physical incapacity involved is nothing like as severe.

INVESTIGATION OF MUSCLE FUNCTION

Table 21.2 summarises the range of tests that might be used to investigate people complaining of weakness or fatigue. These tests fall between two poles. At one end are detailed investigations of the contractile properties of an individual muscle while at the other are assessments of functional ability such as jumping or of endurance whilst exercising at some known proportion of maximum aerobic capacity. In an ideal situation a full investigation of, say, a patient having difficulty climbing stairs might start with a careful documentation of this functional deficit, determining how fast he or she can climb a standard set of steps, followed by checks on balance and eyesight, before proceeding to measurements of strength, range of movement and the fatiguability of

Table 21.2 Possible investigations of muscle function in relation to symptoms of weakness and fatigue

The amount of contractile material	Isometric strength (with or without electrical stimulation)
	Anthropometry; CT, MRI or Ultrasound imaging
Speed of the muscle	Relaxation from an isometric contraction
	The degree of fusion of a sub-maximal tetanus
	Shape of the force/velocity relationship; estimates of maximum velocity of shortening
Power and impulse (speed and strength)	Standing and vertical jump
	Stair running
	Wingate test
	Isokinetic dynamometry
	Isokinetic cycling
Length of a muscle	Angle/force or torque relationship (range of movement)
Fatiguability	Repeated contractions (stimulated or voluntary; isometric or dynamic; with or without an intact circulation)
	Prolonged exercise at fixed percentage of VO_{2max}; 6 or 12 min walk tests
	Rating of perceived exertion (Borg 10 or 20 point scale)
Other investigations	Clinical history
	Biochemistry (CK, inflammatory markers, genetic investigation)
	EMG

individual muscle groups, the expectation being that an abnormality of muscle function might explain the overall functional deficit. A similar sequence could be envisaged for an athlete who was injured or was complaining of loss of form. However, in practice, there is often neither the time nor the facilities to undertake such a full investigation and much will depend on taking a full history and experienced clinical judgement.

The majority of common muscle complaints involve wasting and it is particularly useful in a clinical situation to know the extent of muscle loss. This can be determined directly by one of the imagining techniques, CT scanning, ultrasound or, preferably, MRI. However, measurement of muscle strength provides a useful and convenient alternative since, with some minor reservations about changes in muscle architecture and fibre composition, strength is proportional to the amount of contractile material and therefore size of the muscle. Most major muscle groups can be measured but the quadriceps remains the most useful since it is a large proximal muscle that is affected in most muscle disorders, it is functionally important in everyday life and is very convenient for other investigations such as muscle biopsy and electromyography (EMG). Quadriceps strength can be measured using an isometric testing chair such as described by Edwards *et al.* (1977) or commercial ergometers such as Cybex,

Lido or Kincom that can be used in either isometric or isokinetic modes. The Edward's testing chair has the advantage of simplicity and it is relatively easy to place patients in a standardised position. The equipment also produces records that are generally superior to those of the more complex machines, but is limited to a single muscle group, lacks the versatility of being able to measure force throughout the range of movement as well as the obvious limitation of not being able to record force during movement of the limb. For the purposes of assessing the size and strength of a muscle in order to document the extent of a disease or the progress of treatment or training, isometric testing is quite sufficient and in many ways preferable to isokinetic testing that introduces several complications such as consideration of the speed, length and range of movement of a muscle. Isokinetic testing is of particular value in assessing injuries affecting joints where the range of movement can be impaired or inhibition might occur at a certain position.

Normal values are difficult to define since strength varies widely with age, sex, body shape and size and with habitual activity. Edwards *et al.* (1977) suggest a useful rule of thumb that the quadriceps strength is about 75% of the force of gravity on the body mass so that for a 70 kg subject, strength would be about 530 N. However, a wide range of quadriceps strength is compatible with a normal active lifestyle as is indicated by the spread of data reported by Edwards. Normative data for the isometric strength of several muscles and for body sizes and ages have been published (NIMS, 1996). It is important to realise the normal variation that occurs with age and Figure 21.1 shows the changes during growth and subsequent ageing in females. Figure 21.2 shows how strength relates to the height of a vertical jump (essentially measuring impulse) and it is notable that performance of the jump deteriorates to a greater extent than strength, primarily because there is a preferential loss of fast motor units in the older subjects.

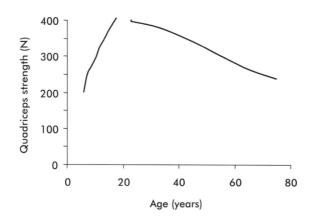

Figure 21.1   Changes in voluntary isometric quadriceps strength with age in healthy females. Mean values, data for children from Round *et al.* (1999) and for the older women from Rutherford and Jones (1992)

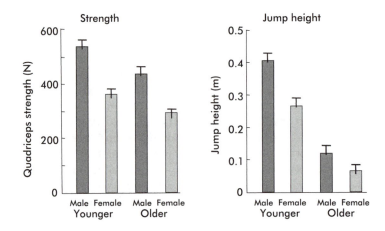

Figure 21.2 Voluntary isometric quadriceps strength and vertical jump height for younger (20–30 years) and older (65–80) healthy males and females. Data are mean ± SEM (unpublished data of Mills and Jones)

Power can be considered the product of the strength and speed of a muscle and is a critical component of performance in many sporting activities. Consequently, it is often of interest to know the speed of a muscle which is largely determined by its fibre type proportions. In theory, muscle function testing can be used to determine speed, either by estimating the maximum velocity of shortening, the rise or relaxation times from twitches or tetani or the extent of oscillation during sub-maximal electrical stimulation. In practice, however, the results are usually disappointing, as it is very difficult to correlate function with fibre type composition except in very extreme cases. This is probably due to the fact that *in vivo* measurements of speed are technically difficult to make and that series compliance of the apparatus and the muscle/tendon complex confuse the issue.

Muscle function testing cannot distinguish the various causes of weakness or fatigue. For this further investigations are required, the most useful of which is muscle biopsy with appropriate histochemical, biochemical and molecular biochemical examinations, together with the full range of standard biochemical and haematological tests for endocrine and inflammatory changes.

The type of patient that is referred to an exercise physiology laboratory depends largely on the speciality of the outpatient clinic. If they are from a rheumatology speciality then patients with polymyositis and other inflammatory diseases are most commonly seen; if attached to an endocrine clinic, the secondary myopathies are relatively common while neurology clinics have frequent referrals of patients with central and peripheral neuropathies. No matter what the speciality, however, probably the most common patients are those with non-specific feelings of fatigue in whom there is no obvious sign of muscle pathology. There has been a tendency in the past to dismiss these patients as malingerers or refer them for psychiatric evaluation, but increasingly it is becoming realised that they have very real, and in some cases disabling, problems and one of the major challenges for the future is to unravel the biochemistry and physiology of this type of exercise intolerance.

REFERENCES

Edwards, R.H.T., Young, A., Hosking, G.P. and Jones, D.A. (1977). Human skeletal muscle function: description of tests and normal values. *Clinical Science and Molecular Medicine*, 52: 283–290.

Jones, D.A., Round, J.M. and de Haan, A. (2004). *Skeletal Muscle from Molecules to Movement*. Edinburgh: Churchill Livingstone.

McComas, A.J. (1996). *Skeletal Muscle: Form and Function*. Champaign, Il: Human Kinetics.

Muscular weakness assessment: use of normal isometric strength data. The National Isometric Muscle Strength (NIMS) Database Consortium. (1996). *Arch Phys Med Rehabil*. 77: 1251–1255.

Round, J.M., Jones, D.A., Honour, J.W. and Nevill, A.M. (1999). Hormonal factors in the development of differences in strength between boys and girls during adolescence: a longitudinal study. *Annals of Human Biology*, 26: 49–62.

Rutherford, O.M. and Jones, D.A (1992). The relationship of muscle and bone loss and activity levels with age in women. *Age and Ageing*, 21: 286–293.

PART 5

SPECIAL POPULATIONS

CHAPTER 22

CHILDREN AND FITNESS TESTING

Gareth Stratton and Craig A. Williams

RATIONALE

There are a number of reasons why guidelines specific for children should be created instead of adopting adult-based ones. These reasons include differences between children and adults in:

- ethics
- informed consent
- the physiological differences due to body size
- the impact of growth and maturation
- the need for a different laboratory environment.

In the last 20 years there has been a proliferation of testing protocols which has resulted in an increasing amount of data related to children's physiology. For the purposes of these guidelines we are delimiting the definition of a child as below 18 years. These guidelines are designed to recommend accurate techniques in measuring physical and physiological parameters in children and can be adopted for sporting or research purposes.

TESTING MODALITIES

Field and laboratory tests of fitness and performance represent the two main modalities available to the paediatric exercise scientist. Both are widely used, although field tests are commonly used as part of fitness education in schools. The choice of test depends on a number of factors such as cost, expedience, accuracy and tester experience. Field tests are limited because they provide no direct physiological data but more accurately assess 'motor performance'.

The advantage of field tests are that they require relatively inexpensive equipment, personnel involved in testing need less training and they can be performed with large sample sizes in readily available facilities, for example, sports halls. Hence field tests are convenient for large epidemiological studies of the population. Laboratory tests however are more expensive, require specialist facilities and staff, but produce more sensitive and precise 'physiological' data and a greater insight into biological mechanisms. Field tests are a useful tool available to coaches, teachers and allied health professionals, and although the tests have been criticised for their use in schools they are useful in tracking changes in whole population studies.

PARTICIPATION OF THE CHILD IN A PROJECT

The Medical Research Council (MRC) have stated that children may participate in research projects which have a therapeutic or a non-therapeutic benefit which does not necessarily benefit the child involved. However, children's involvement in testing must involve 'negligible risk' defined as no greater than risks of harm ordinarily encountered in daily life. The following test procedures are considered negligible risk:

- Observation of behaviour
- Non-invasive physiological monitoring
- Developmental assessments and physical examinations
- Changes in diet
- Obtaining blood and urine samples (Medical Research Council, 1991).

For exercise testing in England and Wales, children under the age of 18 cannot legally consent to participate in exercise tests and therefore parental or guardian's consent is essential. Recently, obtaining children's assent has become accepted practice alongside, but not in place of parental consent, as a safeguard to ensure the child is not being coerced into a project by their parents (Jago and Bailey, 1998; Williams, 2003). Explanation of the details of procedures should allow for the wide range of intellectual capabilities of the participating children. Common to all ethical procedures for research should be the emphasis that the child is free to withdraw at any time.

The Protection of Children Act 1999 (DoH, 2000) requires all activities involving children to have a responsibility to protect their welfare. Where children are involved in testing without the presence of a parent or guardian those responsible for testing are acting 'in loco parentis' (*in the place of the parent*). It is now common procedure that anyone without a Criminal Records Bureau Enhanced Disclosure should not be left in sole charge of children (DfES). It is also recommended that testers are not left in a one to one situation with children including during transport arrangements.

At the location of testing (field or laboratory) it is important to ensure such details as the following have been arranged:

- Participation health questionnaire including, if necessary, detailed information on medical, special educational, cultural and nutritional needs.
- Clear establishment of who is in charge.
- Check your insurance covers working with children.
- Establish acceptable conduct for children, that is, children cannot go off on their own anywhere, what are you going to do if a child becomes uncooperative.
- Details in the event of an emergency, for example, contact details of school, head teacher or classroom teacher, parent/guardian.

ASSESSING MATURATION

The assessment of physiological and physical changes during growth is essential for the valid interpretation of human performance.

Maturation can be assessed in a variety of ways and until recently these have been mainly invasive and ethically questionable. A number of scientists (Greulich and Pyle, 1959; Roche, 1988) developed similar methods for assessing, 'skeletal maturation'. These involved an X-ray of the left wrist and hand where constituent bones were assessed for their stage of ossification against a developmental atlas. Whilst this approach is the gold standard for skeletal maturation it is limited for two important reasons: (1) Measurement requires advanced technical expertise and (2) youngsters receive a dose of radiation during each assessment.

One non-invasive method to assess maturation is 'morphological age' which calculates the percentage of predicted adult stature. This is a simple technique to use but is limited by the need for the exact stature of both biological parents and it is not valid for children under 10 years of age. Furthermore, skeletal age is the only measure of maturation that can be applied from infant to adulthood whereas morphological age is only valid between 10 and 18 years of age. Unfortunately neither skeletal nor morphological age is able to adequately predict pubertal stage.

The most practical approach to assess maturation was developed by Tanner (1962). Tanner developed a 5-point scale to assess 'biological maturity' through observation of secondary sexual characteristics. The scales depicted five or more stages of breast and pubic hair (girls) pubic hair and genitalia development (boys). A limitation is that trained health professionals such as paediatricians and school nurses are typically employed to assess the scales. Subsequently Morris and Udry (1980) developed a self-assessment scale based on Tanner stages and found that children were able to accurately assess their own stage of maturation with correlation coefficients in the range of 60–70% (Matsudo and Matsudo, 1993).

Mirwald and colleagues (2001) developed a technique that uses anthropometrical data to calculate maturity offset and thus avoids ethical and technical complexities found in other techniques. This approach has gained widespread approval, as it only requires decimal age and simple measures of body mass, stature and sitting height. Leg length is also required but is calculated by subtracting sitting height from stature. These data are then substituted into a regression equation and distance in time before or after peak height velocity is calculated. This method has an accuracy of ±0.4 years.

Males

Maturity offset = −9.236 + (0.0002708 × (leg length × sitting height)) + (−0.001663 × (age × leg length)) + (0.007216 × (age × sitting height)) + (0.02292 × (mass by stature ratio)).

Females

Maturity offset = −9.376 + (0.0001882 × (leg length × sitting height)) + (−0.0022 × (age × leg length)) + (0.005841 × (age × sitting height)) + (0.02658 × (age × mass)) + (0.07693 × (mass by stature ratio)).

In these equations age is measured in decimal years, lengths in centimetres and mass in kilograms.

The technique proposed by Mirwald and Bailey is to be recommended, although morphological age and self-assessment of maturity are also acceptable methods.

ANTHROPOMETRY AND BODY COMPOSITION

Anthropometrical measures are important during growth. Typical growth curves of stature and mass are widely used by health professionals to assess a child's growth status against normative values (Child Growth Foundation). The basic principles of anthropometrics are the same for children and adults. The key

Sex	Maturation level	Estimated per cent body fat
Male	Prepubertal	$25.56 (\log S_4) - 22.23$
	Pubertal	$18.70 (\log S_4) - 11.91$
	Post-pubertal	$18.88 (\log S_4) - 15.58$
Female	Prepubertal	$29.85 (\log S_4) - 25.87$
	Pubertal	$23.94 (\log S_4) - 18.89$
	Post-pubertal	$39.02 (\log S_4) - 43.49$

Note
Where S_4 is the log (base 10) of the sum of four skinfolds in mm

differences are related to the approaches of the measurement, analysis and interpretation of data. For example, special regression equations have been used for the conversion of the sum of four skinfolds (biceps, triceps, subscapular and iliac crest) to percentage body fat for circumpubertal children (Deurenburg *et al.*, 1990).

These equations are different to those reported for use with adults (Durnin and Womersley, 1974) as children's body density changes with age from about 1.08 g·ml^{-1} at age 7 to 1.10 g·ml^{-1} at age 18 (Westrate and Deurenberg, 1989).

Clearly changes in body density will affect calculation of per cent body fat when using hydrostatic weighing. Lohman (1984) has reported an alternative to the Siri's equation for 8–12-year-old girls and boys that accounts for this change. Subsequently per cent body fat can be calculated using the following equations:

% fat $= (530/D) - 489$ (Lohman, 1984)

% fat $= ((5.62 - 4.2 \ (\text{age} - 2))/D) - (525 - 4.7 \ (\text{age} - 2))$ (Westrate and Deurenburg, 1989).

Skin folds are still a valid method for assessing adiposity in children. However, changes in the density of subcutaneous fat and other body tissues mitigate converting skinfold measures to percentage body fat. Therefore using the 'sum of skinfolds' technique is the most appropriate way of reporting adiposity data.

BODY MASS INDEX

The Body Mass Index (BMI) has taken on greater emphasis for reporting changes in whole population adiposity. Whereas this measure is not appropriate for use with individuals, its use in tracking population trends in adiposity has been controversial. There are a number of different interpretations of BMI cut points for UK children (Chinn and Rhona, 2002). These are calculated from adult cut points of 25 kg·m^{-2} (overweight) and 30 kg·m^{-2} (obese). BMI cut points for overweight and obese children are included in Table 22.1.

Body Mass Index is not without its critics, but the measure is still the most widely used to report changes in adiposity at a population level. Waist circumference is also being used in field studies where an estimate of visceral adiposity is required. Other more sophisticated measures such as bio-impedance, Dual Electron X-Ray Absorptiometry (DEXA), magnetic resonance imaging (MRI) and air displacement plethysmography (BodPod) are also available but their use is outside the scope of this chapter.

LABORATORY TESTS

Ergometry

Depending on the purpose of the testing, ergometers (treadmill or cycle) should be as child-friendly as possible. This should include either child-sized

Table 22.1   Cut off points for girls and boys between age 5 and 18 years defined to pass through UK BMI 25 and 30 at age 19.5 years

Age (years)	Overweight		Obese	
	Boys	*Girls*	*Boys*	*Girls*
5	16.9	17.3	18.9	19.6
6	17	17.5	19.3	20.1
7	17.3	17.9	20	21
8	17.7	18.4	20.8	22
9	18.2	19.1	21.8	23
10	18.8	19.8	22.8	24
11	19.4	20.5	23.7	25
12	20.1	21.3	24.6	26
13	20.8	22.1	25.5	26.9
14	21.5	22.8	26.4	27.7
15	22.3	23.4	27.2	28.3
16	23	23.9	27.9	28.8
17	23.6	24.3	28.6	29.3
18	24.2	24.6	29.2	29.6

Source: Chinn and Rona, 2002

ergometers or adaptations of the mechanical parts, for example, consideration of different crank lengths for younger children or when measuring $\dot{V}O_2$ appropriate sized mouth-pieces is crucial to account for differences in dead space and ventilation between adults and children. Familiarisation is very important particularly as for many children it might be their first experience of this equipment. As with adult data children's $\dot{V}O_2$ *peak* scores are higher on a treadmill than a cycle ergometer.

AEROBIC PERFORMANCE

Oxygen uptake test

Tests of oxygen uptake are well tolerated by children who have been suitably familiarised and then are capable of reaching limits of voluntary exhaustion. The preferred term when testing children to maximum is $\dot{V}O_2$ *peak* as only a minority of children exhibiting the classic plateau that is used to define $\dot{V}O_{2max}$ in adults. Studies comparing participants who plateau and those who do not plateau have not found a significant difference in final oxygen uptake scores, so it is considered a valid and reliable measure (Armstrong *et al.*, 1996).

Protocol

Both continuous and discontinuous protocols are suitable for children and will depend partially on what other measures are being collected. It is preferable that the younger a child is, that a discontinuous test is performed. This will allow talking and supporting the child during the rest periods and encourage them to maximal effort. This is particularly crucial, as few children will have experienced this level of effort.

For tests on the treadmill children tend to find it harder to run at high speeds therefore it is recommended that increments in intensity is achieved by raising the treadmill gradient. Initial starting speeds can be determined in the warm-up and should seek to elicit <70% heart rate maximum.

For cycle ergometers the principle of increasing intensity is similar to the treadmill, such that increments should not be so large as to induce premature fatigue and consequently these will not be as large as for adults.

Children, on average, reach a steady state in $\dot{V}O_2$ in ~2 min, therefore stage durations of 3 min or longer might only be beneficial if additional measures, for example, blood lactate are being collected.

An example of a discontinuous treadmill protocol is:

1   A warm-up of 3–4 min at 7 km·h^{-1} or 1 km·h^{-1} below the starting speed.
2   Test commences at 8 km·h^{-1} for 2 min duration.
3   A 1 min rest.
4   Repeat with increments of 1 km·h^{-1} every 2 min until the 10 km·h^{-1} stage is completed.
5   Speed remains constant and slope is raised 2.5% every 2 min until voluntary exhaustion.

An example of a continuous cycle protocol is:

1   A warm-up of 3–4 min at 25–50 W.
2   A starting power output of 50 W with increments of 25 W every 2 min until voluntary exhaustion.
3   A pedal cadence of between 60 and 70 rev·min^{-1} is well tolerated by most children.

Finally, in both examples it is important to monitor the child after the test to ensure no ill effects.

CRITERIA FOR $\dot{V}O_2$ PEAK

$\dot{V}O_2$ peak is defined as the highest $\dot{V}O_2$ elicited by the child and usually lacks the demonstration of a plateau. To support the conclusion of maximal effort specific secondary criteria should accompany the $\dot{V}O_2$ peak value. These include an RER >1.0 (treadmill) or 1.06 (cycle), a heart rate which is ≥95% of age predicted maximum and subjective criteria of facial flushing, hypernoea, sweating and unsteady gait. It is not recommended that a blood lactate value be used as an indicator of maximal effort in children, as suggested by some authors (Leger, 1996), as the variability post exercise is too great in children. Perceived exertion is another typical measure taken during a $\dot{V}O_2$ peak test and we recommend using the perceived exertion scale which has been developed for use with children. The Children's Effort rating table (CERT) (Williams *et al.*, 1994) is a numerical scale from 1 to 10 and has verbal exertional expressions that have been developed for children. This scale does not however, appear to be predictive of heart rate.

ANAEROBIC

Anaerobic testing of children is not as well developed as the testing of aerobic performance. The most common test of anaerobic performance is the Wingate test (Bar-Or, 1986) and most protocol guidelines are similar to adults. The most important issue is the load applied most common is 75 g·kg^{-1} body mass (0.74 N·kg^{-1}) although it has been found that loads between 64 and 78 g·kg^{-1} does not significantly alter the peak power obtained. As with adults there is an aerobic contribution to the 30 s Wingate test as high as 36% in some studies, hence shorter tests such as the Force–velocity might be advantageous to assess peak anaerobic power. We would recommend a flying start for the commencement of anaerobic power tests to overcome the inertia of flywheel that is going to be disproportionately higher for children compared to adults. However, software is available to account for these inertial and load corrections. For the youngest children 30 s might be too long as the ensuing fatigue might render the pedal cadence so slow that continuing to turn the pedals becomes extremely difficult. Therefore, a test of 20 s might be more appropriate (Chia *et al.*, 1997).

BLOOD ANALYSIS

The interpretation of children's blood lactate response is not well understood because of the influence of growth and maturation. Differences in methodologies such as venous or capillary samples, whole blood or plasma, and protein-free or lysed blood assays have not helped to clarify these influences (Williams *et al.*, 1992). Although venous sampling has been performed in children for studies investigating cholesterol or free fatty acids, the collection of serum lactates would appear not to be justifiable.

In adults studies the 4 mmol·l^{-1} reference point as an indicator of sub-maximal performance has often been used. However in children, this absolute value is too high and approaches maximal values. More common is a fixed value of 2.5 mmol·l^{-1} (Williams and Armstrong, 1991). For ascertaining peak blood lactate values, a 3-min post-exercise sampling appears to be the most commonly reported. However, it should be noted that this merely reflects the peak value at 3 min and does not necessarily indicate the highest value post exercise.

ISOKINETIC STRENGTH TESTING

Although there is much strength data available for children, much of it is field-based or conducted using purpose-built dynamometers. There is less data on commercially available isokinetic dynamometers, however, children are able to use this equipment if it is adapted. This includes appropriate attention to the back support, length of lever, stabilising straps and the mechanical degree of adjustment for the ergometer. Unlike for adults (Osternig, 1986) there are no set protocols for children when testing for strength (e.g. number of repetitions ranges from 3 to 8) or endurance (number of repetitions ranges from 10 to 50). Suffice that familiarisation and practice will need to be more extensive than for adults. A typical protocol for a maximal isokinetic strength test in children could be:

1   Warm-up 4–5 min including cardiovascular and stretching routine.
2   Practice tests consisting of 5–10 sub-maximal contractions and re-iteration of pre-test instructions.
3   Maximal contractions consisting of 3–6 repetitions.

For a review see de Ste Croix *et al.* (2002).

FIELD MEASURES OF FITNESS/ PERFORMANCE

Coaches, teachers, researchers and allied health professionals commonly use field measures to track the fitness of large populations. During field-testing, fitness is assessed through a battery of tests that are carried out in a predetermined order. The battery usually includes each component of the health (cardiorespiratory, strength, flexibility, body composition, local muscular endurance) and skill (agility, speed, power, balance, reaction time, coordination) related fitness model. These tests have received much criticism over the years because of the limited reliability and validity data and their appropriateness in educational settings. The reliability and validity data that are available have good agreement with criterion and test–retest measures, respectively (see Docherty, 1996 for a review). A better understanding of how to use field tests with youngsters now allows more accurate interpretation and presentation of test results. 'Normative tests' that were popular in the 1970s and 1980s have now been superseded by 'criterion-referenced' tests. Criterion-referenced tests produce performance bands that all children are expected to achieve as opposed to norm tests where percentile scores are attributed to each test. The use of normative referenced tests results in peer comparison that is problematic as results are significantly influenced by physical maturity and genetic endowment whereas criterion-referenced tests use set standards that students can meet and use individually. The other problem with field tests is that there is little empirical evidence to suggest that they are related to any aspect of health or wellness (Riddoch and Boreham, 2000). Given these limitations appropriately designed and delivered field tests of fitness with British

Table 22.2 The EUROFIT fitness test battery

Dimensions	Factor	EUROFIT test	Order of test
Balance	Total body balance	Flamingo balance	1
Speed	Limb speed	Plate tapping	2
Flexibility	Flexibility	Sit and reach	3
Power	Explosive strength	Standing broad jump	4
Strength	Static strength	Hand grip	5
Muscular endurance	Trunk strength	Sit-ups	6
Muscular endurance	Functional strength	Bent arm hang	7
Speed	Running speed agility	Shuttle run 10 m × 5 m	8
Cardiorespiratory fitness	Cardiorespiratory fitness	Endurance shuttle run	9

populations are needed. The largest set of field test fitness data was produced in the Northern Ireland Children's Fitness Survey (Riddoch *et al.*, 1991) and more recently through the Sportlinx project (Taylor *et al.*, 2004). Other than these datasets there is little whole population fitness data available on United Kingdom children. The test most widely used in the United Kingdom is the EUROFIT fitness test battery (Adam *et al.*, 1988). The component of fitness assessed and the order of the tests are outlined in Table 22.2. A detailed description of the tests can be found elsewhere (Adam *et al.*, 1988).

An excellent review of field tests of fitness can be found in Safrit and Wood (1995) and Docherty (1996).

IMPLEMENTATION OF TESTS

When used appropriately fitness testing can be an important aspect of children's education (Cale and Harris, 2005). To achieve a positive testing climate, environments should be inclusive, supportive and conducive to learning where emphasis should be on effort and individual development from test to test. Children should be able to practice the tests before an official measurement starts.

These criteria are important, as field tests have been criticised for de-motivating children who are either unfit or disenfranchised from physical activity. Therefore, care should be taken to ensure that social environments are developed that reward effort as well as performance during fitness testing. For example, setting up an environment where an overweight and physically immature child may be exposed as a failure is clearly bad practice and this should be avoided. When comparisons need to be made these can be done at a group level where boys tend to have better endurance running capacity than girls, heavier children have better grip strength then their lighter peers and girls are more flexible than boys. The uses of field tests by suitably qualified personnel are appropriate at whole population level (for research) or to provide individual feedback about the development of a child's fitness during the growing years.

ADULT CHILD DIFFERENCES

Children will need more time than adults to familiarise themselves with tests. Test results may be more affected by biological age than chronological age making individual comparisons between circumpubescents difficult. Scoring systems in the 20-m multi-stage shuttle run test are different. Instead of using levels (e.g. 7.2) the number of 20-m shuttles are counted, 50 shuttles = 1,000 m.

The use of field tests of fitness to monitor individuals in education, sport and health settings is supported if they are implemented in an appropriate manner by trained individuals who understand their strengths and limitations for use with children.

Key messages for fitness testing in young children:

1   *Individualise* fitness testing.
2   Make fitness testing a *positive* and *fun* experience for *all*.
3   *Teach* concepts during fitness tests. *For example, sit and reach would be linked to flexibility for daily tasks, issues about losing flexibility with age, etc.*
4   Use *developmentally appropriate* tests.
5   Minimise the public nature of testing when you think it may cause embarrassment.
6   Take care to monitor fitness over time and make children aware that sometimes *fitness testing results may be affected by stage of maturation.*
7   Physical activity and fitness test results are *not always* related. A child's fitness may be mainly due to genetic inheritance. This relates to the 'cannot choose my own parents' adage.

PHYSICAL ACTIVITY

Objective and subjective measures

There are over 30 methods of measuring physical activity available but no gold standard is available. Methods can be broadly categorised into objective and subjective areas. Subjective methods include activity diaries, retrospective questionnaires and systematic observation. Objective methods include, pedometers, accelerometers, heart rate monitors and doubly labelled water. The type of monitor chosen will primarily depend on the scientific question being asked but may also be influenced by expediency, accuracy and cost. Paper-based questionnaires whilst being less intrusive are generally thought to be the least robust measure of physical activity particularly in younger children. The most commonly used measures in paediatric populations are accelerometers, pedometers and heart rate telemetry systems. The most important factor to consider when measuring physical activity in children is that 90% of their activity is of high intensity and lasts for 15 s or less (Bailey, 1990). Therefore, scientists need to use sampling rates of 15 s or less if valid results are to be gained. Systems that use sophisticated software also allow detailed analysis of the frequency, duration and intensity of physical activity. The tempo of physical activity is of particular interest for studies that wish to have a detailed measure of behaviour change. For a more detailed description of physical activity measurement see Welk (2002).

REFERENCES

Adam, C., Klissouras, V., Ravazzolo, M., Renson, R. and Tuxworth, W. (1988). *EUROFIT: European Test of Physical Fitness*. Rome: Council of Europe, Committee for the Development of Sport.

Armstrong, N., Welsman, J. and Winsley, R. (1996). Is peak VO_2 a maximal index of children's aerobic fitness? *International Journal of Sports Medicine*, 17: 356–359.

Bailey, R.C., Olson, J., Pepper, S.L., Porszasz, J., Barstow, T.J. and Cooper, D.M. (1995). The level and tempo of children's physical activities: an observational study. *Medicine and Science in Sports and Exercise*, 27: 1033–1041.

Bar-Or, O. (1996). Anaerobic performance. In D. Docherty (ed.), *Measurement in Pediatric Exercise Science*, pp. 161–182. Champaign, IL: Human Kinetics.

Cale, L. and Harris, J. (2005). *Exercise and Young People: Issues, Implications and Initiatives*, pp. 41–80. Basingstoke, UK: Palgrave Macmillan.

Chia, M., Armstrong, N. and Childs, D. (1997). The assessment of children's anaerobic performance using modifications of the Wingate anaerobic test. *Pediatric Exercise Science*, 9: 80–89.

Child Growth Foundation.

Children Act 1999 Craig.

Chinn, S. and Rona, R.J. (2002). International definitions of overweight and obesity for children: a lasting solution? *Annals of Human Biology*, 29: 306–313.

De Ste Croix, M.B.A., Deighan, M.A. and Armstrong, N. (2003). Assessment and interpretation of isokinetic muscle strength during growth and maturation. *Sports Medicine*, 33(10): 727–743.

Department of Health (2000). The Protection of Children Act 1999: a practical guide to the act for all organisations working with children. Department of Health and the NHS Executive, London: Department of Health.

Deurenberg, P., Pieters, J.J. and Hautvast, J.G. (1990). The assessment of the body fat percentage by skinfold thickness measurements in childhood and young adolescence. *British Journal of Nutrition*, 63: 293–303.

Durnin, J.V. and Womersley, J. (1974). Body fat assessed from total body density and its estimation from skinfold thickness: measurements on 481 men and women aged from 16 to 72 years. *British Journal of Nutrition*, 32(1): 77–97.

Docherty, D. (ed.) (1996). *Measurement in Pediatric Exercise Science*. Champaign, IL: Human Kinetics.

Greulich, W.W. and Pyle, S.I. (1959). Radiographic atlas of skeletal development of the hand and wristv (2nd edn) Stanford, CA: Stanford University Press.

Jago, R. and Bailey, R. (2001). Ethics and paediatric exercise science: issues and making a submission to a local ethics and research committee. *Journal of Sports Science*, 19(7): 527–535.

Leger, L. and Gadoury, C. (1989). Validity of the 20 m shuttle run test with 1 min stages to predict VO_{2max} in adults. *Canadian Journal of Sports Science*, 14(1): 21–26.

Lohman, T.G. (1984). Research progress in validation of laboratory methods of assessing body composition. *Medicine and Science in Sports and Exercise*, 16: 596–603.

Matsudo, S.M. and Matsudo, V.R. (1993). Validity of self evaluation on determination of sexual maturation level. In A.C Claessens, J. Lefevre and B. Vanden Eynde (eds), *World Wide Variation In Physical Fitness*, pp. 106–109. Leuven: Institute of Physical Education.

Mirwald, R.L., Baxter-Jones, A.D., Bailey, D.A. and Beunen, G.P. (2002). An assessment of maturity from anthropometric measurements. *Medicine and Science in Sports and Exercise*, 34(4): 689–694.

Morris, N.M. and Udry, J.R. (1980). Validation of a self-administered instrument to assess stage of adolescent development. *Journal of Youth and Adolescence*, 9: 271–280.

Osternig, L.R. (1986). Isokinetic dynamometry; implications for muscle testing and rehabilitation. In K.B. Pandolf (ed.), *Exercise and Sorts Sciences Reviews*, 14: 45–80. New York: Macmillan.

Riddoch, C.J. and Boreham, C. (2000). Physical activity, physical fitness and children's health: current concepts. In A. Armstrong and W. van Mechelen (eds), *Pediatric Exercise Science and Medicine*, pp. 243–252. Oxford, UK: Oxford University Press.

Riddoch, C.J., Mahoney, C., Murphy, N., Boreham, C. and Cran, G. (1991). The physical activity patterns of Northern Irish schoolchildren age's 11–16 years. *Pediatric Exercise Science*, 3: 300–309.

Roche, A.F., Chumlea, W.C. and Thissen, D. (1988). Assessing the skeletal maturity of the hand-wrist: Fels method. Springfield, IL: Charles Thomas.

Safrit, M.J. and Wood, T.M. (1995). *Introduction to Measurement in Physical Education and Exercise Science*, 3rd edn. New York: Mosby.

Tanner, J.M. (1962). *Growth of Adolescents*, 2nd edn. Oxford, UK: Blackwell Scientific.

Taylor, S.R., Hackett, A.F., Stratton, G. and Lamb, L. (2004). SportsLinx: improving the health and fitness of Liverpool's youth. *Education and Health*, 22: 11–15.

Welk, G.J. (2002). *Physical Activity Assessments for Health Related Research*. Champaign, IL: Human Kinetics.

Westrate and Deurenberg (1989).

Williams, C.A. (2003). Ethics in paediatric exercise science. BASES World, March, 10–11.

Williams, J.G., Eston, R. and Furlong, BA.F. (1994). CERT: a perceived exertion scale for young children. *Perceptual and Motor Skills*, 79: 1451–1458.

Williams, J.R. and Armstrong, N. (1991). Relationship of maximal lactate steady state to performance at fixed blood lactate reference values in children. *Pediatric Exercise Science*, 3: 333–341.

Williams, J.R., Armstrong, N. and Kirby, B.J. (1992). The influence and site of sampling and assay medium upon the measurement and interpretation of blood lactate responses to exercise. *Journal of Sports Sciences*, 10: 95–107.

Working Party of Research in Children (1991). *The Ethical Conduct of Research on Children*. London: Medical Research Council.

CHAPTER 23

TESTING OLDER PEOPLE

John M. Saxton

INTRODUCTION

The 2001 census showed that over a fifth of the UK population is now aged over 60. Furthermore, the number of people aged 65 and over is expected to increase at 10 times the overall rate of population growth over the next 40 years and the number of people over the age of 80 is expected to treble in the next quarter of a century (Dean, 2003). The rapid growth of the ageing population, especially amongst the oldest old, means that preventing or delaying the onset of physical frailty and increasing the number of years spent in good health has become an important public health goal.

THE AGE-ASSOCIATED DECLINE IN PHYSIOLOGIC FUNCTION

Ageing is characterised by a decline in cardiorespiratory, muscular, neurological and metabolic capacities (Pendergast *et al.*, 1993). This can severely limit the ability to perform everyday activities, including walking, stair-climbing and even rising from a chair. As many older adults function close to their maximum physical ability level during normal daily activities (Rikli and Jones, 1997), any further decline in physiologic function or small physical set-back could result in the loss of functional independence (Rikli and Jones, 1999a). Shephard (1997) outlined a classification system for the different stages of middle to old age, based on functional status:

- Middle age (40–65 years) – associated with a 10–30% loss of biological function.
- Old age or 'young old age' (65–75 years) – associated with some further loss of biological function, but without any gross impairment of homeostasis.

- Very old age (75–85 years) – characterised by substantial impairment of function in daily activities, but still being capable of functional independence.
- Oldest old age (>85 years) – during which time institutional or nursing care is often required.

The age-associated decline in cardiovascular function is characterised by anatomical and neurological changes affecting the heart and blood vessels, which decrease cardiorespiratory capacity, and hence, aerobic exercise capacity. Aerobic exercise capacity declines at the rate of 7–10% per decade from early adulthood (Fitzgerald *et al.*, 1997; Wilson and Tanaka, 2000), and this can severely reduce sustainable exercise intensity in later years. Changes in arterial structure and vasomotor tone also adversely affect blood pressure, which has a tendency to rise with increasing age in most Western societies and contributes to the age-related increased risk of cardiovascular disorders.

The decline in muscular strength and power with advancing age is judged to have a more profound impact on daily functioning than the decline in cardiorespiratory capacity (Pendergast *et al.*, 1993). The age-related decline in muscular strength occurs sooner and at a faster rate in the lower extremities than in the upper extremities (Frontera *et al.*, 1991), and this can severely affect ambulatory activities. Lower-limb muscle function is considered vital for functional independence and prevention of disability (Pendergast *et al.*, 1993; Guralnik *et al.*, 1995). A direct association between impaired lower-limb physiologic function and everyday activities such as walking and rising from a chair has been demonstrated in the elderly (Judge *et al.*, 1993b; Ferrucci *et al.*, 1997). The decline in leg strength and power with advancing age is also associated with an increased risk of falls and resulting fractures (Whipple *et al.*, 1987; Nevitt *et al.*, 1989; Gehlsen and Whaley, 1990).

FUNCTIONAL FITNESS FOR OLDER ADULTS

Functional fitness for older people has been defined as the physical capacity required to perform normal everyday activities safely and independently without undue fatigue, or with adequate physiologic reserve (Rikli and Jones, 1997). Traditional ergometric tests to volitional exhaustion (developed and validated for younger populations) are generally deemed inappropriate for older adults, as they do not reflect the physical abilities required for common daily activities, including stair climbing, rising from a chair, lifting, reaching and bending. Furthermore, they are likely to be unsafe for the majority of older adults who, on the whole, are likely to be poorly accustomed to exercise ergometers and generally need medical supervision for anything other than light to moderate intensity physical exertion. Traditional ergometer tests are perhaps only suitable for an elite few per cent of the elderly population who are physically fit and/or 'Master' athletes and accustomed to the demands of vigorous exercise. At the other end of the continuum, assessment of functional status in the frail and/or disabled elderly, who constitute ~25% of the elderly population (Rikli and Jones, 1997), requires the use of self-care activity scales, referred to as activities of daily living (Mahoney and Barthel, 1965; Katz *et al.*, 1970; Hedrick, 1995) or instrumental activities of daily living (Lawton and Brody 1969; Lawton *et al.*, 1982).

The physically independent elderly make up the largest sub-group of older people, constituting ~70% of adults over 75 (Spirduso, 1995; Rikli and Jones, 1997). The physically independent elderly exhibit wide variations in physical ability, from those who have enough physical function to participate in voluntary social, occupational and recreational activities, to those who are borderline frail and highly vulnerable to unexpected physical stress or challenge (Spirduso, 1995). Reliable and valid tests that can detect the early stages of functional decline and aid in the prescription of appropriate physical activity interventions in this large heterogeneous sub-group could have the biggest impact on fraily prevention and maintenance of physical independence in older people (Guralnik *et al.*, 1995; Gill *et al.*, 1996; Lawrence and Jette, 1996; Morey *et al.*, 1998).

FUNCTIONAL FITNESS TEST BATTERY ITEMS

A number of functional fitness test batteries have been developed and validated for older adults in the age-range 60 – >90 years, including the American Alliance for Health, Physical Education, Recreation and Dance (AAHPERD) Functional Fitness Assessment Battery (Osness *et al.*, 1990, 1996), the Physical Performance Test (Reuben and Siu, 1990), the MacArthur Physical Performance Scale (Seeman *et al.*, 1994), the Established Populations for Epidemiologic Studies of the Elderly (EPESE) short battery of items to measure strength, balance and gait speed (Guralnik *et al.*, 1994) and the Senior Fitness Test (SFT) (Rikli and Jones, 1999a,b; Rikli and Jones, 2001).

The test items described in this section are typical of those used to assess functional fitness in physically independent older adults of diverse physical ability. Many of the test items have been through extensive validation procedures, although it is recommended that each test centre develop its own test–retest reproducibility data. Normative data for older people on the individual test items can be found in the Allied Dunbar National Fitness Survey (Activity and Health Research, 1992), and in the publications of Osness *et al.* (1996), Rikli and Jones (1999b) and Holland *et al.* (2002). It is recommended that a test battery of functional fitness for older adults should include at least one test item from each of the core physiologic function variables that underpin common everyday activities. These were defined by Osness *et al.* (1990) and Rikli and Jones (1999a) as:

1   Muscle strength/endurance
2   Aerobic endurance
3   Flexibility
4   Balance/agility
5   Body composition.

Muscular strength/endurance

Chair sit-to-stand test

A common method of assessing lower-body muscle function in older adults is the chair sit-to-stand test. Variations of this test exist, but protocols that assess the time it takes to perform a given number of sit-to-stand repetitions (e.g. 5 or 10) have the disadvantage of 'floor' effects because some elderly people might not be able to achieve the number required to complete the test. However, testing the number of repetitions achievable in a set amount of time can overcome this problem. Chair sit-to-stand performance has a good correlation $(r > 0.7)$ with one repetition maximum leg-press strength in elderly men and women (Rikli and Jones, 1999a).

   The equipment requirements for this test are a stopwatch and a foldable or plastic moulded straight-back chair (without arms or seating cushion) with approximate seating height, width and depth dimensions of 0.45, 0.50 and 0.40 m, respectively (Csuka and McCarty, 1985; Jones et al., 1999; Rikli and Jones, 2001). The chair should have rubber tips underneath each leg to prevent slippage. The chair back is placed against the wall to prevent movement and the participant is seated in the middle of the chair, with back straight and feet approximately shoulder width apart at an angle slightly back from the knees; one foot is placed slightly in front of the other to aid balance and the arms are crossed in front of the chest. This test should be performed either barefooted, or in low-heeled shoes. At the signal to 'go', the participant rises to the full standing position before returning to the seated position as many times as possible in 30 s. Participants are instructed to look straight ahead and to stand up with their weight evenly distributed between both feet. The score is the total number of stands performed correctly (full standing position attained and fully seated between stands) in 30 s. If a participant is more than half way up at the end of the 30 s, this is counted as a full stand (Jones et al., 1999).

Arm-curl test

Adequate upper-body strength and endurance are required for many everyday activities, such as cleaning, carrying food shopping and gardening. A test that reflects the strength requirements of these every activities is the arm-curl test (Osness et al., 1990; Rikli and Jones, 2001). In this test, participants curl a standardised weight using the forearm flexors as many times as possible in a set amount of time. As upper-body strength declines with increasing age and in elderly women is ~50% of that in elderly men (Frontera et al., 1991), these considerations need to be taken into account when deciding on the weight to be used for women and men. The AAHPERD test (Osness et al., 1990) states that weights of 4 lb (1.81 kg) and 8 lb (3.63 kg) should be used for women and men, respectively, whereas the SFT (Rikli and Jones, 2001) uses a weight of 5 lb (2.27 kg) for women.

   The equipment requirements for this test are a stopwatch, a foldable or plastic moulded straight-back chair (as for chair sit-to-stand test), and a dumbbell or other suitable weight such as plastic milk cartons filled with sand, water or other material with handles that can be gripped easily. As normative data for the age-ranges 60–94 years are available for the SFT (Rikli and Jones, 2001), weights of 2.27 kg (women) and 3.63 kg (men) are suggested. Velcro wrist straps can be used for individuals with gripping problems resulting from conditions such as arthritis. The participant is seated with back straight and feet flat on the floor, holding the weight in the dominant hand at the side of the body in the fully extended elbow position. The elbow should be braced against the side of the body to stabilise the upper arm. Using good form (the upper arm must remain still throughout the test), the participant curls the weight up and down. The score is the total number of repetitions performed correctly in 30 s. An arm-curl that is more than half way up at the end of 30 s is counted as a full arm-curl (Rikli and Jones, 2001). In the AAHPERD test battery (Osness et al., 1990, 1996), the lower arm must touch the test administrator's hand which is placed on the participant's bicep at termination of the up-phase to be deemed a successful repetition. The number of repetitions achieved in 30 s has a good correlation ($r > 0.77$) with overall upper body strength (as indicated by combined 1TRM biceps, chest press and seated row strength) in elderly men and women (Rikli and Jones, 1999a).

Grip strength

Maximum grip strength can also be included in a functional fitness test battery as an index of upper-limb strength. In this test, a grip-strength dynamometer is gripped between flexed fingers and the base of the thumb with the participant in a seated position, and with the measurement normally being restricted to the dominant hand, unless prevented by injury. The Allied Dunbar National Fitness Survey (Activity and Health Research, 1992) reported a significant decline in hand-grip strength with age, being 30% less in the 65–74 year age group, in comparison to younger adults aged 25–44 years. Handgrip strength of 150 N, or that is equivalent to 20% of body weight, has been suggested as a threshold for performance of everyday tasks requiring a firm grip, as the strength needed to raise body weight onto a raised bus platform is estimated as 17–20% body weight (Activity and Health Research, 1992).

Aerobic endurance

Six-min walk test

Walking is an activity that is fundamental to functional independence. The timed 6-min walk test, which is an adaptation of the 12-min walk-run test originally developed by Cooper (1968) assesses the maximum distance walked in 6 min along a rectangular course (Rikli and Jones, 2001), or up and down a 20–30 m corridor (Simonsick et al., 2001; Steffen et al., 2002). As it is a timed test, walking distance can be obtained for elderly individuals of wide-ranging functional ability. For this test, the 20–30 m corridor or flat 50 m rectangular course (20 m × 5 m) is marked off in 5 m segments with marker cones and foldable or plastic moulded straight-back chairs are positioned at various locations along the course for resting. Participants walk as fast as they can (without running) up and down or around the course, covering as much distance as possible in the 6-min time limit. Standardised encouragement can be given at minutes 1, 3, and 5 to aid pacing (Steffen *et al.*, 2002). At the end of the 6-min time period, participants are told to stop walking and the distance walked, to the nearest meter, is recorded. The timed 6-min walk test has a good correlation ($r > 0.7$) with time to reach 85% predicted maximum heart rate on a progressive treadmill test in elderly men and women (Rikli and Jones, 1998). Alternative tests of lower-limb aerobic endurance (where space is limited) include the 2-min step test (Rikli and Jones, 2001) and the Self-Paced Step Test (Petrella *et al.*, 2001), which were developed for older people.

Flexibility

Lower back and hamstrings flexibility: sit-and-reach test

Impaired flexibility, such as the age-associated decreased range of motion at the hip joint (Roach and Miles, 1991), influences movement dysfunction and disability in the elderly. Variations of the sit-and-reach test have been used for assessing lower back and hamstrings flexibility in older persons, including the conventional 'floor' sit-and-reach test (Osness *et al.*, 1990), a modified sit and reach test (Lemmink *et al.*, 2003) and a seated sit-and-reach test developed by Jones *et al.* (1998).

For this test, the participant sits on the floor in an upright position, with back straight and legs fully extended with the bottom of the bare feet against a sit-and-reach box. The hands are placed one on top of the other and the participant is instructed to slowly reach forward, keeping the hands together and pushing the fingers along the box as far as possible. If participants cannot hold a sitting position on a flat surface with both legs extended, a seated sit-and-reach test can be used (Jones *et al.*, 1998). In this test, the participant sits on the front edge of a chair with one leg extended out in front (knee straight, ankle fully dorsi-flexed, heel resting on the floor) and the other leg bent at the knee with foot flat on the floor. The chair sit-and-reach test has a good correlation ($r > 0.75$) with goniometer-measured hamstring flexibility in elderly men and women (Jones *et al.*, 1998). In both variations of the test, the final position should be held for 2 s and the distance between the finger tips and toes, to the nearest centimetre is recorded. A negative score is assigned to a distance short of reaching the toes and a positive score to a distance reached beyond the toes. Sit-and-reach testing is contra-indicated in participants with extreme kyphosis and in osteoporotic individuals who have previously sustained a vertebral fracture.

Shoulder flexibility: back scratch test

Shoulder flexibility is required for everyday activities such as reaching behind the head and/or lower back to comb hair, to put on, take off or fasten garments, reach into back pockets and wash one's back (Rikli and Jones, 1999a). The back scratch test (Rikli and Jones, 2001) is a convenient way to measure overall shoulder range of motion. This test involves a combination of shoulder abduction, adduction, and internal and external rotation, and measures the distance (or overlap) of the middle fingers behind the back. The only equipment requirement for this test is a 0.5 m ruler or meter stick. The participant places one hand behind the same side shoulder with palm flat on the back and fingers reaching down towards the middle of the back as far as possible. The other hand is placed behind the back (palm facing outwards) and reaches up as far as possible in an attempt to touch or overlap with the fingers of the other hand. Two test trials are allowed and the score is the distance of overlap (positive score) or distance between the middle fingers (negative score), recorded to the nearest centimetre. Both arm combinations can be measured, but normative data are only generally available for the preferred hand combination (i.e. the hand combination that gives the best score), which can be determined during practice trials.

Balance/agility

Static and dynamic balance

A number of different test protocols have been used to assess static and dynamic balance in the elderly. The Berg Balance Scale assesses the ability to successfully accomplish static, dynamic and weight shifting activities, with each of the 14 items being graded 0–4 by the test administrator (Berg et al., 1989; Berg et al., 1992a,b). A common measure of static balance in the elderly is the ability to maintain balance under conditions of reduced base of support with the eyes open or closed. Different stances are commonly used, including the parallel stance (feet touching side-by-side); semi-tandem stance (from the parallel stance, one foot is moved half a length forward); tandem stance (one foot placed in front of the other, heel to toe) and single-leg stance (Iverson et al., 1990; Verfaillie et al., 1997; Brown et al., 2000). The test score is the maximum length of time that a stance can be held, but usually with the test being terminated after a predetermined length of time (e.g. 10–60 s) for practical reasons. A major problem with static balance tests is that a large proportion of the elderly can achieve perfect scores (ceiling effect). However, caution should be taken with eyes-closed tests to reduce the risk of falls.

Dynamic balance has been measured by counting the number of successful steps or stepping errors while subjects walk toe to heel (tandem walk) over a specified distance or to a maximum number of steps (Nevitt et al., 1989; Topp et al., 1993; Dargent-Molina et al., 1996). Dynamic balance can also be assessed by measuring the time taken to walk along a balance beam placed on the floor (Cress et al., 1999; Brown et al., 2000) or by using the functional reach test, which is a test of the maximum forward displacement of the centre of mass and thus, the 'margin of stability' within the base of support (Duncan et al., 1990). In the latter test, the difference between arm's length and maximum forward reach is measured using a meter stick attached to the wall.

Surrogate measures of dynamic balance include the preferred and maximal walking velocities. Preferred walking velocity decreases linearly with advancing age (Cunningham *et al.*, 1982) and slower preferred and maximal walking velocities are characteristic of older adult fallers (Wolfson *et al.*, 1990; Lipsitz *et al.*, 1991; Wolfson *et al.*, 1995). Preferred and maximal walking velocity is usually measured over a set distance of 6–10 m (Reuben and Siu, 1990; Judge *et al.*, 1993a; Buchner *et al.*, 1996). However, preferred gait velocity has also been measured over 100 m on an indoor oval course (Bassey *et al.*, 1976). This approach may be superior to shorter distance tests, as participants have more time to attain and maintain preferred gait velocity (Table 23.1).

Agility

Timed up-and-go tests measure agility and reflect everyday activities such as disembarking from a bus or car in an efficient and safe manner, quickly getting up to answer the door or telephone, or to tend to something in the kitchen (Rikli and Jones, 1999a). A number of such tests have been described in the literature (Mathias *et al.*, 1986; Osness *et al.*, 1990; Rikli and Jones, 2001) and

Table 23.1 Common tests of balance and agility in the elderly

Functional fitness dimension	Protocol	References
Static balance	Ability to balance for 10–60 s in various stances: for example parallel stance; tandem stance; single-leg stance	Brown *et al.* (2000)
		Iverson *et al.* (1990)
		Verfaillie *et al.* (1997)
Dynamic balance	Tandem walk	Nevitt *et al.* (1989)
		Topp *et al.* (1993)
		Dargent-Molina *et al.* (1996)
	Balance beam walk	Cress *et al.* (1999)
		Brown *et al.* (2000)
	Functional reach test	Duncan *et al.* (1990)
	Preferred and maximum	Buchner *et al.* (1996)
	walking velocity	Judge *et al.* (1993a)
		Reuben and Siu (1990)
Combined static and dynamic balance	Berg Balance Scale	Berg *et al.* (1989)
		Berg *et al.* (1992a)
		Berg *et al.* (1992b)
Agility	Timed up-and-go tests	Mathias *et al.* (1986)
		Osness *et al.* (1990)
		Rikli and Jones (2001)

consist of a timed course, which can be set-up using minimal equipment and space. Variations of timed up-and-go tests involve participants walking as quickly as possible around cones located 2–3 m in front of, or diagonally to the rear of a seated starting position, before returning quickly to the seated position.

Body composition: body mass index

There is evidence of a link between body composition and ability to perform common everyday activities in community-dwelling elderly people and elderly individuals with a high or low body mass index (BMI) are more likely to be disabled in later years than people with normal BMI scores (Galanos *et al.*, 1994). Low BMI is also associated with increased risk of mortality in the elderly, particularly in individuals who lose 10% or more of body weight between the age of 50 and old age (Losonczy *et al.*, 1995). Thus, the inclusion of BMI as a simple index of body composition in a functional fitness test battery for the elderly seems appropriate.

PRE-TEST CONSIDERATIONS FOR ELDERLY PERSONS

The functional fitness test items described should be safe for most community-residing physically independent older adults to perform without medical screening or supervision, as they bear no more risk than common everyday activities. Nevertheless, test administrators (and testing centres, if appropriate) should have a well-defined emergency plan to deal with unexpected medical emergencies and accidents, and have 'first aiders' on hand to manage such situations as they arise. Test administrators should also be vigilant of warning signs that are indicative of undue physiological stress (e.g. excessively high heart rate, nausea, dyspneoa, pallor and pain).

Pre-test procedures should include adequate training and practice sessions for the test administrator(s) and an appropriate gentle warm-up for the participants. The warm-up should provide a period of cardiovascular and metabolic adjustment, followed by mobility exercises in which relevant joints are moved through their comfortable ranges of motion. All tests should be preceded by a full demonstration of the procedure and 1–2 practice trials. Pre-test documentation to be administered should include:

- A 'user-friendly' information sheet, including details of the pre-test instructions (e.g. the need to avoid strenuous exercise, alcohol, heavy meals in the hours preceding the test and the importance of suitable attire).
- A Physical Activity Readiness Questionnaires (PAR-Q) to identify individuals who require a General Practitioner's examination and approval before performing the test battery. Older individuals who have

previously experienced chest pain, irregular, rapid or fluttery heart beats or severe shortness of breath should seek the advice of their General Practitioner before undergoing an assessment of functional fitness.

- An informed consent form explaining the risks and responsibilities associated with the testing procedures and informing prospective participants of their right to discontinue testing at any time.

REFERENCES

Activity and Health Research. (1992). *Allied Dunbar National Fitness Survey: Main Findings*. Sports Council and Health Education Authority, London.

Bassey, E.J., Fentem, P.H., MacDonald, I.C. and Scriven, P.M. (1976). Self-paced walking as a method for exercise testing in elderly and young men. *Clinical Science and Molecular Medicine*, 51(Suppl.): 609–612.

Berg, K., Wood-Dauphinee, S., Williams, J.I. and Gayton, D. (1989). Measuring balance in the elderly: preliminary development of an instrument. *Physiotherapy Canada*, 41: 304–311.

Berg, K.O., Maki, B.E., Williams, J.I., Holliday, P.J. and Wood-Dauphinee, S.L. (1992a). Clinical and laboratory measures of postural balance in an elderly population. *Archives of Physical Medicine and Rehabilitation*, 73: 1073–1080.

Berg, K.O., Wood-Dauphinee, S.L., Williams, J.I. and Maki, B. (1992b). Measuring balance in the elderly: validation of an instrument. *Canadian Journal of Public Health*, 83 (Suppl. 2): S7–S11.

Brown, M., Sinacore, D.R., Ehsani, A.A., Binder, E.F., Holloszy, J.O. and Kohrt, W.M. (2000). Low-intensity exercise as a modifier of physical frailty in older adults. *Archives of Physical Medicine and Rehabilitation*, 81: 960–965.

Buchner, D.M., Guralnik, J.M. and Cress, M.E. (1996). The clinical assessment of gait, balance, and mobility in older adults. In L.Z. Rubenstein, D. Wieland and R. Bernabei (eds). *Geriatric Assessment Technology: The State of Art*, pp. 75–89. Milan: Kurtis Editrice.

Cooper, K.H. (1968). A means of assessing maximal oxygen intake. Correlation between field and treadmill testing. *Journal of the American Medical Association*, 203: 201–204.

Cress, M.E., Buchner, D.M., Questad, K.A., Esselman, P.C., deLateur, B.J. and Schwartz, R.S. (1999). Exercise: effects on physical functional performance in independent older adults. *Journals of Gerontology. Series A, Biological Sciences and Medical Sciences*, 54: M242–M248.

Csuka, M. and McCarty, D.J. (1985). Simple method for measurement of lower extremity muscle strength. *American Journal of Medicine*, 78: 77–81.

Cunningham, D.A., Rechnitzer, P.A., Pearce, M.E. and Donner, A.P. (1982). Determinants of self-selected walking pace across ages 19 to 66. *Journal of Gerontology*, 37: 560–564.

Dargent-Molina, P., Favier, F., Grandjean, H., Baudoin, C., Schott, A.M., Hausherr, E., Meunier, P.J. and Breart, G. (1996). Fall-related factors and risk of hip fracture: the EPIDOS prospective study. *Lancet*, 348: 145–149.

Dean, M. (2003). *Growing Older in the 21st Century*. Swindon: Economic and Social Research Council.

Duncan, P.W., Weiner, D.K., Chandler, J. and Studenski, S. (1990). Functional reach: a new clinical measure of balance. *Journal of Gerontology*, 45: M192–M197.

Ferrucci, L., Guralnik, J.M., Buchner, D., Kasper, J., Lamb, S.E., Simonsick, E.M., Corti, M.C., Bandeen-Roche, K. and Fried, L.P. (1997). Departures from linearity in the relationship between measures of muscular strength and physical performance of the lower extremities: the Women's Health and Aging Study. *Journals of Gerontology. Series A, Biological Sciences and Medical Sciences*, 52: M275–M285.

Fitzgerald, M.D., Tanaka, H., Tran, Z.V. and Seals, D.R. (1997). Age-related declines in maximal aerobic capacity in regularly exercising vs. sedentary women: a meta-analysis. *Journal of Applied Physiology*, 83: 160–165.

Frontera, W.R., Hughes, V.A., Lutz, K.J. and Evans, W.J. (1991). A cross-sectional study of muscle strength and mass in 45- to 78-yr-old men and women. *Journal of Applied physiology*, 71: 644–650.

Galanos, A.N., Pieper, C.F., Cornoni-Huntley, J.C., Bales, C.W. and Fillenbaum, G.G. (1994). Nutrition and function: is there a relationship between body mass index and the functional capabilities of community-dwelling elderly? *Journal of the American Geriatrics Society*, 42: 368–373.

Gehlsen, G.M. and Whaley, M.H. (1990). Falls in the elderly: Part II, Balance, strength, and flexibility. *Archives of Physical Medicine and Rehabilitation*, 71: 739–741.

Gill, T.M., Williams, C.S., Richardson, E.D. and Tinetti, M.E. (1996). Impairments in physical performance and cognitive status as predisposing factors for functional dependence among nondisabled older persons. *Journals of Gerontology. Series A, Biological Sciences and Medical Sciences*, 51: M283–M288.

Guralnik, J.M., Simonsick, E.M., Ferrucci, L., Glynn, R.J., Berkman, L.F., Blazer, D.G., Scherr, P.A. and Wallace, R.B. (1994). A short physical performance battery assessing lower extremity function: association with self-reported disability and prediction of mortality and nursing home admission. *Journal of Gerontology*, 49: M85–M94.

Guralnik, J.M., Ferrucci, L., Simonsick, E.M., Salive, M.E. and Wallace, R.B. (1995). Lower-extremity function in persons over the age of 70 years as a predictor of subsequent disability. *New England Journal of Medicine*, 332: 556–561.

Hedrick, S.C. (1995). Assessment of functional status: activities of daily living. In L.Z. Rubenstein, D. Wieland and R. Bernabei (eds), *Geriatric Assessment Technology: The State of the Art*, pp. 51–58. Milan: Editrice Kurtis.

Holland, G.J., Tanaka, K., Shigematsu, R. and Nakagaichi, M. (2002). Flexibility and physical functions of older adults: a review. *Journal of Aging and Physical Activity*, 10: 169–206.

Iverson, B.D., Gossman, M.R., Shaddeau, S.A. and Turner, M.E., Jr. (1990). Balance performance, force production, and activity levels in noninstitutionalized men 60 to 90 years of age. *Physical Therapy*, 70: 348–355.

Jones, C.J., Rikli, R.E., Max, J. and Noffal, G. (1998). The reliability and validity of a chair sit-and-reach test as a measure of hamstring flexibility in older adults. *Research Quarterly for Exercise and Sport*, 69: 338–343.

Jones, C.J., Rikli, R.E. and Beam, W.C. (1999). A 30-s chair-stand test as a measure of lower body strength in community-residing older adults. *Research Quarterly for Exercise and Sport*, 70: 113–119.

Judge, J.O., Lindsey, C., Underwood, M. and Winsemius, D. (1993a). Balance improvements in older women: effects of exercise training. *Physical Therapy*, 73: 254–262.

Judge, J.O., Underwood, M. and Gennosa, T. (1993b). Exercise to improve gait velocity in older persons. *Archives of Physical Medicine and Rehabilitation*, 74: 400–406.

Katz, S., Downs, T.D., Cash, H.R. and Grotz, R.C. (1970). Progress in development of the index of ADL. *Gerontologist*, 10: 20–30.

Lawrence, R.H. and Jette, A.M. (1996). Disentangling the disablement process. *Journals of Gerontology. Series B, Psychological Sciences and Social Sciences*, 4: S173–S182.

Lawton, M.P. and Brody, E.M. (1969). Assessment of older people: self-maintaining and instrumental activities of daily living. *Gerontologist*, 9: 179–186.

Lawton, M.P., Moss, M., Fulcomer, M. and Kleban, M.H. (1982). A research and service oriented multilevel assessment instrument. *Journal of Gerontology*, 37: 91–99.

Lemmink, K.A., Kemper, H.C., de Greef, M.H., Rispens, P. and Stevens, M. (2003). The validity of the sit-and-reach test and the modified sit-and-reach test in middle-aged to older men and women. *Research Quarterly for Exercise and Sport*, 74: 331–336.

Lipsitz, L.A., Jonsson, P.V., Kelley, M.M. and Koestner, J.S. (1991). Causes and correlates of recurrent falls in ambulatory frail elderly. *Journal of Gerontology*, 46: M114–M122.

Losonczy, K.G., Harris, T.B., Cornoni-Huntley, J., Simonsick, E.M., Wallace, R.B., Cook, N.R., Ostfeld, A.M. and Blazer, D.G. (1995). Does weight loss from middle age to old age explain the inverse weight mortality relation in old age? *American Journal of Epidemiology*, 141: 312–321.

Mahoney, F.I. and Barthel, D.W. (1965). Functional evaluation: the barthel index. *Maryland State Medical Journal*, 14: 61–65.

Mathias, S., Nayak, U.S. and Isaacs, B. (1986). Balance in elderly patients: the 'get-up and go' test. *Archives of Physical Medicine and Rehabilitation*, 67: 387–389.

Morey, M.C., Pieper, C.F. and Cornoni-Huntley, J. (1998). Physical fitness and functional limitations in community-dwelling older adults. *Medicine and Science in Sports and Exercise*, 30: 715–723.

Nevitt, M.C., Cummings, S.R., Kidd, S. and Black, D. (1989). Risk factors for recurrent nonsyncopal falls. A prospective study. *Journal of the American Medical Association*, 261: 2663–2668.

Osness, W.H., Adrian, M., Clark, B., Hoeger, W., Raab, D. and Wiswell, R. (1990). *Functional Fitness Assessment for Adults Over 60 Years (A Field Based Assessment)*. Virginia: The American Alliance for Health, Physical Education, Recreation and Dance.

Osness, W.H., Adrian, M., Clark, B., Hoeger, W., Raab, D. and Wiswell, R. (1996). *Functional Fitness Assessment for Adults Over 60 Years (A Field Based Assessment)*. Dubuque, IA: Kendall/Hunt.

Pendergast, D.R., Fisher, N.M. and Calkins, E. (1993). Cardiovascular, neuromuscular, and metabolic alterations with age leading to frailty. *Journal of Gerontology*, 48: Spec No. 61–67.

Petrella, R.J., Koval, J.J., Cunningham, D.A. and Paterson, D.H. (2001). A self-paced step test to predict aerobic fitness in older adults in the primary care clinic. *Journal of the American Geriatrics Society*, 49: 632–638.

Reuben, D.B. and Siu, A.L. (1990). An objective measure of physical function of elderly outpatients. The Physical Performance Test. *Journal of the American Geriatrics Society*, 38: 1105–1112.

Rikli, R.E. and Jones, C.J. (1997). Assessing physical performance in independent older adults: issues and guidelines. *Journal of Aging and Physical Activity*, 5: 244–261.

Rikli, R.E. and Jones, C.J. (1998). The reliability and validity of a 6-minute walk test as a measure of physical endurance in older adults. *Journal of Aging and Physical Activity*, 6: 363–375.

Rikli, R.E. and Jones, C.J. (1999a). Development and validation of a functional fitness test for community-residing older adults. *Journal of Aging and Physical Activity*, 7: 129–161.

Rikli, R.E. and Jones, C.J. (1999b). Functional fitness normative scores for community-residing older adults. *Journal of Aging and Physical Activity*, 7: 162–181.

Rikli, R.E. and Jones, C.J. (2001). *Senior Fitness Test Manual*. Champaign, IL: Human Kinetics.

Roach, K.E. and Miles, T.P. (1991). Normal hip and knee active range of motion: the relationship to age. *Physical Therapy*, 71: 656–665.

Seeman, T.E., Charpentier, P.A., Berkman, L.F., Tinetti, M.E., Guralnik, J.M., Albert, M., Blazer, D. and Rowe, J.W. (1994). Predicting changes in physical performance in a high-functioning elderly cohort: MacArthur studies of successful aging. *Journal of Gerontology*, 49: M97–108.

Shephard, R.J. (1997). *Aging, Physical Activity and Health*, p. 4. Champaign, IL: Human Kinetics.

Simonsick, E.M., Montgomery, P.S., Newman, A.B., Bauer, D.C. and Harris, T. (2001). Measuring fitness in healthy older adults: the Health ABC Long Distance Corridor Walk. *Journal of the American Geriatrics Society*, 49: 1544–1548.

Spirduso, W.W. (ed.) (1995). Physical functioning and the old and oldest-old. In *Physical Dimensions of Aging*, pp. 329–365. Champaign, IL: Human Kinetics.

Steffen, T.M., Hacker, T.A. and Mollinger, L. (2002). Age- and gender-related test performance in community-dwelling elderly people: six-minute walk test, berg balance scale, timed up & go test, and gait speeds. *Physical Therapy*, 82: 128–137.

Topp, R., Mikesky, A., Wigglesworth, J., Holt, W., Jr and Edwards, J.E. (1993). The effect of a 12-week dynamic resistance strength training program on gait velocity and balance of older adults. *Gerontologist*, 33: 501–506.

Verfaillie, D.F., Nichols, J.F., Turkel, E. and Hovell, M.F. (1997). Effects of resistance, balance, and gait training on reduction of risk factors leading to falls. *Journal of Aging and Physical Activity*, 5: 213–228.

Whipple, R.H., Wolfson, L.I. and Amerman, P.M. (1987). The relationship of knee and ankle weakness to falls in nursing home residents: an isokinetic study. *Journal of the American Geriatrics Society*, 35: 13–20.

Wilson, T.M. and Tanaka, H. (2000). Meta-analysis of the age-associated decline in maximal aerobic capacity in men: relation to training status. *American Journal of Physiology*, 278: H829–H834.

Wolfson, L., Whipple, R., Amerman, P. and Tobin, J.N. (1990). Gait assessment in the elderly: a gait abnormality rating scale and its relation to falls. *Journal of Gerontology*, 45: M12–M19.

Wolfson, L., Judge, J., Whipple, R. and King, M. (1995). Strength is a major factor in balance, gait, and the occurrence of falls. *Journals of Gerontology. Series A, Biological Sciences and Medical Sciences*, 50: Spec No. 64–67.

CHAPTER 24

TESTING THE FEMALE ATHLETE

Melonie Burrows

INTRODUCTION

Over the last 30 years, physiological testing of the female athlete has grown dramatically, particularly in assessing the physiological predictors of performance (Lynch and Nimmo, 1999; Burrows and Bird, 2005). However, such testing has brought with it many controversies due to the variety of methodological flaws and inconsistencies in the preparation and testing of the female athlete (Burrows and Bird, 2000). Therefore, this chapter aims to cover pertinent issues regarding assessment of the female athlete.

THE MENSTRUAL CYCLE

Unique to the female athlete is the exposure to rhythmic variations in endogenous hormones during the menstrual cycle (Figure 24.1). The textbook length of the menstrual cycle is 28 days. However, the 'normal' menstrual cycle length varies greatly between women from 22 to 36 days between the ages of 20 and 40 years (Vollman, 1977). The cycle is typically divided into three phases, the menses phase, the follicular phase and the luteal phase, during which the levels of gonadotrophins vary considerably. This variation in menstrual cycle hormones and affect on performance has been extensively studied (Burrows *et al.*, 2002; Sunderland and Nevill, 2003; Bambaeichi *et al.*, 2004; Burrows and Bird, 2004), however there is no universal agreement as to the hormonal effects, so precaution needs to be exercised; with hormonal levels and menstrual phases classified and identified prior to, and during, testing of the female athlete. Such classification is essential to ensure that any significant differences found in testing are down to the intervention, and not the variations in hormonal levels at the time of testing. Suitable methods to classify the menstrual cycle phases have been discussed in the literature, of which the main ones are outlined below.

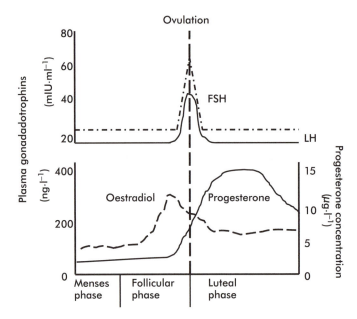

FSH = Follicle stimulating hormone; LH = Luteinsing hormone

Figure 24.1 Diagrammatic representation of the menstrual cycle

MENSTRUAL CYCLE DIARIES AND QUESTIONNAIRES

Menstrual cycle diaries have been used to identify females' menstrual phases by means of a menstrual calendar, in which the female details the dates of menses commencement and cessation. From such information one can estimate the day of ovulation as day 14 from the start of menses (assuming a 28 day text book cycle), and thus the end of the follicular phase and the beginning of the luteal phase (Figure 24.2). Although such a method is non-invasive and easy to administer over consecutive menstrual cycles, the variability of the 'normal' menstrual cycle (22–36 days), makes such a method highly inaccurate (Bauman, 1981). Thus, although the menses phase can be determined very accurately, the end of the follicular phase and the beginning of the luteal phase would lack precision. In addition, no assessment of ovulation can directly take place.

Menstrual cycle questionnaires have also been utilised to report the onset and cessation of menses and thus the occurrence of the follicular and luteal phases, by asking the female to remember past menses. Such questionnaires can assess the female for menstrual history since menarche, age at menarche, menstrual flow in days and cycles experienced per year, so providing useful information on past regularity and irregularity of the females cycle. This may aid in identifying the females menstrual irregularity in the coming months during the testing period as well as highlighting a history of irregularity which may affect current testing results. However, one must keep in mind that such questionnaires provide retrospective data and so the inherent flaws need to be taken into account. Further, no identification of ovulation can take place.

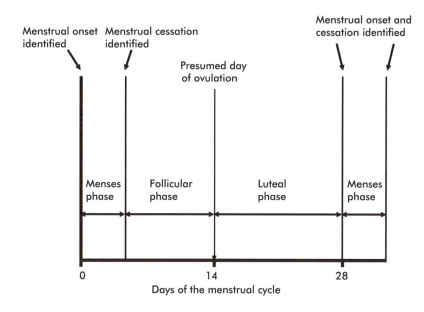

Figure 24.2   The use of menstrual cycle diaries to identify the menstrual phases

Note
The estimation of ovulation on day 14 is based on assuming a 28-day cycle, so the phases of the menstrual cycle can be identifies as seen above. The start of the next menstrual cycle can be assessed by menstruation onset and cessation identified through a menstrual diary

BODY TEMPERATURE

The cyclical core body temperature (CBT) changes across the menstrual cycle are characterised by a pre-ovulatory rise in temperature and a post-menstrual fall followed by a return to baseline (Birch, 2000). Previous research has indicated that CBT is not an accurate predictor of luteal phase onset, even though there is little doubt that rises in progesterone cause a rise in CBT in the luteal phase of the cycle. The lack of accuracy could be due to the fact that in many studies the timing and collection protocols for CBT have not been tightly controlled (Eston, 1984). When the collection procedures are strictly controlled, a relationship may be found between body temperature and ovulation (Guida *et al.*, 1999). If females follow a strict protocol for CBT collection it increases the chance of gaining a clear CBT profile. Such a controlled method would be:

- Using a valid and reliable digital thermometer.
- Taking CBT every morning upon awakening (at the same time of day if possible), prior to getting out of bed.
- Placing the thermometer under the tongue for the time taken for the digital thermometer to register the temperature, after which immediately recording the value in a menstrual diary.
- Recording any missed temperature readings, late nights, alcohol usage, cold-symptoms and any factors that they feel might have affect the temperature readings in the menstrual diary.

- Analysing the CBT readings using the Cumulative Sum (CUSUM) method of Lebenstedt *et al.* (1999).

However, it has been reported that 12–22% of apparently 'normal' women do not exhibit a luteal rise of body temperature (Bauman, 1981), and as such these women would not gain a true identification of luteal phases. Additionally, CBT does not provide direct evidence of ovulation.

DIRECT PROGESTERONE ASSESSMENT

Well-controlled research papers have focused on identifying the menstrual phases by classifying the surge of endogenous progesterone or LH around the middle of a 'normal' ovulatory cycle via urine (Ecochard *et al.*, 2001), plasma, serum (Serviddio *et al.*, 2002), or saliva samples (Stikkelbroeck *et al.*, 2003). The medium which has received most attention in the exercise literature to date is the assessment of salivary progesterone concentrations, due to the collection procedures being non-invasive, stress-free, and requiring minimal supervision, allowing multiple participant collections and storage at home (Tremblay *et al.*, 1996l; Chatterton *et al.*, 2005).

When using saliva a strict collection protocol must be followed to ensure clear samples, a low risk of contamination and adequate sample size for analysis. The salivette method of collection has been reported to decrease the possibility of gingival bleeding that is associated with the chewing and spitting methods of saliva collection, and thus lends itself to providing clear samples (Kruger *et al.*, 1996). However, it has received some criticism due to the cotton and polyether rolls affecting saliva composition (Leander-Lumikari *et al.*, 1995; Strazdins *et al.*, 2005). Thus, currently the dribbling method of saliva collection is most popular (Nieman *et al.*, 2005). A strict collection protocol would be as follows:

- Saliva samples should be taken prior to the brushing of teeth and application of make-up (to avoid any contamination in the sample).
- Hands should be washed to ensure no contamination upon handling.
- The mouth should be rinsed with water a few times to remove any debris and then the female should swallow 2–3 times to remove old saliva.
- The females should rest for 2 min prior to taking the sample.
- Unstimulated collection should take place for 4 min by expectoration into a plastic, sterilised vial.
- The female should be urged to pass as much saliva as possible.
- Samples should be immediately frozen and stored in a freezer at −80°C for later analysis.
- There are various assays for the measurement of salivary progesterone and a full review of these is unwarranted here. Please refer to reviews by O'Rorke *et al.* (1994) and Moghissi (1992).
- Total protein should be quantified.
- All samples should be taken at the same time of day.

Saliva samples need to be taken regularly over the menstrual cycle to optimise the identification of the progesterone peak. Although there has been shown to be a strong correlation between progesterone values and ovulation if the plasma concentrations of the hormone exceed 25 nmol·l^{-1} (Abdulla et al., 1983), or 200 pmol·l^{-1} (Simpson et al., 1998), one can never be sure whether the actual peak values are being measured if daily samples are not taken. Daily saliva sampling removes the concern of 'timing' samples to measure the true progesterone peak that exists if venous blood sampling is used. Indeed, the invasiveness of venipuncture means that the amount of samples taken over one month is limited and as a result, many studies have relied on one sample collected on a day estimated to correspond to the middle of the luteal phase, or 2–3 samples around the presumed day of ovulation, to classify menstrual regularity (Sunderland and Nevill, 2003). However, by utilising a low number of blood samples the chance of missing the progesterone peak increases and the likelihood of accurately identifying the luteal phase and ovulation decreases. Thus, although blood samples for the analysis of progesterone concentrations have great validity they are limited by the inconvenience of frequent venipuncture and cost of analysis. Whereas, daily samples of saliva provide a comprehensive profile of the cycle and thus any menstrual irregularities that may be present. Females have a large variation in salivary progesterone measures, thus, the CUSUM method of Lebenstedt et al. (1999) should be used for the objective determination of luteal phase onset as it allows for large variations in salivary progesterone concentrations by analysing significant rises from individual's follicular baseline measures. However, the rise in endogenous progesterone is not a direct measure of ovulation with increases in progesterone being reported in anovulatory cycles (Soules et al., 1989). Therefore, the only direct method to document ovulation is the detection of an ovum from ultrasonography or the occurrence of pregnancy in the participant (Israel et al., 1972).

ULTRASONOGRAPHY

Ultrasonography is a direct method of assessing ovulation and thus whether any female is anovulatory. The method uses transvaginal ultrasound, sending out high frequency sound waves into the pelvic region, which bounce of the structures, enabling identification of an ovum if present. The image is of high quality and is a direct measure, and as such is one of the gold standards for assessment of ovulation. However, the method is unavailable in most physiology laboratories due to the expertise and expense required to utilise it. As such, the indirect methods of hormonal classification and diary assessment are often utilised.

Menstrual cycle regularity

What is becoming increasingly clear is that when assessing the female athlete, menstrual cycle status can change from month to month along with the cycle

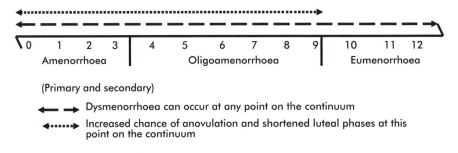

| 0 | 1 | 2 | 3 | 4 | 5 | 6 | 7 | 8 | 9 | 10 | 11 | 12 |

Amenorrhoea   Oligoamenorrhoea   Eumenorrhoea

(Primary and secondary)

← → Dysmenorrhoea can occur at any point on the continuum

◄·····► Increased chance of anovulation and shortened luteal phases at this point on the continuum

Figure 24.3 The continuum of menstrual cycle irregularities

Table 24.1 Definitions for menstrual terms in female athletes

Term	Definition
Eumenorrhoea	'Normal' cycle: 10–13 menstrual bleeds per year inclusive
Oligoamenorrhoea	4–9 menstrual bleeds per year inclusive, or menstrual cycles longer than 35 days
Amenorrhoea	0–3 menstrual bleeds per year inclusive[a]
Primary amenorrhoea	A female who has never had menstrual bleeding
Secondary amenorrhoea	Females who have had at least 1 episode of menstrual bleeding before loss of the cycle
Delayed menarche	The onset of menses after 16 years old
Dysmenorrhoea	Lower abdominal pain radiating to the lower back or legs, headache, nausea and vomiting across the cycle
Shortened luteal phases	A luteal phase shorter than 10 days
Anovulation	No ovum released at ovulation

Note
a Definitions of amenorrhoea vary greatly so to standaridsed future reports the IOC defined amenorrhoea as 'one period or less in a year'. However, this definition is more rigid than that used in other gynaecological or endocrine literature, and such a definition excludes many athletes with altered endocrinology (Carbon, 2002). Thus, 0–3 cycles per year inclusive is used instead to provide a more encompassing definition

hormone levels. Indeed females may not stay within one category of menstrual regularity, but move between them as the month's progress (Figure 24.3). Due to this variation, when assessing the menstrual cycle phases and ovulation, monitoring of one menstrual cycle may not be adequate to gain an accurate picture. A number of menstrual cycles may be required and a few studies to date have started to assess three menstrual cycles prior to testing the female, continuing the assessment throughout the testing period; gaining a more accurate picture of menstrual regularity (Burrows *et al.*, 2002). Table 24.1 provides some clear definitions of menstrual irregularities to aid identification and standardised interpretation.

SUMMARY

In summary, it would seem that the most accurate, reliable and practical methods to assess the menstrual cycle are a combination of menstrual cycle diaries to assess menses onset and cessation, menstrual cycle questionnaires to assess menstrual history, and salivary progesterone measurement to directly assess hormonal status. Although ultrasonography is a direct measure of ovulation, it is often inapplicable and unavailable in many contexts due to the expertise and expense required. Therefore, saliva progesterone values could offer a more readily available and cheaper method of detecting luteal phase onset and ovulation if the limitations are kept in mind. Longitudinal assessment of menstrual functioning is required over 3+ cycles prior to testing and during the testing period to ensure accurate luteal phase onset and prediction of ovulation across menstrual cycles and thus the occurrence of any menstrual irregularity (Loucks *et al.*, 1992). Such methodology and protocols can be expensive and very time consuming, but it is the only way to ensure the validity and reliability of the testing results from the female athlete.

OTHER IMPORTANT FACTORS TO CONSIDER

Once the menstrual cycle has been accurately identified and classified, other important issues need to be addressed with specific reference to the female athlete. These are circadian rhythms, pregnancy, age, contraceptive use and mood states.

Circadian rhythms

Once the menstrual cycle has been classified and the phases identified, the timing of testing needs to be arranged. As with many physiological variables, the menstrual cycle hormones follow circadian rhythms and thus testing should take place at the same time of day across the menstrual phases. However, in addition to looking across the menstrual cycle phases, the variation of hormones within each phase needs to be taken into account. As such, testing should not only take place at a specified time of day, but on a specified day or days within each of the menstrual phases.

Pregnancy

Pregnancy, in females of reproductive age, must be the first issue discounted prior to testing and/or when assessing menstrual status. Pregnancy can be assessed through a simple urine dipstick test with results available in 5 min. Specific confidentiality issues need to be considered when one is conducting a pregnancy test. If you are testing a female athlete above 18 years of age the results should be given to the adult, along with suggestions to gain advice from the GP. However, if one is working with female athletes below the age of

18 years the confidentiality issues become clouded. Under such conditions it is advisable to solicit advice from the ethical committee or lead physiologist under whom such testing is taking place.

Age

When working with female athletes age needs to be considered. The age of the female will directly affect the regularity of the menstrual cycle. The menstrual cycle should be more regular between the ages of 20–45 years, and thus a large amount of testing on females has been conducted between this age range. Once one tests outside this age range, menstrual cycle irregularity may increase, and present problems with accurately identifying hormonal levels and menstrual phases (Astrup *et al.*, 2004). Obviously, once you go over 45 years, the chance of females progressing towards, or going through, the menopause increases and this needs to be taken into account in the test design or screened for. If working with a minor, the ethical issues that come about with working with children should be followed (see the appropriate section in these guidelines).

Contraceptive use

When testing the female athlete the issue of contraceptive use needs to be addressed. Currently, there are numerous forms of contraceptive agents available to the female, that is, the contraceptive pill, the contraceptive injection and hormonal implants. Due to this array of contraceptives, research is limited into the effects of such agents on the hormones of the menstrual cycle and the concomitant affects on physiological variables. Therefore, when testing the female athlete, one should screen out for any use of contraceptive agents. However, if this is not possible the following issues need to be considered:

1   The type of contraceptive agent the females are taking may affect the test results. If in a research study, all females should be on the same agent, such as the contraceptive injection, implants or the pill. If in a physiological testing service, then over time any changes in contraception should be noted and the test results interpreted accordingly.

2   Whichever agent the females are using should be of the same type. For example, if in a research study, all the females on the contraceptive pill should be using either the Monophasic or Triphasic pills. In addition, all females should be on a similar dose pill, that is, high or low doses of progestrone and/or oestrogen.

3   The duration the female has been on the contraceptive agent should be taken into account prior to testing and controlled for (Lynch and Nimmo, 1998).

4   Any missed pills should be recorded in a diary noting how many pills have been missed, on what day(s) of the packet, and the reason for not taking the pill.

Such information can be gained from well-designed questionnaires, with contraceptive use monitored through a diary. Testing would then need to take place on the same pill day for all females to minimise any hormonal variation. Please refer to a review by Burrows and Peters (2006) for a more detailed discussion on oral contraceptives and performance in female athletes.

Mood states

Mood states should be assessed using a previously validated, prospective mood state questionnaire, prior to and during testing, to ensure any significant changes in variables being assessed are not down to alterations in mood states but the intervention (Choi and Salmon, 1995; Terry, 1995). Participants should complete the questionnaire at an appropriate time, such as prior to the testing session, and follow the appropriate questionnaire instructions.

BONE HEALTH

Bone health is an area of interest that is rapidly growing, particularly with reference to the female athlete. When assessing bone health in the female certain issues need to be addressed, such as the equipment to use, the variables to measure, timing of the measurement and data analysis.

Bone densitometry has been shown to provide a reliable and valid measure of bone mineral content and future fracture risk at all body sites that is far superior to other available methods that have error rates of 30–50% (Cummings *et al.*, 1993). Bone mineral content should be measured over a range of body sites taking into account both cortical and trabecular bone remodelling. However, if time is a limiting factor enabling only one or two body sites to be assessed, the major sites to be measured are the femoral neck and lumbar spine for they are highly correlated with future fracture risk (National Osteoporosis Society, 2002). Prior to any scanning, females should be screened for osteoporosis risk factors, such as long-term corticosteroid use, smoking and alcoholism to aid interpretation of the scan results. Pregnancy should also be assessed using the 28-day rule (i.e. a menses period within the last 28 days), or a negative pregnancy urine test.

When designing a scanning protocol, it should take into account the fact that bone-remodelling cycles (activation–resorption–formation) take about 3–4 months to complete (Eastell *et al.*, 2001). As such, any repeat assessment within this time-span is highly questionable. Indeed, the determination of when to repeat a scan should take into account the sample size and the precision error of the DEXA scanner (Precision error = CV of machine $\times$ 2.8), as well as the intervention. As a result, other short-term measures to assess bone remodelling may be required, and bone biochemical markers may prove useful. A full discussion of these markers is beyond the scope of this chapter so the reader is referred to Eastell *et al.* (2001) for further information. Suffice to say though, that such markers could provide a short-term indication of the global bone response to an intervention, and be utilised in conjunction with DEXA on a long-term scale.

The interpretation of DEXA scans needs to be accurate, and as bone is a 3D parameter, bone area and volume should be taken into account

(Nevill *et al.*, 2002). Such scaling is particularly important in young females who are still growing and various adjustments for bone size and area are required. Refer to the National Osteoporosis Society guidelines on bone densitometry in children for advice on such scaling issues (National Osteoporosis Society, 2004). All scanning should adhere to Ionising Radiation in Medical Exposure Regulations (2000), and only one trained operator should perform all scans for each distinct study as well as across testing sessions. The analysis procedures should conform to the DEXA manufacturer guidelines.

CONCLUSIONS

This chapter has provided an insight into the many issues that need to be addressed when testing the female athlete and given across some information on specific protocol points. It is up to the physiologist working with the female athlete to decide on the most appropriate course of action for the female at that particular point in time. Although working and researching with the female athlete requires a lot of planning and preparation, it is an area where the complicated physiological mechanisms behind health and sports performance are unclear and as such requires further attention. It is imperative that, as exercise and sports physiologists, we have the evidence-based knowledge to understand the impact of exercise on the females' health and performance. The only way to gaining such evidence is through implementing well-designed and controlled research studies and testing sessions. The extra time and planning needed to achieve this should not be a factor in determining the research conducted in this important area.

REFERENCES

Abdulla, U., Diver, M.J., Hipkin, L.J. and Davis, J.L. (1983). Plasma progesterone levels as an index of ovulation. *British Journal of Obstetrics and Gynaecology*, 90, 543–548.

Astrup, K., Olivarius, N.F., Moller, S., Gottschau, A. and Karlslund, W. (2004). Menstrual bleeding patterns in pre- and perimenopausal women: a population-based prospective diary study. *Acta Obstetrics and Gynaecology in Scandinavia*, 83: 197–202.

Bambaeichi, E., Reilly, T., Cable, N.T. and Giacomoni, M. (2004). The isolated and combined effects of menstrual cycle phase and time-of-day on muscle strength of eumenorrhoeic females. *Chronobiology International*, 21: 645–660.

Bauman, J.E. (1981). Basal body temperature: unreliable method of ovulation detection. *Fertility and Sterility*, 36: 729–733.

Birch, K.M. (2000). Circamensal rhythms in physical performance. *Biological Rhythm Research*, 31: 1–14.

Burrows, M. and Bird, S.R. (2000). The physiology of the highly trained female endurance runner. *Sports Medicine*, 30: 281–300.

Burrows, M. and Bird, S.R. (2004). Velocity at $VO_{2\,max}$ and peak treadmill velocity are not influenced within or across the phases of the menstrual cycle. *European Journal of Applied Physiology*, Dec 3 (Eprint ahead of publication).

Burrows, M. and Bird, S.R. (2005). Velocity at $\dot{V}O_{2max}$ and peak treadmill velocity are not influenced within or across the phases of the menstrual cycle. *European Journal of Applied Physiology*. 93(5–6): 575–80.

Burrows, M. and Peters, C.E. (2006). The influence of oral contraceptives on athletic performance in female athletes. *Sports Medicine* (in press).

Burrows, M. Bird, S.R. and Bishop, N. (2002). The menstrual cycle and its effect on the immune status of female endurance runners. *Journal of Sports Sciences*, 20: 339–344.

Chatterton, R.T., Jr, Mateo, E.T., Hou, N., Rademaker, A.W., Acharya, S., Jordan, V.C. and Morrow, M. (2005). Characteristics of salivary profiles of oestradiol and progesterone in premenopausal women.*Journal of Endocrinol*, 186(1):77–84.

Choi, P.Y. L. and Salmon, P. (1995). Symptom changes across the menstrual cycle in competitive sportswomen, exercisers and sedentary women. *British Journal of Clinical Psychology*, 34: 447–460.

Cummings, S.R., Black, D.M., Nevitt, M.C., Browner, W., Cauley, J., Ensrud, K., Genant, H.K., Gluer, C.C., Hulley, S.B., Palmero, L., Scott, J. and Vogt, T. (1993). Bone density at various sites for prediction of hip fractures. *Lancet*, 341: 72–75.

Eastell, R., Baumann, M., Hoyle, N.R. and Wieczorek, L. (2001). *Bone Markers: Biochemical and Clinical Perspectives*. London: Dunitz.

Ecochard, R., Boehringer, H., Rabilloud, M. and Marret, H. (2001). Chronological aspects of ultrasonic, hormonal, and other indirect indices of ovulation. *British Journal of Obstetrics and Gynaecology*, 108: 822–829.

Eston, R.G. (1984). The regular menstrual cycle and athletic performance. *Sports Medicine*, 1: 431–445.

Guida, M., Tommaselli, G.A., Palomba, S., Pellicano, M., Moccia, G., Carlo, C. and Nappi, C. (1999). Efficacy of methods for determining ovulation in a natural planning program. *Fertility and Sterility*, 72: 900–904.

Ionising Radiation (Medical Exposure) Regulations. (2000). *Documents of the National Radiological Protection Board*. Her Majesty's Stationary Office. Didcot, England.

Israel, R., Mishell, D.R., Stone, S.C., Thorneycroft, I.H. and Moyer, D.C. (1972). Single luteal phase serum progesterone assay as an indicator of ovulation. *American Journal of Obstetrics and Gynaecology*, 15: 1043–1046.

Kruger, C., Ulrike, B., Jutta, B.S. and Helmuth, G.D. (1996). Problems with salivary 17-Hydroxyprogesterone determinants using the salivette device. *European Journal of Clinical and Chemical Biochemistry*, 34: 927–929.

Lebenstedt, M., Platte, P. and Pirke, K.M. (1999). Reduced resting metabolic rate in athletes with menstrual disorders. *Medicine and Science in Sports and Exercise*, 31: 1250–1256.

Lenander-Lumikari, M., Johansson, I., Vilja, P. and Samaranayake, L.P. (1995). Newer saliva collection methods and saliva composition: a study of two salivette kits. *Oral Diseases*, 1: 86–91.

Loucks, A.B. and Horvath, S.M. (1992). Exercise-induced stress responses of amenorrhoeic and eumenorrhoeic runners. *Journal of Clinical Endocrinology and Metabolism*, 59: 1109–1120.

Lynch, N.J. and Nimmo, M.A. (1999). Effects of menstrual cycle phase and oral contraceptive use on intermittent exercise. *European Journal of Physiology*, 78: 565–572.

Matthews, K.A., Santoro, N., Lasley, B., Chang, Y., Crawford, S., Pasternak, R.C., Sutton-Tyrrell, K. and Sowers, M. (2006). Relation of cardiovascular risk factors in women approaching menopause to menstrual cycle characteristics and reproductive hormones in the follicular and luteal phases. *Journal of Clinical Endocrinology and Metabolism*, 91(5):1789–95.

Moghissi, K.S. (1992) Ovulation detection, *Endocrinology and Metabolism Clinics of North America*, 21(1): 39–55.

National Osteoporosis Society. (2002). *Position Statement on the Reporting of DEXA Bone Mineral Density Scans. NOS*, August.

National Osteoporosis Society. (2004). *Position statement: A practical guide to bone densitometry in children. NOS*, November 2004.

Nevill, A.M., Holder, R.L., Maffulli, N., Cheng, J.C., Leung, S.S., Lee, W.T. and Lau, J.T. (2002). Adjusting bone mass for differences in projected bone area and other confounding variables: an allometric perspective. *Journal of Bone Mineral Research*, 17: 703–708.

Nieman, D.C., Henson, D.A., Austin, M.D. and Brown, V.A. (2005). Immune response to a 30-minute walk. *Medicine and Science in Sports and Exercise*, 37: 57–62.

O'Rorke, A., Kane, M.M., Gosling, J.P., Tallon, D.F. and Fotrell, P.F. (1994). Development and validation of a monoclonal antibody enzyme immunoassay for measuring progesterone in saliva. *Clinical Chemistry*, 40: 454–458.

Serviddio, G., Loverro, G., Vicino, M., Prigigasllo, F., Grattagliano, I., Altomare, E. and Vendemiale, G. (2002). Modulation of endometrial redox balance during the menstrual cycle: relation with sex hormones. *Journal of Clinical Endocrinology and Metabolism*, 87: 2843–2848.

Simpson, H.W., McArdle, C.S., Griffiths, K.M., Turkes, A. and Beastall, G.H. (1998). Progesterone resistance in women who have breast cancer. *British Journal of Obstetrics and Gynaecology*, 105: 345–351.

Soules, M.R., Mclachlan, R.I. and Ek, M. (1989). Luteal phase deficiency: characterisation of reproductive hormones over the menstrual cycle. *Clinical Endocrinology and Metabolism*, 69: 804–812.

Stikkelbroeck, N.M., Sweep, C.G., Braat, D.D., Hermus, A.R. and Otten, B.J. (2003). Monitoring of menstrual cycles, ovulation, and adrenal suppression by saliva sampling in female patients with 21-hydroxylase deficiency. *Fertility and Sterility*, 80: 1030–1036.

Strazdins, L., Meyerkort, S., Brent, V., D'Souza, R.M., Broom, D.H., Kyd, J.M. (2005). Impact of saliva collection methods on sIgA and cortisol assays and acceptability to participants. *Journal of Immunological Methods*, 307(1–2): 167–171.

Sunderland, C. and Nevill, M. (2003). Effect of the menstrual cycle on performance of intermittent, high-intensity shuttle running in a hot environment. *European Journal of Applied Physiology*, 88: 345–352.

Terry, P. (1995). The efficacy of mood state profiling with elite performers: a review and synthesis. *Sport Psychology*, 9: 309–324.

Tremblay, M.S., Chu, S.Y. and Mureika, R. (1996). Methodological and statistical considerations for exercise-related hormones evaluations. *Sports Medicine*, 20: 90–108.

Vollman, N. (1977). *The Menstrual Cycle: Major Problems in Obstetrics and Gynaecology*, 7. Philadelphia, PA: WB Saunders.

CHAPTER 25

TESTING AN AESTHETIC ATHLETE: CONTEMPORARY DANCE AND CLASSICAL BALLET DANCERS

Matthew Wyon

INTRODUCTION

This chapter will focus on an unusual 'athlete' in that they participate in non-competitive performances. The physical demands of the performance is determined by a choreographer and each piece can have widely varying physiological demands for the dancer from pedestrian movement to high-intensity intermittent exercise.

DEVELOPING A TESTING PROTOCOL FOR DANCE

In developing a testing protocol for the physiological assessment of elite dancers, one needs to consider the nature of dance performance, as well as examining previously reported maximal physiological variables. It must be mentioned that some of the data reported might not be truly maximal as dancers are not used to exercising maximally due to the high skill level within dance (Chatfield *et al.*, 1990).

THE NATURE OF DANCE PERFORMANCE AND TRAINING

Unlike most sport teams, dance companies have a series of performance blocks of between 1 and 6 weeks with up to 8 performances a week, accumulating in a total performance season of 24–32 weeks (the commercial dance world often asks dancers to perform 6–7 shows a week for 40 weeks). Principal dancers within ballet companies have a less rigorous schedule, though the roles they undertake are physically more demanding than that of the dancers in the corps (Schantz and Astrand, 1984).

The physiological classification of dance has proven to be an area of contention mainly due to the fact that dancers' see themselves as artists and not athletes and that physiological training is only a symptom of a primary require-ment, the search for the aesthetic. Cohen (1984) noted, 'dance is quick bursts of energy interspersed with steady state activities' which seems to suggest a form of intermittent exercise (Rimmer *et al.*, 1994). Class has for centuries focused on increasing the dancer's movement vocabulary, improving musicality, and phras-ing and developing creativity and expression; in summary the focus has been on the mastery of the art form (Krasnow and Chatfield, 1996). The aerobic com-ponent of dance is very limited due to the structure of the primary training forum, the dance class. The dance class has two distinct section the warm-up and the centre; the former is identified by the dancer remaining mainly static and exercising at low intensities whilst, in the latter, the dancer traverses the studio at higher intensities. The dance warm up, either at the bat, on the floor or in the centre (depending on the dance style of the class) aims to warm-up the body, increase joint articulation and improve limb alignment. The work time during the warm-up phase is more continuous though the intensity is low. The 'centre' phase of the class is generally at a higher intensity but the exercise periods are shorter than during the warm-up period. Dance has a high skill requirement with a great emphasis on precision; this has a direct influence on work economy. Skilled/professional dancers will therefore be able to perform sequences at much lower heart rates than their less skilled or trained counterparts and therefore the metabolic training effect is reduced. Even within professional dancers fitness levels will vary due to the different demands placed upon them (Wyon *et al.*, in press). Within classical ballet, soloists were aerobically fitter than corps members (Schantz and Astrand, 1984). This disparity is not often seen within modern dance due to a reduced hierarchical company structure.

The demands of performance are forever increasing and diversifying as choreographers strive for the new. This has led to a gap in the skills and tech-nique taught in class and the performance requirements of the choreographer (Rist, 1994). Budgetary funding means that only major companies have the financial ability for comprehensive rehearsal periods that allow their dancers' bodies to adapt to the physical and mental requirements of new choreography. The end result is that dancers often have to perform when they are both men-tally and physically tired and their bodies still in the process of adapting to the new stress placed upon them.

WHAT PHYSIOLOGICAL COMPONENTS ARE IMPORTANT

There has been little research on the physiological demands of dance performance and due its diverse nature only generalisations are possible. Performance analysis has classified dance as high-intensity intermittent exercise with a mean percentage exercise time of 60% and a reliance on the fast glycolytic and aerobic energy systems (Wyon, 2004). From this foundation participants are required to demonstrate extreme ranges of movement (either statically or dynamically), lifts (involving near body weight resistance rarely following optimal biomechanical kinetics), jumps (where the height needs to be optimised to fit in extra skills), balance (while holding a pose) and falls (onto wooden surfaces) whilst giving the impression that this exertion is effortless. This is even more remarkable when research has shown that professional dancers' fitness parameters are often comparable to age-matched sedentary healthy individuals (Koutedakis and Jamurtas, 2004).

STRENGTH

Compared to athletes, dancers generally have lower strength indices (Kirkendall and Calabrese, 1983). Contemporary dancers are stronger than their classical counterparts mainly due to their multidisciplinary backgrounds and diversity of choreography they are exposed to. Though there is a gender difference (Westbald et al., 1995) all reported data is on leg strength. Present choreographic demands within both genres and an increase in upper body injuries suggest more attention needs to be paid to the upper body; this is especially true for female contemporary dancers. Although physiotherapists have noted up to 50% bilateral difference in muscular tone (using manual muscle testing techniques), though this has not been seen in the literature (Westbald et al., 1995). There is still a fear of strength training within the dance community due to the myth that it would destroy their aesthetics. Literature has noted the opposite in fact that strength gains are beneficial in the reduction of injury rates and balance between antagonistic muscles (Koutedakis et al., 1997).

Protocol

Concentric force measurements for the quadriceps and hamstrings using isokinetic dynamometry have been reported in the literature, generally at $60°·s^{-1}$ (Table 25.1). The use of free-weights (isoinertia) is another option, though the technical proficiency of the dancers to carry out safe lifts must be examined initially. This will allow the monitoring of closed-kinetic chain movements targeting the lower limbs (squat), shoulders (shoulder press) or whole body (clean and jerk).

Isokinetic dynamometry protocol

The most common assessment protocol is concentric peak torques of the knee flexors (hamstrings) and extensors (quadriceps). Participants are recommended to warm-up on a cycle ergometer for 5-min at a low–moderate intensity. The participant should be positioned on the dynamometer so that their hips

Table 25.1   Peak strength values for quadriceps and hamstrings in dancers

Study	Sex	Style/sport	Angular velocity	Knee extension (mean value?)	Knee flexion (mean value?)
Brinson and Dick (1996)	M	Contemporary	$60°·s^{-1}$	196 Nm	94 Nm
	F	Contemporary	$60°·s^{-1}$	133 Nm	68 Nm
	M	Ballet	$60°·s^{-1}$	181 Nm	89 Nm
	F	Ballet	$60°·s^{-1}$	118 Nm	59 Nm
Chatfield et al. (1990)	F	Contemporary	$30°·s^{-1}$	1.32 $Nm·kg^{-1}$	0.25 $Nm·kg^{-1}$
	F	Contemporary	$180°·s^{-1}$	0.98 $Nm·kg^{-1}$	0.13 $Nm·kg^{-1}$

and knees are flexed at 80° and 90° respectively (Koutedakis and Sharp, 2004) and electronic stops set at 0° and, 90° to prevent hyperextension and hyperflexion. The pivot point of their knee (distal lateral protrusion of the femur) is in line with the fulcrum of the dynamometer's arm. The lower limb should be strapped onto the dynamometer's arm ~4 cm above the lateral malleolus. Gravitational corrections should be made and the individual undergo a familiarisation series of concentric flexion–extension cycles at the test angular velocity several days prior to the testing procedure. It is recommended that three maximal extension–flexion cycles be carried out for each leg with 5-min rest between each cycle.

Isoinertia protocol

After a whole body warm-up, the participant should under take two sets of eight repetitions at 50% of the estimated one repetition maximum (1-RM) of the chosen lift. Any stretching should take place between the general warm-up and the practice sets so as not to affect the test scores (Kokkonen et al., 1998; Young and Behm, 2002). It is recommended that participants attempt 3–5 RM and the 1-RM can then be estimated from tables. Each participant should rest for a minimum 5 min between attempts to allow for complete recovery of the utilised energy systems. Testers should be proficient 'spotters' and be able to give feedback on the participant's technique to help reduce the chances of injury through loss of control of the bar.

ANAEROBIC POWER

In dance it is anaerobic 'endurance' rather than power than is utilised the most during adagios and sequences, these generally last between 30 and 60 s and

Table 25.2 Indices of anaerobic power in dancers and comparative indices from other sports

Study	Sex	Style/sport	Mean peak power (W)	Mean power (W)	Fatigue (%)
Chatfield *et al.* (1990)	Females	Modern	310	152	
Rimmer *et al.* (1994)	Males	Ballet	725.3		44.3
	Females	Ballet	503.5		43.0
Brinson and Dick (1996)	Males	Contemporary	740	580	
	Females	Contemporary	465	359	
	Males	Ballet	680	580	
	Females	Ballet	410	329	
	Males	Students	650	510	
	Females	Students	477	374	
Ueno *et al.* (1987)	Males	Rugby	985.3		
	Males	Gymnasts	852.8		38.4
	Females	Gymnasts	439.9		35.7
Heller *et al.* (1995)	Males	Football	914		

involve multiple jumps, though anaerobic power is vital to grande allées. Lactate values post-performance are comparable to that recorded during field and racquet sports (10–12 mmol·l^{-1}) (Brinson and Dick, 1996; Koutedakis, Agarwal and Sharp, 1999; Koutedakis, Myszkewycz, Soulas *et al.*, 1999), though power indices are under-developed compared to similar athletic populations and values for comparison can be found in Table 25.2.

Protocol

It is recommended that either a 30-s or 6 × 10-s Wingate be used for monitoring anaerobic capabilities in dancers. The former will allow comparison with previous reported data and also give an indication of anaerobic endurance by calculating the fatigue index. The later, though not reported previously in the literature, might provide a more dance-specific insight in the dancers ability to carry out repeated high-intensity activity. A 30-s rest period between bouts is recommended, though this can be adapted, as can the length of exercise bout, to match the choreographic requirements of the piece. The exact protocols are reported elsewhere within this book.

AEROBIC CAPACITY

The results from previous studies suggest that the aerobic capacities of dancers are similar to non-endurance trained athletes (Cohen *et al.*, 1982;

Table 25.3 Maximal aerobic uptake of dancers, other selected sports and untrained individuals

Study	Sex	Style	$ml\cdot kg^{-1}\cdot min^{-1}$ (mean value?)
Aerobic Power			
Chmelar *et al.* (1988)	Female	Ballet	42.2
	Female	Modern	49.1
Chatfield *et al.* (1990)	Female	Modern	43.6
Rimmer *et al.* (1994)	Male	Ballet	50.5
	Female	Ballet	44.5
Brinson and Dick (1996)	Male	Modern	55.7
	Female	Modern	43.5
	Male	Ballet	53.2
	Female	Ballet	39.1
Kirkendall and Sharp (1999)	Males	Untrained	42.0
	Females	Untrained	38.0
Neumann (1989)	Males	Figure skating	50–55
	Females	Figure skating	45–50
	Males	Gymnastics	45–50
	Females	Gymnastics	40–45

Dahlstrom *et al.*, 1996), though data in Koutedakis and Sharp (1999) place the scores closer to totally untrained individuals. Data from other intermittent exercise sports and for technical acrobatic sports show similar aerobic capacity results (Table 25.3).

The mode of testing has proven difficult and previous research has used a variety of methods. The use of a treadmill would be optimal, though there is great resistance to dancers running due their enhanced external rotation at the hips making this activity difficult. From experience, there are few biomechanical problems with dancers running, though post exercise they often experience soreness as they have used underconditioned muscles and the greatest resistance is from hearsay and the fact few have exercised on a treadmill previously. The use of cycle ergometers has also proven difficult with local muscular fatigue often being the termination criteria rather than cardiorespiratory parameters.

Protocol

It is suggested that the main parameter that needs monitoring is VO_{2max}, therefore a rapid increase in workload is recommended. A 1 $km\cdot h^{-1}$ increase every 1-min has proven successful on a 1° incline. This allows maximal data to be recorded without causing too much trauma to the participant. Termination criteria should exclude RER values as it has been noted that RER values have reached >1.3 before VO_2 values stopped rising during maximal VO_{2max} tests.

FLEXIBILITY

Dancers are renown for their large range of movement (ROM), though little absolute data have been published. Desfor (2003) suggested that although extreme joint mobility (hypermobility) is an asset within the dance profession it may put them at risk of injury (McCormack et al., 2004). The profession requires extensive ROM in the hips in all planes, including rotation, the ankles and in the lower back. Turn-out is a controversial topic as often the profession's 'ideal' of 180° is often considered to be anatomical impossible (Mahendranath, 2004). Dancers generally practice passive stretching with focus on the development of strength within the agonist muscles. This has lead to a significant difference in hip flexion between active and passive ROM especially in male dancers though no bilateral differences were noted (Redding and Wyon, 2004). The use of the sit-and-reach test is pointless within this population and therefore the use of fluid goniometers and photography is recommended, this will allow dance-specific ranges of movement be assessed (Table 25.4).

Protocol

It is suggested that both active and passive ROM are measured within the selected joints. The hip should be measured in multiple planes (frontal: flexion and extension; saggital: flexion; transverse: rotation) and care needs to be taken that the hips remain horizontal (hip on the testing leg often rises) and the back stays flat (no increase in the natural lordosis).

Hip flexion in the saggital plane (à la seconde)

The participant should carry out a general warm-up that includes cardiovascular and stretching exercises. For passive ROM the participant, standing unsupported, lifts the test leg with their hand (or an assistant lifts the leg) as high as

Table 25.4 Reported ranges of movement in dancers

Study	Sex	Style	ROM (deg) (mean value?)
Chatfield et al. (1990)	F	Contemporary	117 (Forward hip flexion)
	F	Contemporary	29 (Hip hyperextension)
Redding and Wyon (2004)	M	Ballet	141 (Lateral hip flexion – passive)
	F	Ballet	160 (Lateral hip flexion – passive)
	M	Ballet	95 (Lateral hip flexion – active)
	F	Ballet	131 (Lateral hip flexion – active)

possible, care must be taken that the hips remain in a neutral position and the leg is not internally rotated before the angle is measured or the photograph is taken (Figure 25.1). The active ROM test is similar except that the hip flexors are used to move the limb through its ROM rather than an external force (Figure 25.2).

Spine extension

Lying face down, the participant is asked to push their upper body as high as possible using their arms, keeping their hips on the floor. The participant can either be photographed or the distance between the clavicle notch and the floor be measured. For active flexibility the participant again starts face down on the floor with their hands by their sides and the movement is repeated using the back extensors to gain ROM. In both tests an external object should not fix the legs.

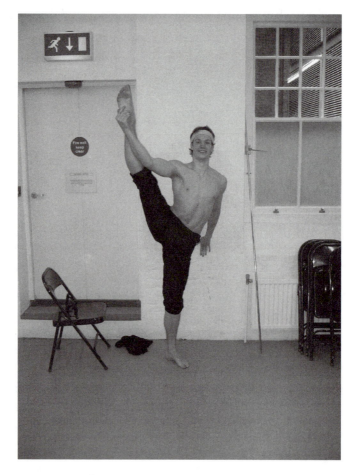

Figure 25.1   Passive range of movement test

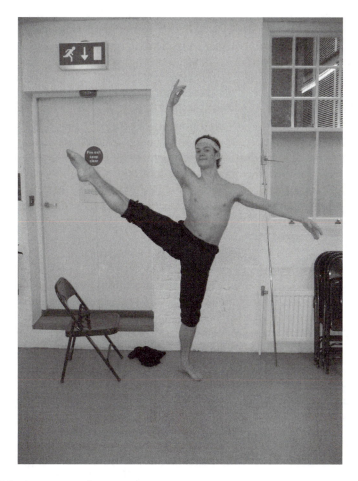

Figure 25.2 Active range of movement test

Turn-out

The participant should be in the prone position with the upper legs strictly parallel and the knees bent 90°. The lower leg can therefore be moved medially or laterally thereby indicating rotation ROM at the hips (Rietveld, 2001); normal ROM is 40°.

BODY FAT/ANTHROPOMETRIC

In any environment where body fat is an issue this is a sensitive area and there is a long history within dance of eating disorders and weight abuse in an attempt to maintain a required aesthetic and body weight (Braisted *et al.*, 1985; Hamilton, 1986; Brooks-Gunn, 1987; Holderness *et al.*, 1994; Geeves, 1997). The problem mainly arises in the fact that dance class and rehearsal are not at a high-enough work intensity to promote weight loss; and when it is the exercise duration periods are very short (Wyon *et al.*, 2004); therefore weight is manipulated by nutritional methods. The artistic director rather than the physical demands of dance often determines the physical characteristics of the dancer; but generally ballet dancers are meso-ectomorphs and contemporary dancers ecto-mesomorphs (Claessens *et al.*, 1987). Wilmerding *et al.* (2003) reviewed the assessment of body fat within the dance community using a number of different methods and noted that due to the very low body fat in both sexes certain methods and their accompanying calculations have resulted in inaccurate values. The author recommends that skinfold measurements be kept as millimetre values and the data are used to monitor variations due to changes in workload rather than report estimated body fat values. Table 25.5 has reference percentage body fat values but they should be viewed with caution.

Protocol

It is recommended that seven sites are used; subscapular, suprailiac, bicep, tricep, thigh, calf and abdomen. Each site should be marked and three readings taken with appropriate rest in between to allow intercellular fluid to return (30 s). When testing classical ballet dancers, difficulty may occur with the suprailiac and thigh sites due to the low body fat levels of this population.

FIELD TESTS

Field-testing allows those without access to laboratory equipment the ability to measure baseline fitness levels and training adaptations. However, the newness of dance science means that few appropriate and specific field tests have been developed.

Table 25.5 Anthropometric data for dancers

Study	Sex	Style	Body fat (mean value?) (%)
Chatfield *et al.* (1990)	F	Contemporary	18
Chmelar *et al.* (1988)	F	Ballet	14
	F	Contemporary	12
Evans *et al.* (1985)	F	Contemporary	22.4
Brinson and Dick (1996)	M	Ballet	10
	F	Ballet	17
	M	Contemporary	12
	F	Contemporary	20

THE MULTISTAGE DANCE AEROBIC FITNESS TEST

This test is a continuous incremental five-stage aerobic fitness test that uses dance-specific movements (Wyon *et al.*, 2003). It has specific stages that correspond to the mean oxygen requirement of dance class (stage 3) and dance performance (stage 5) (Wyon *et al.*, 2004). The movement sequence of each stage was designed so that both novice and elite dancers of the same gender would work at the same relative oxygen requirement ($ml \cdot kg^{-1} min^{-1}$). The test is able to observe changes in a dancer's aerobic fitness by their ability to either to dance at a higher stage or by recording lower heart rates during each stage during a repeat test thereby indicating an improvement in their aerobic power (Wyon and Redding, in press). This test can be used as an indicator of whether a participant is capable of coping with the physical requirements of dance class or performance.

JUMP TESTS

The vertical jump test is a well recognised test of anaerobic power (Vandewalle *et al.*, 1987), and can be easily adapted for dance. It is suggested that arms remain in bras-bar (arms slightly in front of the body) for all jumps and rather than a squat countermovement jump, the participant should carry out a demi-plié with the heels remaining on the ground. Single leg hops should also be carried out on both legs starting in a turned-out position and the non-active leg's foot positioned behind the ankle of the test leg. Bilateral differences have been noted at student level but this discrepancy is not noted at professional level. In all tests, after a general warm-up, three attempts should be carried out and the highest value recorded.

Koutedakis *et al.* (2004) have developed a repetitive jump test that measures anaerobic endurance and aesthetic qualities. Participants perform a specially choreographed dance sequence using two pairs of concentric circles (60 and 70 cm, and 55 and 65 cm in diameter for males and females, respectively) drawn on the studio's floor. Dancers will be required to perform with reference to the circles' centre 'travelling' away from them followed by 'returns' towards the centre of the circles. The marking procedures are the same as those used in sports such as gymnastics and ice-skating, as well as dance-technique criteria utilised during auditions. Performance is calculated from the number of complete repetitions (physical component) and the technical/artistic competence (aesthetic component).

SUMMARY

Few dance companies or individual dancers recognise the importance or relevance of regular fitness testing, even though Dance UK has been advocating this strategy for the last 10 years. Elite dancers are extremely skilled practitioners but this has also been their downfall as their economy of movement is very good which has had a negative influence on their underlying physiological fitness. This, accompanied by an environment that does not promote beneficial supplemental training, has lead to a situation where injury is rife within the profession; ~80% of dancers will get an injury that will mean taking off at least four consecutive days a year (Brinson and Dick, 1996). The supplemental training that is promoted is generally Pilates or Gyrotonics based, which does help rectify any muscular imbalances, but does not put enough force or overload through the dancer for them to adapt.

REFERENCES

Braisted, J.R., Mellin, L., Gong, E.J. and Irwin, C.E. (1985). The adolescent ballet dancer: nutritional practices and characteristics associated with anorexia nervosa. *Journal of Adolescent Health Care*, 6: 365–371.

Brinson, P. and Dick, F. (1996). *Fit to Dance?* London: Calouste Gulbenkian Foundation.

Brooks-Gunn, J., Warren, M.P. and Hamilton, L.H. (1987). The relation of eating problems and amenorrhea in ballet dancers. *Medicine and Science in Sport and Exercise*, 19(1): 41–44.

Chatfield, S.J., Brynes, W.C., Lally, D.A. and Rowe, S.E. (1990). Cross-sectional physiologic profiling of modern dancers. *Dance Research Journal*, 22(1): 13–20.

Chmelar, R.D., Schultz, B.B., Ruhling, R.O., Shepherd, T.A., Zupan, M.F. and Fitt, S.S. (1988). A physiologic profile comparing levels and styles of female dancers. *The Physician and Sportsmedicine*, 16(7): 87–94.

Claessens, A.L.M., Beunen, G.P., Nuyts, M.M., Lafevre J.A. and Wellens, R.I. (1987). Body structure, somatotype, maturation and motor performance of girls in ballet schooling. *Journal of Sports Medicine*, 27: 310–317.

Cohen, A. (1984). Dance – aerobic and anaerobic. *Journal of Physical Education, Recreation and Dance*, March: 51–53.

Desfor, F.G. (2003). Assessing hypermobility in dancers. *Journal of Dance Medicine and Science*, 7(1): 17–23.

Evans, B.W., Tiburzi, A. and Norton, C.J. (1985). Body composition and body type of female dance majors. *Dance Research Journal*, 17(1): 17–20.

Geeves, T. (1997). Safe Dance II – National injury and lifestyle survey of Australian adolescents in pre-professional dance training. Australian Dance Council – Ausdance.

Hamilton, W.G. (1986). Physical prerequisites for ballet dancers. *The Journal of Musculoskeletal Medicine*, November: 61–67.

Heller, J., Bunc, V., Buzek, M., Novotny, J. and Psotta, R. (1995). Anaerobic power and capacity in young and adult football (soccer) players. *Acta Universitatis Carolinae. Kinanthropologica*, 31(1): 73–83.

Holderness, C.C., Brooks-Gunn, J. and Warren, M.P. (1994). Eating disorders and substance use: a dancing vs a nondancing population. *Medicine and Science in Sport and Exercise*, 26(3): 297–302.

Kirkendall, D.T. and Calabrese, L.H. (1983). Physiological aspects of dance. *Clinics in Sports Medicine*, 2(3): 525–537.

Kokkonen, J., Nelson, A.G. and Cornwell A. (1998). Acute muscle stretching inhibits maximal strength performance. *Research Quarterly for Exercise and Sport,* 69(4): 411–415.

Koutedakis, Y. and Jamurtas, A. (2004). The dancer as a performing athlete: physiological considerations. *Sports Medicine*, 34(10): 651–661.

Koutedakis, Y. and Sharp, N.C.C. (1999). *The Fit and Healthy Dancer*. Chichester, UK: John Wiley & Sons.

Koutedakis, Y. and Sharp, N.C.C. (2004). Thigh-muscles strength training, dance exercise, dynamometry, and anthropometry in professional ballerinas. *Journal of Strength and Conditioning Research*, 18(4): 714–718.

Koutedakis, Y. and Tsartsara, E. (2004). *Is fitness associated with professional dance*. San Fransisco, CA: International Association of Dance Medicine and Science. (IADMS). IADMS.

Koutedakis, Y., Frischnecht, R. and Murphy, M. (1997). Knee flexion to extension peak torque ratios and\lower-back injuries in highly active individuals. *International Journal of Sport Medicine*, 18: 290–295.

Koutedakis, Y., Agrawal, A. and Sharp, N.C.C. (1999). Isokinetic characteristics of knee flexors and extensors in male dancers, Olympic oarsmen, Olympic bobsleighers, and non-athletes. *Journal of Dance Medicine and Science*, 2(2): 63–67.

Koutedakis, Y., Myszkewycz, L., Soulas, D., Papapostolou, V., Sullivan, I. and Sharp, N.C.C. (1999). The effects of rest and subsequent training on selected physiological parameters in professional female classical dancers. *International Journal of Sports Medicine*, 20(6): 379–383.

Krasnow, D.H. and Chatfield, S. J. (1996). Dance science and the dance technique class. *Impulse*, 4: 162–172.

McCormack, M., Briggs, J., Hakim, A. and Grahame, R. (2004). Joint laxity and the benign joint hypermobility syndrome in student and professional ballet dancers. *Journal of Rheumatology*, 31(1): 173–178.

Mahendranath, K.M. (2004). The performing arts medicine: the disease of excellence.... is it the curse of performing artists or the proce of creativity? *APLAR Journal of Rheumatology*, 7(2): 137–140.

Neumann, G. (1989). Informational value and limits of sport medical functional diagnostics. *Theorie und Praxis der Koerperkultur*, 6: 198–205.

Redding, E. and Wyon, M.A. (2004). *Differences between active and passive flexibility in dancers' extension a la seconde in classical ballet and contemporary dancers*. International Association of Dance Medicine and Science, San Francisco, CA St Francis Hospital.

Rietveld, A.B.M. (2001). Sports, Dance- and Musicians' Medicine. *Orthopedie*. Bohn, Stafleu en Van Loghum: 103–121.

Rimmer, J. H., Jay, D. and Plowman, S.A. (1994). Physiological characteristics of trained dancers and intensity level of ballet class and rehearsal. *Impulse*, 2: 97–105.

Rist, R. (1994) Children and exercise: training young dancers, a dance medicine perspective. *Sportcare Journal*, 1(6) 5–7.

Schantz, P.G. and Astrand, P.-O. (1984). Physiological characteristics of classical ballet. *Medicine and Science in Sport and Exercise*, 16(5): 472–476.

Vandewalle, H., Peres, G. and Monod, H. (1987). Standard anaerobic exercise tests. *Sports Medicine*, 4(4): 268–289.

Westbald, P., Tsai-Fellander, L. and Johansson, C. (1995). Eccentric and concentric knee extensor muscle performance in professional ballet dancers. *Clinical Journal of Sport Medicine*, 5: 48–52.

Wilmerding, M., Gibson, A., Mermier, C. and Bivins, K. (2003). Body composition analysis in dancers. *Journal of Dance Medicine and Science*, 7(1): 24–31.

Wyon, M. (2004). Cardiorespiratory demands of contemporary dance. *School of Life and Sport Sciences*. London: University of Roehampton Surrey.

Wyon, M.A. and Redding, E. The physiological monitoring of cardiorespiratory adaptations during rehearsal and performance of contemporary dance. *Journal of Strength and Conditioning Research* 19(3): 611–614 (in press).

Wyon, M.A., Abt, G., Redding, E., Head, A. and Sharp, N.C.C. (2004). Oxygen uptake during of modern dance class, rehearsal and performance. *Journal of Strength and Conditioning Research*, 18(3): 646–649.

Wyon, M., Redding, E., Abt, G., Head, A. and Sharp, N.C.C. (2003). Reliability and validity of a multistage dance specific aerobic fitness test (DAFT). *Journal of Dance Medicine and Science*, 7(2): 80–84.

Young, W.B. and Behm, D. (2002). Should static stretching be used during a warm-up for strength and power activities. *Strength and Conditioning Journal*, 24(6): 33–37.

INDEX

Note: Page numbers in italics refer to figures and tables.